1000 HOME REMEDIES

METRO BOOKS
New York

An Imprint of Sterling Publishing
387 Park Avenue South
New York, NY 10016

This 2013 edition published by Metro Books by arrangement with Anova Books.

All images reproduced courtesy of istockphoto.com apart from pages 6, 14, 22, 23 (Lucinda Symons), pages 16, 17 (Caroline Molloy).

ISBN 978-1-4351-4719-5

For information about custom editions, special sales, and premium and corporate purchases, please contact Sterling Special Sales at 800-805-5489 or specialsales@sterlingpublishing.com.

Manufactured in China

2 4 6 8 10 9 7 5 3 1

www.sterlingpublishing.com

1000 HOME REMEDIES

Safe and sensible treatments for everyday ailments

METRO BOOKS
New York

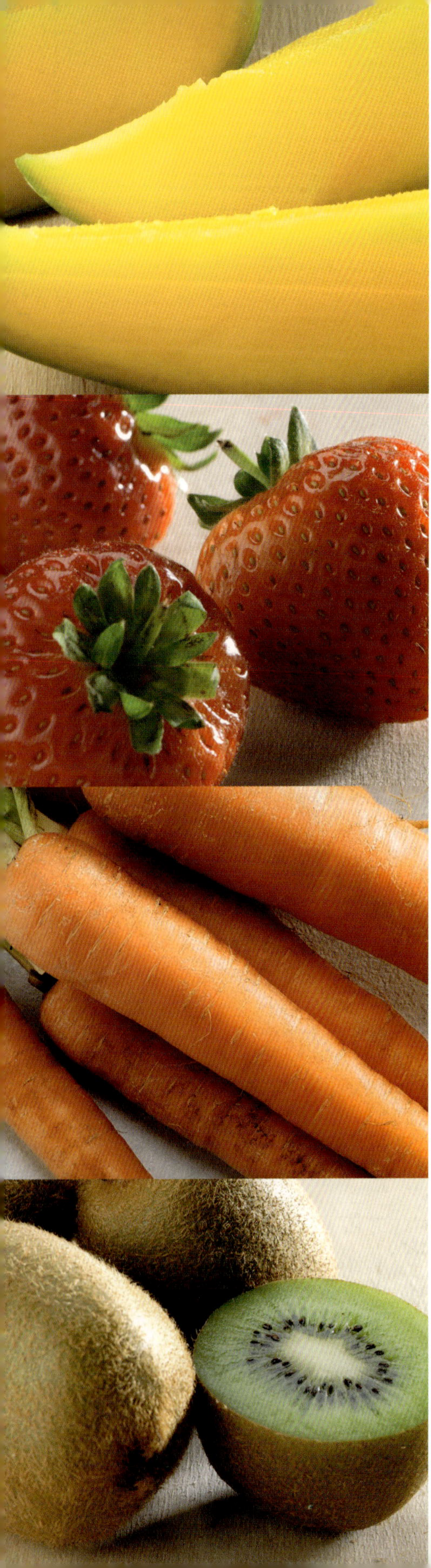

Contents

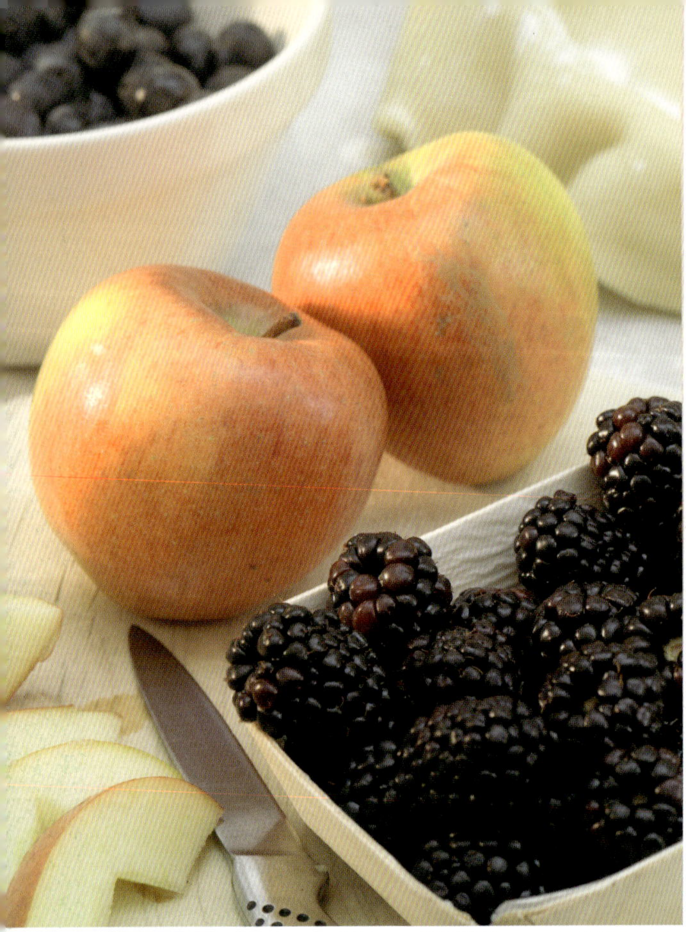
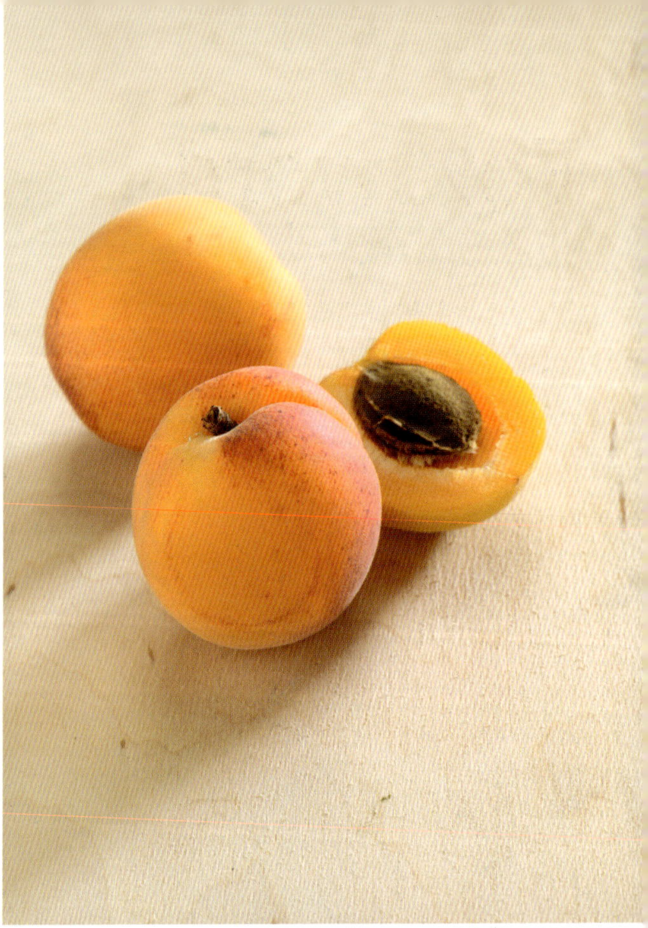
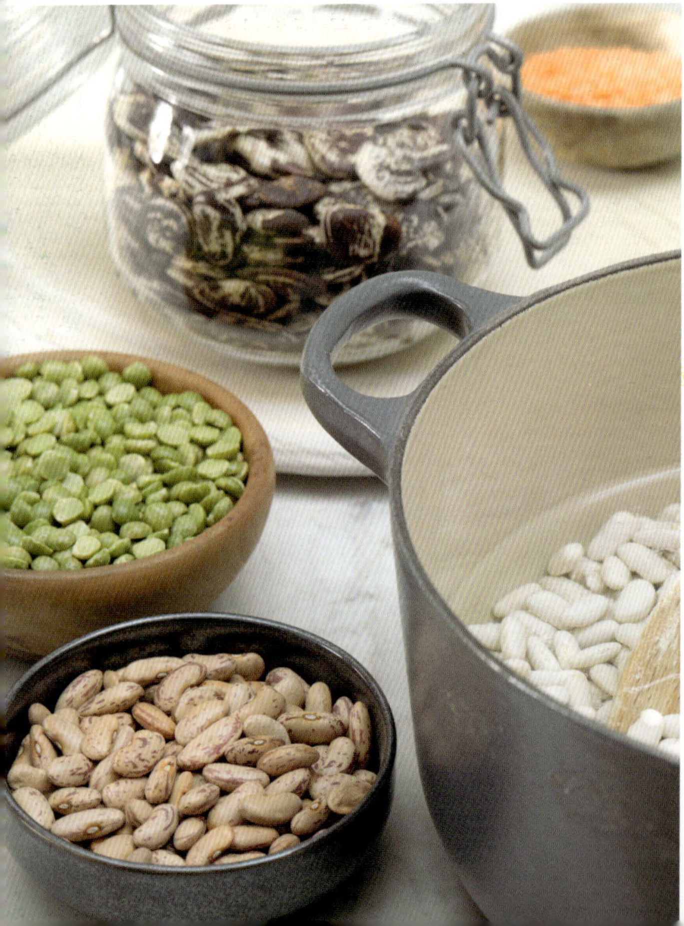
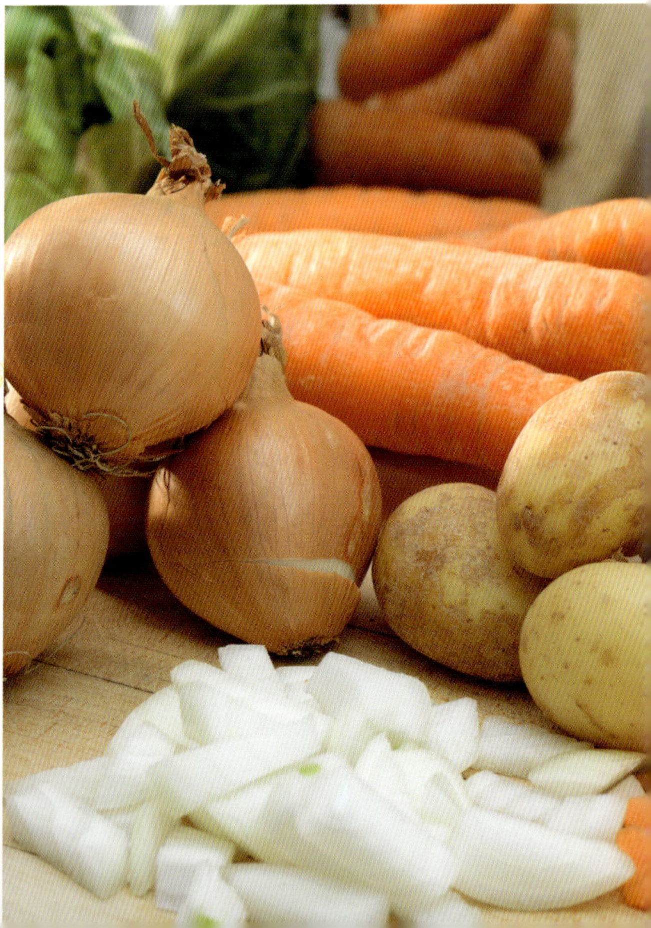

Foreword

We live in a fast-paced, high-technology world. The boundaries of medicine seem to be being pushed back at an awesome speed and there has never been a greater range and availability of medicines available to both physicians and patients alike. Laser treatments, gene therapy, and body scanning are becoming almost commonplace, yet the growth in interest in natural treatments continues to grow at an even faster rate. This increasing popularity of complementary and alternative medicine (CAM) has meant that health practitioners should take notice as to why about 38 percent of Americans are now willing to consider using natural treatments. More physicians than ever before are training in the use of complementary medicine to complement their conventional scientific background, allowing them to practice integrated medicine in which conventional and complementary treatments are used to achieve a full holistic range of therapy in a wide range of common medical conditions.

This book looks at the key areas of women's and men's health—such as medical, circulatory, urinary, and skin problems, nervous disorders, and first aid—from both a conventional and natural viewpoint. Laid out in easy-to-find sections, with color coding and concise advice in all areas, each topic looks at symptoms, prevention, available treatments, and when to seek medical advice, either as an emergency or as a routine appointment. There are also "quick-fix" tips, which will be a revelation to many people, and fascinating "Did You Know?" boxes to increase your understanding of each area of health. Its aim is to help demystify complementary treatments and allow anyone to evaluate their state of well-being as well as providing the most complete answers to common medical questions. It can be read as a textbook from start to finish, or dipped into as and when required.

More than 2,000 years ago, the great physician Galen, the father of modern medicine, said that "the doctor is only Nature's assistant." That quotation is as true today as it was then, and it reminds us that it is by looking at the widest range of treatments available to us that we stand the greatest chance of remaining as healthy as possible. If we also remind ourselves that health is actually a state of complete physical, mental, and social well-being rather than the absence of disease or infirmity, then we should surely add home remedies to the armory of conventional medical treatments at our disposal.

As a family physician whose patients frequently ask for my advice on complementary treatments, I have long believed that the best physicians have an open mind but not one that is closed to science. This book is a major step forward in helping people to take a holistic approach to their well-being and, in doing so, promote optimum health for all—the holy grail for physicians and patients.

Common Herbal Remedies

ALOE VERA Clear gel from leaves is used for skin problems, acne, burns, insect bites, and cuts.

BASIL Improves digestion and reduces excess mucous.

BURDOCK Cleanses the blood and is used to treat arthritis, fever, infections, boils, and sores.

CAYENNE Improves circulation, helps digestion, normalizes blood pressure, and is also used to treat stiff joints.

CHAMOMILE Traditionally used to induce sleep but also for digestive problems, poor appetite, colds, fever, flu, and for anxiety and stress due to its calming effect. Also good for sleeping problems, colic, and teething in babies and young children.

CHICKWEED Used as a diuretic to stimulate the kidneys as well as for treating wounds and itchy or inflamed skin.

CLOVES Improves digestion and clears mucous in lungs (asthma, colds, and coughs) as well as relieving toothache.

COLTSFOOT Used as a cough remedy; the leaves can be made into a poultice for bites and stings.

COMFREY Soothes coughs, and heals wounds and burns, promoting new healthy tissue growth.

CRAMP BARK Used to treat menstrual cramps, asthma, and heart palpitations.

DANDELION A powerful diuretic that is used to treat a wide range of conditions, including liver, gallbladder and kidney problems, constipation, dyspepsia, skin disease, and rheumatism.

ECHINACEA This natural antibiotic herb is used for colds, coughs, sore throat, influenza, and fever, as well as acne, athlete's foot, thrush, and urinary tract infections.

GARLIC Promotes good digestion, lowers blood cholesterol, strengthens the immune system, and fights respiratory infections, colds, and influenza.

GINGER Calms the digestive system, stimulates circulation, and is used to treat arthritis, muscular cramps, colds, chills, nausea, vomiting, and motion sickness.

GOLDENSEAL Treats respiratory infections, digestive ailments (nausea, colitis, gastroenteritis, irritable bowel), urinary tract infections, and boils. Combined with echinacea, it is a natural antibiotic.

GOTU KOLA An Asiatic herb used to cleanse the blood and to strengthen nerves; treats fevers and skin problems.

LAVENDER A sedative, calming herb that is used for treating headaches, migraine, stress, insomnia, indigestion, and burns.

LEMON BALM A calming herb for many nervous problems, depression, upset stomach, fever, premenstrual symptoms, and treating insect bites; a natural insect repellent.

LICORICE Promotes hormonal balance and used for some pregnancy and menopausal problems, as well as treating coughs and congestion.

MARIGOLD As an ointment or cream (calendula), treats cuts, grazes, burns, insect bites, stings, eczema, and skin problems; also used for fevers, gum disease, and to regulate menstruation.

MARSHMALLOW Good for soothing inflammations and treating boils, abscesses, infections, coughs, congestion, irritable bowel, and colitis.

MEADOWSWEET A source of natural aspirin; good for headaches, arthritis, rheumatism, urinary infections, and digestive problems.

MINTS Stimulating, energizing, and calming; aids digestion, colic, and flatulence; good for catarrh and bronchitis, and soothes headaches.

NETTLE (STINGING) A good blood cleanser, regulator, and strengthener, used to treat anemia and bleeding; also for arthritis, rheumatism, and asthma.

PARSLEY Improves digestion, eases menstrual cramping and tension headaches, and is also a good diuretic herb.

PLANTAIN Good for treating wounds, abrasions, burns, insect bites and stings, and skin problems, including eczema; also for urinary infections, thrush, irritable bowel syndrome, fever, and gum disease.

ROSEMARY A herb used for many common health

problems, including headaches, migraine, colds, fever, influenza, congestion, stomach ache, indigestion, constipation, and premenstrual symptoms, as well as for treating arthritis and rheumatism.

SAGE Excellent for sore throats, clearing excess mucous, and also for alleviating hot flashes during menopause.

SLIPPERY ELM All-round herb for treating wounds, ulceration, congestion, digestive problems (diarrhea, constipation, colitis, irritable bowel syndrome, gastroenteritis), sore throat, bronchitis, and asthma.

ST. JOHN'S WORT Effective antidepressant used commonly for treating anxiety, stress, nervous tension, depression, and night terrors in children; also used for neuralgia, sciatica, rheumatism, and period pain as well as cuts, abrasions, and burns.

THYME A good expectorant for coughs and bronchitis, and also used for treating colds, influenza, and sore throat.

YARROW An ancient herb used for treating wounds and infection; also good for the digestion, treating colds and influenza, and easing cramps and heavy bleeding.

Aromatherapy Essential Oils

BASIL Clears the sinus and a good study aid, helping to focus the mind.

BERGAMOT Calming, uplifting, and mood enhancing; used to treat anxiety, stress, and depression, and also abscesses and boils.

CLOVE Oil is commonly used for relieving toothache.

CYPRESS Used for treating respiratory problems, especially coughs, sore throat, bronchitis, and asthma; also for rheumatism and foot odor.

EUCALYPTUS Effective in treating many respiratory ailments, including colds, sinusitis, and congestion, but also good for relieving muscular pain.

FRANKINCENSE A calming, soothing oil, which is used for anxiety and inducing meditation; also for asthma and lung infections.

GERANIUM Good for women's health problems and balancing hormones, especially premenstrual symptoms and during menopause; also used for acne, fluid retention, and nervous tension.

GINGER Warming and good for digestive problems, nausea, and motion sickness, as well as muscular aches and pains and arthritis.

JASMINE Uplifting and antidepressant, this is used for painful periods and to ease labor pain.

JUNIPER Cleansing and detoxifying, this is useful for treating respiratory infections, sciatica, gout, and rheumatism.

LAVENDER Relaxing, sedative, and calming, used to treat insomnia and headaches; also colds, sore throat, and bronchitis, and insect bites and stings, cuts, and minor burns.

LEMON Good for oily skin and acne as well as warts and verrucas.

LEMONGRASS Excellent for fatigue and tired, aching muscles as well as restless legs; an effective insect repellent and a digestive tonic.

MANDARIN A calming, relaxing oil, and it is suitable for babies; used to treat rheumatic aches and pains, nervous tension, cellulite, and water retention.

MARJORAM Calming oil for nervous tension, headaches, and stress; induces sleep; eases respiratory problems, such as colds, sinusitis, and bronchitis; and good for muscular pain, stiffness, and sport-related injuries.

MELISSA A good antidepressant for treating shock, anxiety, and depression; it is also used for irregular periods and cold sores.

NEROLI Good for stress, panic attacks, and insomnia as well as stress-related irritable bowel syndrome.

ORANGE An uplifting tonic that is used for heartburn, indigestion, constipation, and colic.

PEPPERMINT A good digestive, used for treating flatulence, indigestion, and colic; decongestant and effective relief for colds, blocked sinus, and influenza.

ROMAN CHAMOMILE An excellent, gentle oil for soothing young children; also can be used to treat skin inflammations, acne, eczema, and psoriasis; muscular aches and sprains and joint problems; digestive ailments (indigestion, flatulence, and colic); and premenstrual symptoms, stress-related headaches, anxiety, and insomnia.
ROSE Antidepressant and used to treat stress and grief; relieves premenstrual symptoms, headaches, and hangovers.
ROSEMARY An invigorating skin toner and good for shiny hair and treating dandruff; used for treating colds, congestion, rheumatism, headaches, and indigestion.
SANDALWOOD Soothing for sore throat, laryngitis, and bronchitis; good for dry skin, eczema, and acne; and useful in treating anxiety and depression.
TEA TREE Extremely beneficial for skin problems, including acne, cuts, cold sores, stings, and minor wounds; also for treating athlete's foot, corns, callouses, warts and verrucas, as well as coughs, congestion, sinusitis, and sore throats.

Homeopathic Remedies

APIS MELLIFICA Often known as Apis and prepared from the honey bee, this homeopathic remedy is used for treating many skin conditions, rheumatism and swollen joints, throbbing headaches, dry coughs, and irregular periods.
ARGENTUM NITRICUM Made from silver nitrate, this can treat hay fever, asthma, anxiety, depression, chronic fatigue syndrome, and nervous disorders; digestive problems, such as gastritis and irritable bowel; and burns and warts.
ARNICA MONTANA The most commonly used remedy for bruising and muscular pain; can also be used for treating fatigue.
ARSENICUM ALBUM Useful for treating skin problems, especially eczema and psoriasis; digestive ailments, such as vomiting, diarrhea, food poisoning, gastritis; hay fever, asthma, sore throat, conjunctivitis, and dandruff.
BELLADONNA Sourced from deadly nightshade, this is good for treating fever, especially in the early stages, as well as rubella; and severe headaches, arthritis, tonsillitis, and neuralgia.
BRYONIA ALBA Made from the climbing bryony plant, this is good for arthritis, rheumatism, sciatica, and back pain as well as digestive disorders (diarrhea, gastritis, indigestion), headaches, and chest infections.
CALCAREA CARBONICA Derived from calcium carbonate, this can be helpful in treating a wide range of ailments, including colds, coughs, and headaches.
CANTHARIS Used for urinary system and skin conditions as well as treating diarrhea and canker sores.
CHAMOMILLA Sourced from the chamomile plant, this is especially good for relieving toothache, teething pain, and earache; colic and painful periods; and arthritis and sciatic pain.
CIMICIFUGA RACEMOSA Sourced from the North American black cohosh plant, this is used for neck and back pain, headaches, and rheumatism.
COLOCYNTHIS A remedy made from the bitter cucumber plant, used for sciatica, neuralgia, colic, and stomach pain.
FERRUM PHOSPHORICUM A remedy sourced from iron phosphate, frequently used for treating fever, headaches, and nosebleeds as well as indigestion and heavy periods.
GELSEMIUM Used for mental and emotional problems, especially anxiety, fear of the dentist, or similar, and chronic fatigue, and influenza.
HEPAR SULPHURIS CALCAREUM Also known as Hepar sulph, can be used for skin conditions, boils, abscesses, and acne; sore throat, earache, coughs, and bronchitis.

IGNATIA Used to treat acute grief, bereavement, and depression; and headaches, coughs, and digestive problems (diarrhea, stomach cramps, and flatulence).

IPECACUANHA Also known as Ipecac, made from the dried root of a Brazilian plant, good for relief of nausea and vomiting, asthma, and heavy periods.

KALI CARBONICUM Derived from wood ash, this is used for treating indigestion and nausea, asthma and puffy eyelids (as in allergies), catarrh and phlegm, and lumbago.

LACHESIS Made from the venom of a South American snake, this constitutional medicine is good for menopausal symptoms (hot flashes), heavy periods, sore throat, asthma, depression, back pain, and sciatica.

LYCOPODIUM Widely used for digestive disorders, especially bowel problems, irritable bowel syndrome, and heartburn; migraine, headaches, and urinary tract infections.

MERCURIUS SOLUBILIS Often referred to as Mercurius, used for colds, tonsillitis, sore throat, and ear infections; arthritis and digestive problems, such as colitis.

NATRUM MURIATICUM Better known as sodium chloride or common salt, this treats canker sores and cold sores; eczema and psoriasis; headaches and premenstrual symptoms; back pain, asthma, and irritable bowel syndrome.

NUX VOMICA Mainly used for digestive problems (colic, peptic ulcers, irritable bowel); stress, fatigue, headaches, insomnia, and sleeping problems; hay fever and asthma.

PHOSPHORUS Sourced from bone ash, this can treat digestive ailments, such as gastritis, colitis, peptic ulcers; dry, hacking coughs and bronchitis; nosebleeds and haemorrhage; and angina.

PULSATILLA Often used in pregnancy for morning sickness and nausea; period and women's hormonal problems; digestive ailments, especially irritable bowel syndrome; hay fever, cystitis, asthma, and arthritis.

RHUS TOXICODENDRON Although derived from poison ivy, this is used for treating skin rashes, eczema, shingles, and chickenpox; rheumatism, arthritis, sprains, stiff neck, and influenza.

SABINA Good for treating arthritis and gout as well as nose bleeds, back pain, and painful periods.

SANGUINARIA CANADENSIS Usually used for treating allergies, especially hay fever and asthma; shoulder pain and joint conditions; menopausal hot flashes, migraine, and coughs.

SEPIA Made from cuttlefish ink, this is helpful for treating fatigue, exhaustion, depression, premenstrual symptoms, and headaches, especially during a period or menopause; also used for cystitis, back pain, warts, and nausea in pregnancy.

SILICEA This is helpful for people who lack physical stamina; often used for treating abscesses and headaches.

STAPHYSAGRIA Good for emotional problems and ailments related to grief or suppressed anger, especially depression, psoriasis, and insomnia; also warts, cystitis, and premenstrual symptoms.

SULFUR Especially useful for skin problems, including eczema, abscesses, acne; and digestive ailments, such as diarrhea; conjunctivitis, migraine, tonsillitis, asthma, dandruff, arthritis, and hot flashes in menopause.

Skin and Hair Problems

The appearance of your skin and hair reflects your state of health and is an important barometer of your general well-being. In fact, skin and hair problems should be taken seriously because they are sometimes signs of underlying illness. Natural blemish-free skin and shiny, healthy hair depend as much on good nutrition and a healthy lifestyle as the conventional and natural products and remedies you use on them.

Your skin is the largest organ in your body (more than 15 percent of your body weight), and it continuously renews itself during a four-week cycle. It protects the skeletal system, muscles, and organs; it helps maintain a constant body temperature; and its specialized cells perform essential functions. Vitamin D is produced when it is exposed to sunlight; and its nerve endings sense pain, itching, pressure, heat, and cold. Rashes, pimples, boils, inflammation, blisters, and redness can all be symptoms of allergic reactions, hormonal changes, or illness.

Your body is covered in hair with the exception of the palms of your hands and the soles of your feet. Most of it is soft and downy, but it grows more profusely on your head and its condition is affected by your diet, environment, and general health. On average, 100 to 150 of the 300,000 hairs on your scalp are shed every day and are replaced by new hairs as part of the natural growth cycle.

Caring for your skin and hair will keep them looking good and help you to notice the telltale signs of underlying health problems, allowing for you to treat them effectively before they get worse.

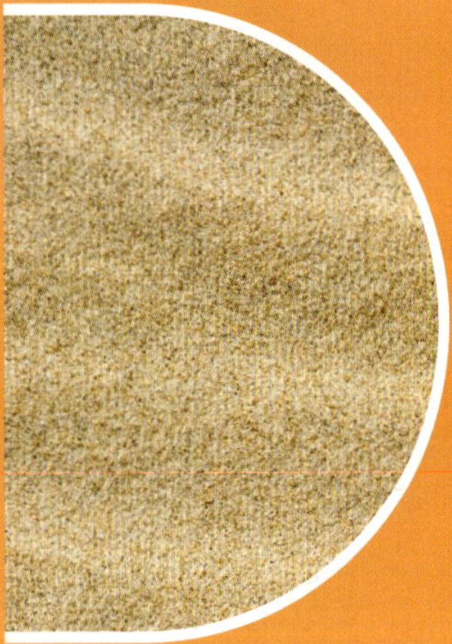

Dry Skin

The skin is the largest organ in your body, accounting for more than 15 percent of your body weight. Its appearance reflects your age, health, and general well-being. Dry skin tends to be fine, but it can flake easily and feel tight, and it is more predisposed to developing fine lines and wrinkles than other skin types.

SYMPTOMS

- Dry, close-textured and fine
- Flaky patches
- Tightness across cheeks and forehead
- Chaps easily
- Skin feels cracked and rough
- Thread veins, facial lines, and wrinkles
- Prone to itching and irritation

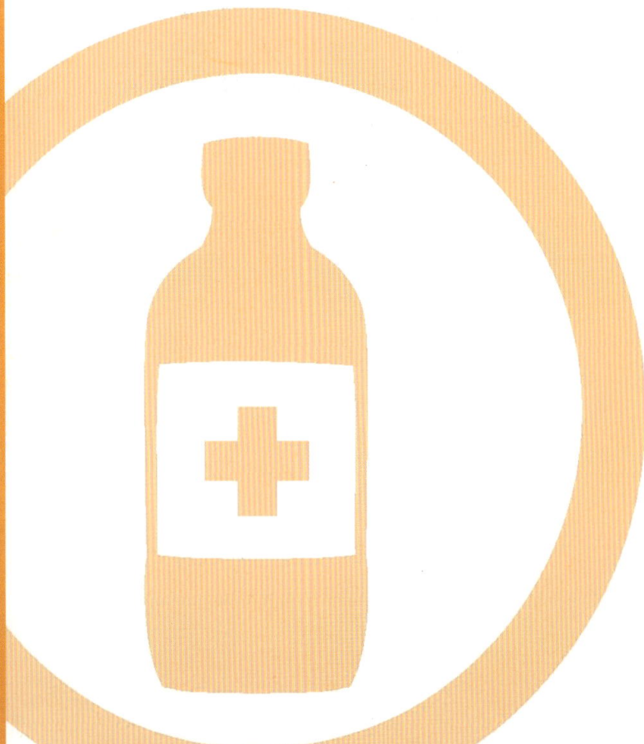

PREVENTION

Using a moisturizer daily locks in natural moisture. Other prevention measures include:

- Use gentle cleansers and alcohol-free toners on your face
- Try to avoid soap, which tends to be drying—liquid soaps and special cream- or oil-base soaps are gentler than conventional ones
- Always use a night cream
- Use a moisturizing face mask once a week
- Protect your skin in extreme cold, heat, and windy conditions
- Do not shower or take a bath more than once a day, if possible, and for no longer than 10 to 15 minutes
- Eat a healthy, well-balanced diet
- Drink plenty of liquids—the recommended daily intake is eight 8-fluid-ounce glasses of water
- Limit alcohol and caffeinated drinks, such as tea and coffee—they have a diuretic effect
- Quit smoking
- Fill your home with houseplants to add moisture, and place a humidifier in your bedroom in winter
- Protect your skin against the sun—always wear a sunscreen lotion.

CONVENTIONAL TREATMENTS

The conventional treatment for dry skin is to use a moisturizer to replace sebum—a natural skin lubricant that keeps it moist. There are so many products to choose from that you may find it difficult selecting the right one. They range from very expensive creams and serums made by international beauty companies to medicated brands to more natural, cruelty-free moisturizers.

NATURAL REMEDIES

Healthy skin is not so much a matter of what you use as what you do. Your lifestyle, environment, level of exercise, and diet will all affect your skin and how it looks. For homemade remedies you can make yourself, see pages 52–53.

HERBAL REMEDIES Try applying some soothing aloe vera gel—it removes dead skin cells and helps moisturize and soften really dry skin. Make herbal tea with dandelion, chamomile, or peppermint and drink a cup once every day.

AROMATHERAPY Tea tree essential oil penetrates deep into the skin—just add a couple of drops to a carrier oil and massage gently into dry areas. When taking a bath, add a few drops of lavender oil to the water.

EXERCISE

Regular exercise has many beneficial effects on your skin: it increases your oxygen intake, removes toxins that can clog up your skin, boosts healthy cell renewal, and helps the efficient absorption of nutrients by your body. You don't have to be a fitness fanatic or join a gym—even a brisk 20-minute walk every day can make a positive difference to your skin.

NUTRITIONAL MEDICINE

A healthy, varied diet that supplies all the essential nutrients is your skin's best friend. Too few vitamins and minerals can leave your skin dehydrated and dull. You need the following:

VITAMIN A Carrots and dark green and yellow vegetables

VITAMIN B Whole-grain cereals, meat, fish, eggs, dairy products, green leafy vegetables, beans and legumes, and yeast

VITAMIN C Citrus fruits and leafy green vegetables

VITAMIN E Whole-grain cereals and eggs

ZINC Meat and dairy products

SELENIUM Meat, fish, and whole-grain cereals.

CALL YOUR DOCTOR

Persistent dry skin that does not respond to a healthy diet and moisturizers may need a different approach. It can even be a symptom of an underlying, more serious health problem, such as diabetes. If the condition does not improve and you experience redness, crustiness, severe rashes, or other irritating skin conditions, consult your doctor.

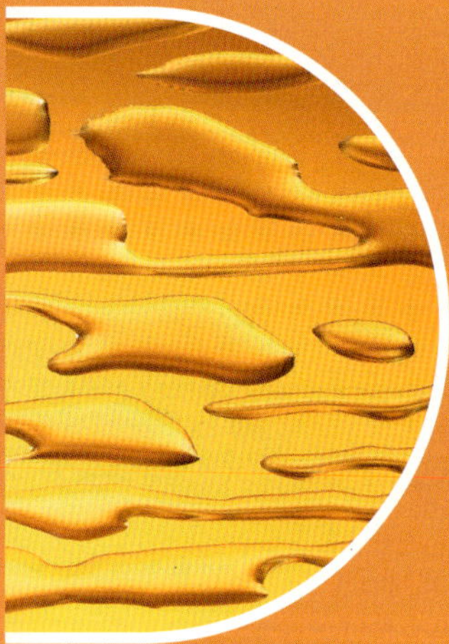

Oily Skin

This skin type looks shiny and has a tendency to develop pimples but, on the plus side, it does have a tendency to age better than other skin types. As with dry skin (see page 14), eating a healthy diet will help to improve its texture and appearance. The increased sebum production is caused by the male hormone testosterone, which is also present, to a lesser extent, in women.

SYMPTOMS

- Enlarged visible and open pores
- Overall shine
- Tendency to blemishes
- Prone to pimples and blackheads
- Skin feels greasy

PREVENTION

If you have a natural tendency to oily skin, it is difficult to prevent it. However, there are positive steps you can take to prevent it from getting worse and becoming "problem" skin.

- Never use harsh cleansers, which can strip away the skin's natural oils.
- Use a mild pH-balanced liquid soap or cleanser.
- Use an oil-free moisturizer.
- Deep-cleansing face masks and facial scrubs can be beneficial.
- Eat a healthy diet with plenty of fresh fruit and vegetables and less fried foods, chocolate, refined flour, and sugar products.
- Drink herbal teas in preference to regular tea and coffee.
- Invest in some flaxseed oil and take one level tablespoon daily.
- Don't forget to protect your skin against the sun—always wear a sunscreen lotion.

Did You Know?

If you take an oral contraceptive pill, your skin may have a tendency to be oily. Some women also find that their skin becomes more oily in late pregnancy because of higher progesterone levels in their body. However, after giving birth, it usually reverts to its normal type.

CONVENTIONAL TREATMENTS

The traditional way of dealing with oily skin was to use harsh astringent toners to dry it out. However, we now know that this approach can be damaging and make the problem even worse by stripping away the natural oils and overstimulating oil production. Instead, use gentle cleansers and toners that have been formulated specially for oily skin.

NATURAL REMEDIES

For homemade remedies you can make yourself, turn to pages 52–53.

HERBAL REMEDIES Make your own gentle toner by steeping some sage or peppermint leaves in hot water for half an hour before straining and cooling. Apply to oily skin with a cotton ball. Alternatively, put some eucalyptus, rosemary, or thyme in a heatproof bowl, pour some boiling water over the herb, and then, with a towel over your head, lean over the bowl and inhale the steam.

AROMATHERAPY Sage and lemongrass essential oils may help to slow down the oil production in the skin, whereas basil, eucalyptus, and lavender oils can help normalize the condition.

NUTRITIONAL MEDICINE

Poor diet and junk food can make naturally oily skin even worse, leading to an increased tendency to developing pimples and acne. Try cutting out all fried, greasy, and high-fat foods, such as potato chips and French fries, and also reduce your consumption of chocolate, sugary cookies, and cakes. Eat more salads, fruit, and fresh vegetables.

CALL YOUR DOCTOR

Oily skin should not usually necessitate a visit to your doctor. However, if you have outbreaks of pimples or a tendency to acne, it would be worth consulting your phsysician and getting some professional advice. You may be prescribed a topical cream or some antibiotics.

Quick Fix

Blot any excess oil on your face with loose face powder, not pressed, which may contain oil. Keep a little packet of alcohol wipes in your purse and use when required.

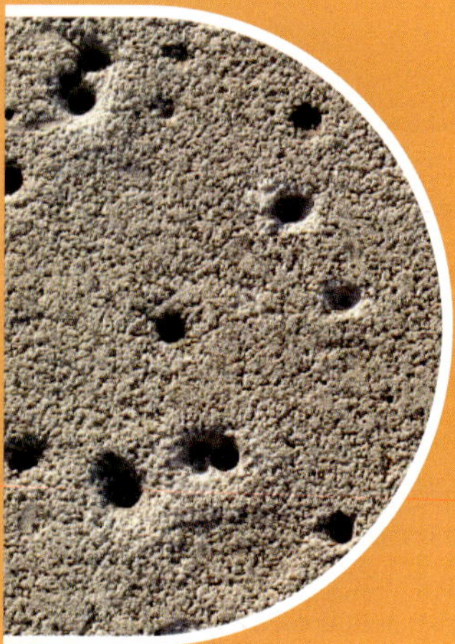

Acne

This distressing condition affects more than 70 percent of young people at some point during their adolescence. The blemishes are caused by an excessive production of sebum, which is secreted through pores in the skin. The pores become plugged, leading to blackheads or whiteheads, or infected, causing pus-filled spots.

SYMPTOMS

- Blackheads—dark-pigmented blocked pores
- Whiteheads—small lumps with a white center
- Skin feels greasy
- Pimples filled with pus on face, neck, chest, shoulders, and back
- Pitted, scarred skin

Did You Know?

Acne can be made worse by the following: taking oral contraceptives, corticosteroids, and some antiepileptic medicines; and when experiencing stress and anxiety.

PREVENTION

Acne is triggered during puberty by an increase in the hormone testosterone and is, therefore, impossible to prevent, especially if it runs in your family. However, you can take positive action to improve it or, at least, to prevent it from getting worse.

- Always wash your hands before touching your face.
- Never squeeze or pick at pimples—this can cause scarring.
- Cleanse your face twice a day—first thing in the morning and before going to bed.
- Use a medicated soap or cleanser or tea tree oil skin wash to remove bacteria.
- Use an oil-free, water-base moisturizer.
- Never use oil-base makeup.
- Eat a healthy diet with plenty of fresh fruit and vegetables and less fried foods, chocolate, potato chips, candies, and cookies.
- Drink plenty of water.
- Regular exercise improves circulation and is beneficial for the skin.
- Tie long hair back off your face and wash greasy hair frequently.

CONVENTIONAL TREATMENTS

Over-the-counter creams, gels, and lotions are all available, and these may be effective in treating mild acne. Prescription medicines for more severe cases may be topical (applied directly to skin) or oral, including antibiotics and retinoids.

NATURAL REMEDIES

Self-help measures and natural remedies can make a difference, especially in improving milder outbreaks of pimples on the face.

HERBAL REMEDIES Facial steam baths can be beneficial because they help open the pores in the skin—just cover some chamomile, rosemary, thyme, or sage leaves with boiling water and, with a towel over your head, "bathe" your face. Alternatively, dab the pimples with a moist, warm chamomile tea bag. Drink one cup of herbal tea made with echinacea, burdock, dandelion, or marigold three times a day.

AROMATHERAPY Bergamot, lavender, and tea tree oils are relaxing, calming, and antibacterial. You can apply a few drops of these essential oils to your bathtub water or use in a compress. Dab a drop of neat lavender oil onto pimples.

NUTRITIONAL MEDICINE

Contrary to popular belief, acne is not caused by poor diet and eating greasy foods, but healthy nutrition can help to combat it. Reduce your intake of animal fats, sugar, and high-fat convenience foods, and try to eat more whole-grain cereals, fruit, and vegetables.

HOMEOPATHIC REMEDIES

Consult a qualified homeopath or, for less severe outbreaks, try the following:

Sulfur 6C: Take one tablet twice daily to relieve chronic acne with itchy, red, sore pimples that are often infected and pus filled

Kali bromatum 6C: Take one tablet twice daily to relieve bluish red spots on the face, cheeks, forehead, neck, and shoulders, which leave scars

CALL YOUR DOCTOR

If your acne is persistent and does not respond to over-the-counter treatments or self-help remedies within two months or becomes worse and distressing, visit your doctor. You may be prescribed antibiotics or be referred to a dermatologist if the condition is bad or you have scarring.

Healing Sunlight

Many people find their acne is worse in the winter, when there is less natural light, and that it improves in the summer, when their skin is exposed to more ultraviolet light. However, do be careful not to sunbathe in the middle of the day, when the sun is at its strongest and you may get burned.

Quick Fix

Whenever you notice a new pimple, just dab it with some witch hazel before applying your concealer in the usual way.

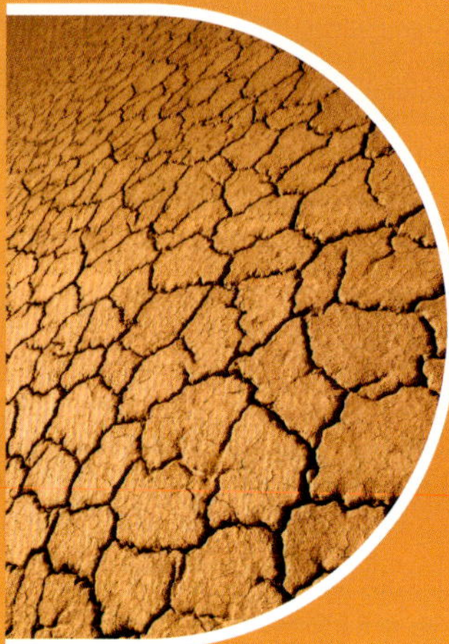

Eczema

Eczema, also referred to as dermatitis, often occurs on the fronts of the elbows, backs of the knees, ankles, wrists, neck, and face. There are different types of eczema, with atopic eczema (the eczema that runs in families) being the most common. There are various conventional and natural treatments you can try to help keep outbreaks of eczema under control.

SYMPTOMS

- ▷ Areas of red, inflamed skin
- ▷ Patches of dry, scaly, or cracked skin
- ▷ Itching
- ▷ Thickening of the skin
- ▷ Flaky scalp
- ▷ Sore, blistering, weeping, wet, or bleeding skin

Did You Know?

Eczema is more common in childhood, and although many children grow out of it, some people continue to live with it into adulthood. Many people with eczema also experience hay fever or asthma.

PREVENTION

One of the most important things you can do to prevent eczema is to stop your skin from drying out by moisturizing regularly.

- Don't use soap—it will dry out your skin. Use an emollient cream instead.
- Avoid overwashing your skin or using water that is too hot, which will strip your skin of its natural oils.
- Use alcohol-free and fragrance-free toiletries to reduce irritation.
- Some materials, such as synthetic fibers or wool, can irritate your skin. Always wear natural fibers, such as cotton.
- Try to avoid any extremes of temperature. Cold weather dries the skin, whereas getting hot and sweaty can cause inflammation.
- Don't scratch—scratching will make the condition worse and may lead to bleeding or infection. Keep your nails short to minimize damage.
- Try to avoid stress, because this can cause outbreaks of eczema. Getting regular exercise and practicing relaxation techniques will help you to cope with stressful situations.

CONVENTIONAL TREATMENTS

Emollients, such as aqueous cream, soften and rehydrate the skin. Corticosteroid creams reduce redness and inflammation, and antihistamines can help to ease itching. If your eczema is persistent, you may be referred to a dermatologist for ultraviolet light therapy. If you have severe eczema, a healthcare provider may show you how to apply a special type of dressing.

NATURAL REMEDIES

Here are some natural remedies that you may want to consider for treating your eczema:

NUTRITIONAL MEDICINE Eczema may be associated with a zinc deficiency. Good sources of zinc include oysters, dairy products, beans, nuts, seeds (especially pumpkin seeds), and fortified breakfast cereals.

HERBAL REMEDIES Applying a cream containing St. John's Wort (hypericum) to any affected areas of skin may provide some relief from eczema symptoms.

ACUPUNCTURE This treatment addresses heat imbalances within the body to treat outbreaks of eczema and provide long-term relief.

HELPFUL THERAPIES

Many people find that their eczema gets better in the summer and flares up again during the winter months, so, therefore, your skin may benefit from a little sun exposure, but without getting sunburned. Sunshine promotes the synthesis of vitamin D, which is necessary for healthy skin.

IMMEDIATE RELIEF

A saltwater compress may help to relieve itching. Dissolve a teaspoon of pure, natural sea salt (not table salt) in one cup of warm water, soak a clean washcloth in it, and apply to itchy areas of your skin.

CALL YOUR DOCTOR

If your current method of treating eczema does not seem to be working, consult your doctor; it may be necessary to change treatments. You should also call your doctor if:

- Your skin becomes crusty or starts oozing, blistering, or bleeding. This could be a sign of infection
- Your self-confidence is low, you feel depressed, or your quality of life is suffering because of your eczema.

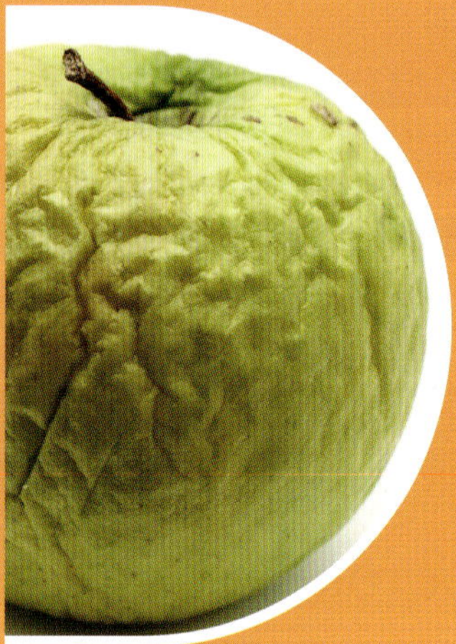

Wrinkles

As you age, your skin's natural moisture content will decrease—it becomes drier, and fine lines and wrinkles start to appear. However, you can take positive action to protect your skin from premature aging and adapt your skincare routine accordingly. In fact, the sooner you start, the better—don't wait until you are in your fifties.

SYMPTOMS

- ▷ Fine lines around the corners of the eyes and down the sides of the mouth
- ▷ Dry skin
- ▷ Skin starts to sag with loss of firmness and elasticity
- ▷ Uneven and dull skin tone

Did You Know?

Antioxidants can help to prevent skin damage and aging by neutralizing free radicals—the electrically charged oxygen molecules that attack healthy cells in your skin.

PREVENTION

You cannot prevent wrinkles totally—they are part of the aging process—but you can do a lot to slow them down and minimize the impact of the ones that appear.

- Apply a soothing eye gel or a little wheat germ oil around the eyes first thing in the morning and at bedtime.
- Moisturize day and night to replace the loss of natural oils in your skin.
- Always wear a sunscreen or sunblock lotion on your face to protect your skin from harmful, aging ultraviolet light.
- Never use tanning beds.
- Always wear sunglasses in bright sunlight.
- Use a soap-free cleanser on your face—soap is too drying.
- Apply a moisturizing mask once weekly.
- Eat a healthy diet with plenty of fruit and vegetables, and reduce your consumption of refined and processed foods.
- Drink plenty of water.
- Quit smoking and reduce your consumption of alcohol.
- Breathe deeply to increase the amount of oxygen supplied to the skin.
- Regular exercise improves circulation and is nourishing for the skin.

CONVENTIONAL TREATMENTS

An astonishing array of antiaging, antiwrinkle creams, serums, and moisturizers is available in your local pharmacy or from the beauty counters in large stores. Or you can even try such treatments as Botox injections, chemical peels, or a facelift.

NATURAL REMEDIES

Luckily, you don't have to spend a fortune on really expensive beauty products when there are so many natural remedies for combating aging skin, fine lines, and wrinkles.

HERBAL REMEDIES Apply aloe vera gel to wrinkles or, better still, take a fresh aloe vera leaf and peel back the outer skin to extract the clear gel within.

AROMATHERAPY Try diluting lavender, patchouli, tea tree, lemon, cranberry, or eucalyptus essential oils in a carrier oil or cream and then massaging it gently into wrinkles.

NUTRITIONAL MEDICINE Eating a varied diet that contains all the essential nutrients your skin needs for good health will help to keep it looking youthful. Make sure that you eat oily fish, which is rich in omega-3 fatty acids, at least twice a week. You can choose from salmon, tuna, mackerel, herring, and sardines.

HOMEMADE REMEDIES

- You can make a nourishing face mask for dry skin by mashing the flesh of a ripe avocado with a drop of lemon juice and smoothing it over your face. Let sit for at least 15 minutes.
- Make an exfoliating mask that helps reduce the appearance of wrinkles by peeling a ripe papaya and mashing the flesh. Blend three tablespoons with one tablespoon oatmeal and smooth it over your face. Let sit for 15 minutes, then rub vigorously into your skin and rinse off thoroughly.

Facial Exercises

Exercising your facial muscles will make them stronger to support the skin and help minimize lines and wrinkles.

- For lines around the nose and mouth, curl your upper and lower lips inward around your teeth. Press your lips together and, with your mouth closed, blow hard. Repeat three times.
- To tone up your cheek and chin muscles, smile with your mouth closed, raising the corners of your lips as you do so. Hold for a count of five and then push your jaw forward. Hold for a count of five. Repeat three times.

Harness the Power of AHAs

AHAs are alpha hydroxy acids, which occur naturally in sugar cane, sour milk, apples, and acidic fruits. They help promote the shedding of dead skin cells and fight free radicals (see box opposite) as well as encouraging skin renewal and collagen growth. Many moisturizing skin products you can buy contain AHAs, or you can even apply some milk, lemon juice, or apple juice directly to your skin.

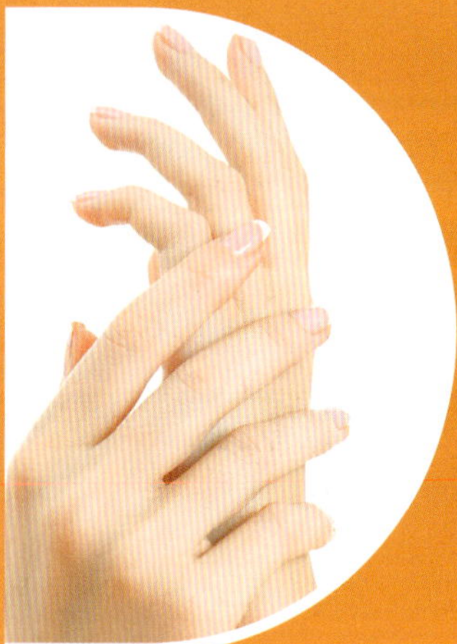

Psoriasis

Psoriasis is a chronic skin disease that is most often characterized by inflamed, red, flaky patches of skin, known as plaques. These plaques form due to excessive numbers of skin cells collecting together on the surface of the skin. The cause of psoriasis is still not fully understood, but genes are known to be partly involved because the condition often runs in families.

SYMPTOMS

- Dry, red crusty patches of skin, with silver scales that flake easily
- Dandrufflike flakes on the scalp
- Itchy skin or scalp
- Pitted or discolored nails
- Sore or painful skin
- Cracked or bleeding skin
- Joint pain and stiffness

Did You Know?

Old skin cells are normally replaced with new ones approximately once every 28 days, but in psoriasis, new skin cells are produced more quickly than usual, before they are needed.

PREVENTION

Psoriasis is unpredictable, coming and going as it pleases, but there are some things that you can do to help prevent it from flaring up.

- Eat a balanced diet to support your general health and well-being.
- Be extra careful to avoid skin injuries, such as cuts, scrapes, bruises, and burns, which can lead to outbreaks of psoriasis.
- Moisturize your skin regularly to counteract dryness, and use an emollient instead of soap.
- Psoriasis can often flare up in times of stress. Some useful ways of managing stress include getting physical exercise, and relaxation and meditation techniques.
- Some medicines, such as ibuprofen and beta blockers, are known to make psoriasis worse. If you are taking any medication, ask your doctor if it will aggravate your psoriasis.
- Moderate your alcohol consumption and don't smoke.

CONVENTIONAL TREATMENTS

If your psoriasis is mild to moderate, your doctor may recommend a corticosteroid, coal tar, emollient, or vitamin D cream to put on your skin, and a shampoo for your scalp. If you have a more persistent case of psoriasis, you may be referred to a dermatologist for ultraviolet light therapy. For more severe cases of psoriasis, there are oral medicines and injections available to help control the inflammation.

NATURAL REMEDIES

You might want to try the following natural methods to see if they improve your psoriasis.

NUTRITIONAL MEDICINE EPA (a type of omega-3 fatty acid found in oily fish) may help to reduce inflammation associated with psoriasis. Try taking a daily supplement.

AROMATHERAPY Helichrysum essential oil is known for its anti-inflammatory effects. Add a few drops to a carrier oil, such as jojoba or sweet almond oil, and massage it into your skin.

ACUPUNCTURE This treatment is a great way of reducing stress, which, in turn, can help alleviate the symptoms of psoriasis.

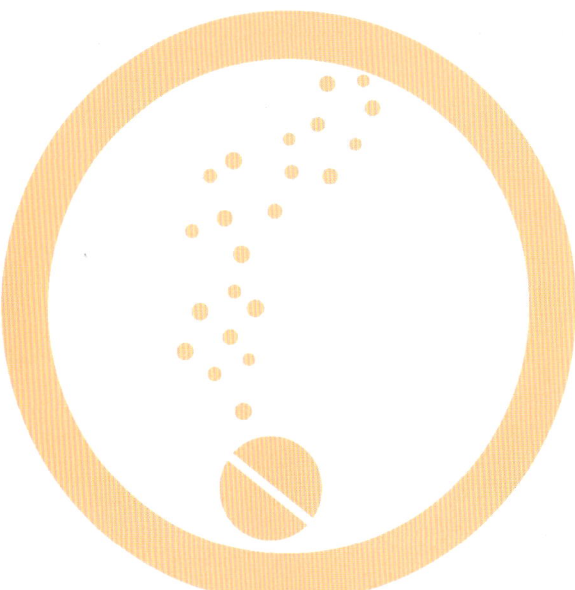

HEALING FOODS

A diet containing foods that are rich in beta-carotene may help reduce the risk of psoriasis. Good sources include green leafy vegetables, carrots, red bell peppers, mangoes, and apricots. The body converts beta-carotene into vitamin A, which is important for healthy skin.

CALL YOUR DOCTOR

You should consult your doctor if:

- Your current method of controlling your psoriasis does not seem to be working
- Your skin becomes inflamed all over, pus-filled spots develop on your skin, or there are signs of infection
- You develop stiff or painful joints
- Your psoriasis is greatly interfering with your everyday activities at home, work, or school
- You become depressed or anxious about the appearance of your psoriasis and it affects your social relationships.

IMMEDIATE RELIEF

Try soaking in a warm, soothing oatmeal bath for 15 minutes to relieve itching and soften your skin. Apply a good moisturizer afterward to lock in moisture.

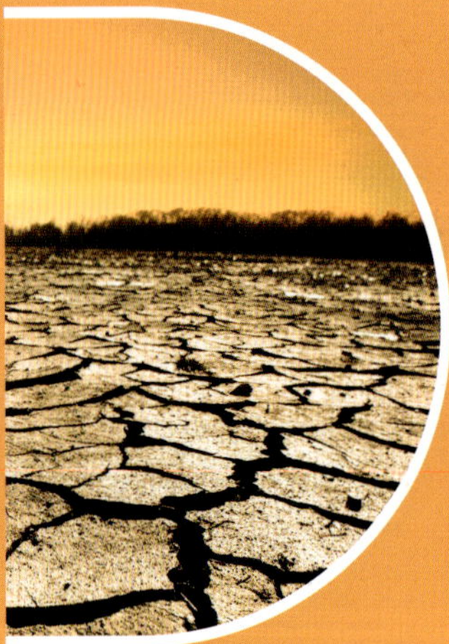

Dermatitis

Dermatitis is inflammation of the skin, most often affecting the hands and face. It occurs when the skin comes into contact with either an irritant (irritant contact dermatitis) or a substance that triggers an allergic reaction (allergic contact dermatitis). Atopic dermatitis, or eczema, runs in families and it often occurs alongside hay fever and asthma.

SYMPTOMS

- Red rash
- Skin inflammation
- Thickened patches of skin
- Dry or cracked skin
- Blisters
- Itching
- Stinging, burning, or sore skin

Did You Know?

If you have allergic contact dermatitis, areas of your skin that did not come into contact with the allergen may be affected as well as the areas that did. Symptoms of allergic dermatitis may take several days to appear.

PREVENTION

The best way to avoid irritant or allergic contact dermatitis is to identify the offending irritant or allergen and avoid coming into contact with it. It could be something in your day-to-day life, or something you come into contact with at work. Some common substances that cause dermatitis include nickel, makeup, hair dye, skin creams, perfumes, latex, adhesives, detergents, oils, solvents, acids, alkalis, dust, soil, and some plants.

- Wash your skin as soon as possible after coming into contact with the substance that triggers your dermatitis.
- Wear gloves or other protective clothing when necessary to protect your skin.
- Avoid immersing your hands in water for long periods of time.
- Avoid products containing alcohol or soap, because these dry out the skin.
- Prevent your skin from drying out with a good moisturizer or an emollient, such as aqueous cream.
- Use fragrance-free products.
- Avoid scratching dermatitis; scratching will make the condition worse and may lead to infection.

CONVENTIONAL TREATMENTS

Although it is best to avoid the substance that is causing your dermatitis, it is not always practical or possible. Most people find they are able to improve the symptoms of dermatitis by using an emollient. Emollient creams soothe and soften the skin, and they should be used frequently throughout the day, if necessary. Your doctor may prescribe a corticosteroid cream to reduce inflammation. A medication known as alitretinoin is used to treat severe cases of dermatitis.

NATURAL REMEDIES

Some natural options for treating dermatitis include the following remedies.

NUTRITIONAL MEDICINE Omega-3 fatty acids have an anti-inflammatory effect and help prevent skin itchiness and dryness. Some good sources include cold-water fish, such as salmon and mackerel, flaxseeds, walnut oil, pumpkin seeds, and green leafy vegetables.

HERBAL REMEDIES Skin creams containing chamomile or witch hazel can help to soothe itching and burning and aid healing.

ACUPUNCTURE The anti-inflammatory effects of acupuncture may relieve the itching caused by dermatitis and help to heal skin lesions.

HOMEOPATHIC REMEDIES

Here are some homeopathic medicines that may ease the symptoms of dermatitis.

Rhus toxicodendron 6C: Take one tablet four times daily for a poison ivy type rash that itches and burns or that has swelling and blisters.

Sulfur 6C: Take one tablet three times daily for red, burning, itching, scaling skin that is irritated by heat and water.

Urtica urens 6C: Take one tablet three times daily for an itchy, stinging, blotchy rash, and cracked skin.

CALL YOUR DOCTOR

You should see your doctor if:

- Your current method of treating your dermatitis is not working
- You are having difficulty avoiding the substance causing your dermatitis
- Your dermatitis flares up more than usual, becomes painful, starts weeping, or crusts over; you may have an infection that needs treatment with antibiotics
- Your dermatitis is making you depressed, or is significantly affecting the quality of your day-to-day life.

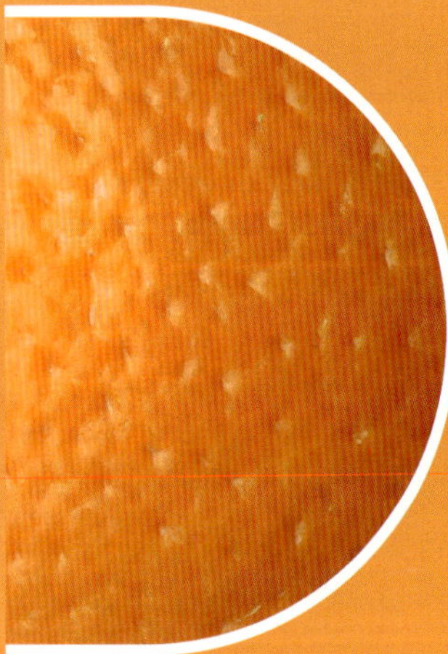

Cellulite

Cellulite is the name given to the visible pockets of fat, fluid, and toxins trapped in tissue beneath the skin, and it is the bane of many women's lives (although men can get it, too). Cellulite appears most often on the buttocks, thighs, stomach, lower back, and upper arms, and it gives the skin a dimpled, wobbly appearance.

SYMPTOMS

- Dimpling of the skin
- An "orange peel" effect
- Cottage cheeselike lumps visible beneath the skin

Did You Know?

It is not just overweight people who develop cellulite; anyone can get it regardless of size. As well as diet, exercise, and other lifestyle factors, genetics can also play an important part in determining whether or not you will develop cellulite.

PREVENTION

The prevention of cellulite focuses on maintaining good blood circulation and preventing the buildup of fluid and toxins. This is achieved by adopting a healthy lifestyle, as listed below.

- Exercise regularly to improve circulation and encourage lymphatic drainage (the removal of fluid from tissues). Aim for about 30 minutes of aerobic activity five times a week.
- Eat a healthy diet with plenty of fiber, fruits, and vegetables, and limit junk food.
- Reduce the amount of saturated fat in your diet. This causes cholesterol to clog up the walls of your blood vessels and hinders blood circulation.
- Avoid excess salt. Too much salt can lead to fluid retention and make cellulite look worse. Eat no more than 1,500 mg (about two-thirds of a teaspoon) of salt per day. Remember that salt is already added to a lot of processed foods.
- Drink at least eight cups of water every day. This will help to prevent water retention, encourage the removal of toxins, and improve the appearance of your skin.
- Minimize your daily consumption of caffeine, alcohol, and nicotine; these all encourage the buildup of toxins.

CONVENTIONAL TREATMENTS

The appearance of cellulite can be improved with diet and exercise. Alternatively, specially formulated cellulite creams may make your skin smoother and improve the appearance of cellulite. Body wrap treatments made from mineral salts and clay may tighten and firm the skin. Endermologie is a type of massage that uses suction and rollers to improve circulation, remove toxins, and soften the skin.

NATURAL REMEDIES

Cellulite can be treated from the inside or outside. Try the following natural remedies and medicines.

NUTRITIONAL MEDICINE Increase your intake of omega-3 fatty acids (found in oily cold-water fish, such as salmon and mackerel, and flaxseeds and walnuts), because they reduce inflammation and hydrate the skin cells.

AROMATHERAPY Mix three drops each of juniper, rosemary, and lavender essential oils with one tablespoon jojoba oil. Massage regularly into your skin to improve the skin tone and circulation.

HERBAL REMEDIES Gotu kola has anti-inflammatory properties, encourages circulation, and improves skin firmness. Take one to two 250-milligram tablets daily.

HELPFUL THERAPIES

Dry skin brushing for a few minutes each day can improve circulation and encourage the removal of toxins. Use a brush with soft, natural bristles to brush your skin in the direction of your heart.

EXERCISE

Try the following exercise for firming up your thighs and buttocks.

1 Stand with your feet hips' width apart.

2 Lunge back with your left leg, squeezing your buttocks as you do so.

3 Hold for one second, and then step forward with your left leg, raising your left knee in front of you.

4 Step back to the standing position and repeat with the other leg. Perform 15 repetitions on each side five times a week.

Quick Fix

You can try vigorously rubbing some used ground coffee over your cellulite-inflicted areas while you are in the shower.

Caution

Liposuction is a medical procedure that vacuums away fatty deposits from underneath your skin. However, it can cause complications, such as circulatory problems and lymphatic system damage, and may make your cellulite look worse than before.

Blisters

Blisters are pockets of clear fluid between the layers of skin. They are usually caused by friction, burns, or skin conditions, such as eczema or shingles. Although not serious, they may be painful and take time to heal.

SYMPTOMS

- Clear fluid (sebum) beneath the skin
- Blister may be tinged with blood
- Friction blisters on hands and feet

PREVENTION

You can prevent blisters from forming by taking the following simple measures:

- Don't wear tight, badly fitting shoes, and wear socks with new shoes
- Wear thick socks—or even two pairs—on hikes and long walks
- Keep your feet dry with powder or antiperspirants; blisters are more likely to form on damp skin
- Wear gloves when you are doing manual work, such as gardening
- Check the grip on your sports rackets
- Wear a protective sunscreen lotion to prevent sunburn and blistering.

CONVENTIONAL TREATMENTS

The conventional treatment depends on where the blisters occur. Do not lance or drain them; keep them clean and, if it's probable that they will rub or be banged into, apply some antiseptic lotion or cream before covering with a bandage; or smear with petroleum jelly or dab with antiseptic lotion and keep open to the air to heal.

NATURAL REMEDIES

To speed up healing and reduce itching and soreness, try one of the following therapies.

HERBAL REMEDIES Apply a little aloe vera gel or calendula cream to the blister and cover with a bandage or dressing.

AROMATHERAPY Dab a little lavender essential oil onto the blister.

CALL YOUR DOCTOR

Most blisters do not merit medical attention, but if you have a extremely large one or it becomes infected or does not heal within a few days, consult your doctor. Seek medical advice for blisters caused by conditions such as eczema, impetigo, chickenpox, and shingles.

Draining a Blister

Resist popping a blister, if possible, because doing so can introduce infection. However, if you do need to drain one, use only a sterilized needle to break the skin. To do this, hold the needle with tweezers over a naked gas flame until really hot and then cool before using. Dab the blister with antiseptic and squeeze out the fluid gently. Apply a soothing antiseptic cream before covering with a bandage, dressing, or special "Second Skin" blister dressing.

Chapped Lips

Your lips do not contain natural moisturizing agents, so they can get dry, sore, and cracked in cold or windy conditions or in hot sunshine. You need to protect them against extreme weather and moisturize them inside and out.

SYMPTOMS

- ▷ Dry lips that crack easily
- ▷ May be sore and itchy

PREVENTION

You can help to keep your lips smooth and moist by doing the following:

- Apply a little petroleum jelly every night at bedtime and wear it under lipstick during the day
- Always wear a protective lip screen in hot weather to prevent sunburn
- Use a creamy, moisturizing lipstick
- Apply a lip salve in cold weather
- Drink plenty of water (ideally, eight glasses a day) to prevent dehydration
- Eat a healthy diet with plenty of whole-grain cereals, leafy green vegetables, fresh fruit, seeds, and nuts
- Don't lick your lips too often.

CONVENTIONAL TREATMENTS

You can buy conventional lip salves and balms in most pharmacies—some are flavored, colored, or frosted. However, be sure you check the labels if you tend to have sensitive skin—a minority of people can be allergic to some ingredients.

Don't Lick Your Lips

It's very tempting to keep licking sore, dry lips, but, unfortunately, this will only make them worse, because saliva dries them out more.

NATURAL REMEDIES

There are many tried-and-tested home remedies for soothing chapped lips. Try one of the following natural treatments.

- Rub a little honey onto sore, chapped lips—it is a natural moisturizer.
- Apply some natural beeswax lip balm.
- Break open a vitamin E capsule and apply the oil to sore lips.
- Smooth in some cocoa butter, coconut oil, or olive oil.

HERBAL REMEDIES Apply a little aloe vera gel to your lips several times a day.

CALL YOUR DOCTOR

Most chapped lips don't necessitate a visit to the doctor, but if your lips are persistently cracked and even bleeding, then get them checked. You may have an allergic reaction to something or a yeast infection.

Cold Sores

Cold sores are painful blisters that appear on the skin around the mouth and lips. They are commonly spread between people through skin-to-skin contact and are caused by the herpes simplex virus.

SYMPTOMS

- ▷ Tingling sensation on the lips
- ▷ Fluid-filled blisters
- ▷ Redness and swelling
- ▷ Yellow crusty scabs

PREVENTION

In the first instance, cold sores are caught through skin-to-skin contact. They can be prevented by avoiding kissing anyone with cold sores and not sharing objects they have used, such as razors or lip gloss. Flare-ups are triggered by various factors, including stress, tiredness, being run down, illness, a weakened immune system, menstruation, and exposure to sun or wind.

- Take antioxidant vitamins, such as C and E, to boost your immune system.
- Take ginseng to improve your body's tolerance to stress.
- Avoid exposure to strong wind or sunlight.
- Get more sleep.
- Avoid coffee, alcohol, and sugar, because they can reduce the immune response.

CONVENTIONAL TREATMENTS

Cold sores are treated with over-the-counter or prescribed antiviral ointments, plus painkillers for pain or discomfort. Antibiotics may be needed if cold sores become infected.

NATURAL REMEDIES

There are various natural remedies you can try. The main ones are listed below.

NUTRITIONAL MEDICINE Eat foods that are rich in the amino acid lysine, such as eggs, meat, fish, and kidney beans, because it may help to suppress the herpes simplex virus.

HERBAL REMEDIES Take the herb echinacea to boost your immune system. Use licorice gel to ease inflammation and lemon balm cream to aid healing.

CALL YOUR DOCTOR

If your symptoms don't ease or your cold sores become infected, consult your doctor.

Did You Know?

Once you've caught the herpes simplex virus, it remains in your body for the rest of your life. Although you can't get rid of the virus, you can take practical steps to reduce the likelihood of getting cold sores again.

Boils

A boil is an infection that occurs in the hair follicles of the skin. It forms as a small red lump, filled with pus. Boils can develop on any area of the skin, but are particularly common on the neck, thighs, face, or in the armpits.

SYMPTOMS

- A small red lump on the skin, which may grow
- When pus forms inside, the head of the boil develops a white or yellow dot
- Boils that get larger can become painful

PREVENTION

To help prevent the likelihood of boils, you can do the following:

- Regularly wash your skin and keep it clean—use an antibacterial soap if you want
- If you have cuts, grazes, or wounds on your skin, keep them covered with a bandage until they heal
- Exercise regularly and eat a healthy diet.

CONVENTIONAL TREATMENTS

You can have single boils, or small clusters, and they can grow bigger, but they're generally harmless. Usually, boils don't require treatment, because they burst on their own and then heal. However, on occasion, your doctor may need to lance the boil, which involves draining out the pus with a sterilized needle. If there's risk of infection, antibiotics may be prescribed.

NATURAL REMEDIES

You can try using natural remedies to treat boils if they appear.

HOMEOPATHIC REMEDIES For a sudden, inflamed, red, and painful boil, try Belladonna 6C.

AROMATHERAPY Lightly dab a boil with one drop of tea tree oil on a cotton ball. Repeat until the boil goes.

CALL YOUR DOCTOR

If a boil does not heal after two weeks, it's particularly large or painful, you develop a fever, or you have a weak immune system, you should consult your doctor.

Quick Fix

Boils respond well to heat and it also helps the healing process, so try putting a warm washcloth or other clean cloth onto the boil for 10 to 20 minutes, twice a day.

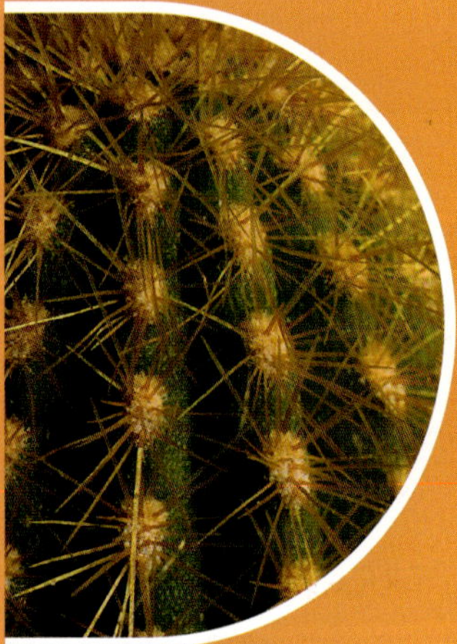

Hives and Heat Rash

Two skin conditions that can suddenly occur are hives (urticaria) and heat rash (also called prickly heat). With hives, red swollen weals suddenly appear on the skin and are itchy. In many cases, they disappear after a few hours, but sometimes they can go on for longer. Unlike hives, heat rash is not an allergic reaction but is caused by blocked sweat glands in hot conditions.

SYMPTOMS

HIVES

- Red, pink, or white raised weals
- A ring of red skin
- Itchiness
- Flat, red marks left on the skin after an attack

HEAT RASH

- Itchy skin
- Red rash
- Small red or clear spots
- Prickling sensation
- Tiredness

PREVENTION

- Avoid using a concoction of soaps and shower gels—stick to a mild or sensitive soap and use it only once a day.
- Try to avoid hot climates or, if you have to be in the heat, acclimatize yourself slowly to the temperature. Always wear loose-fitting and lightweight clothing.
- Stay out of the sun if you're taking antibiotics, because some medicines can increase the risk of heat rash.
- Avoid having hot showers or baths, eating spicy food, and drinking hot drinks.
- If you've managed to identify a potential allergen for your hives, then avoid it where possible.
- If you have chronic hives, avoiding stress and alcohol can prevent them from getting worse.

Did You Know?

Hives can often be caused by an allergic reaction to lifestyle or dietary factors, such as the washing product you are using. Diet is also important. An elimination diet, worked out with a qualified nutritionist, can help to identify the potential cause of hives.

CONVENTIONAL TREATMENTS

Antihistamines may be prescribed for hives, because they usually reduce the itching and help allergic reactions. Some types of antihistamines can be bought over the counter, too, but try and avoid any pills that make you sleepy. For severe symptoms, steroids may be required, alongside an antihistamine. Heat rash can be eased by cooling creams, such as calamine lotion or those containing menthol.

NATURAL REMEDIES

Try the following natural remedies for alleviating the symptoms of hives and heat rash.

AROMATHERAPY Make a compress of lavender or chamomile oil (a few drops will be sufficient) and apply to a heat rash. Or add a few drops of one of the oils into a warm bath and soak in it.

FLOWER REMEDIES Take four drops of Rescue Remedy or the flower remedy Impatiens to relieve itchy skin caused by heat rash or hives. Apply neat to the tongue or add two drops to a small glass of water and sip it.

NUTRITIONAL MEDICINE Vitamin C has a natural antihistamine effect, but it's more effective if combined with bioflavonoids, such as quercetin or rose hip. Take one tablet daily to reduce the symptoms of hives and prevent future attacks.

HERBAL REMEDIES

- Soothe irritated, inflamed, itchy, or burning skin with some aloe vera gel, stinging nettle juice, or calendula cream.
- Drink yarrow and chamomile tea to help ease the symptoms of hives. Make your own tea by adding one tablespoonful of each herb to a teapot and pouring boiling water over the top. Steep for 10 minutes before straining and drinking.

HOMEOPATHIC REMEDIES

Remedies vary depending on the symptoms you have. If they don't work within 24 to 36 hours, you should consult your doctor.

Apis 30C: Take one tablet every two hours, up to a maximum of eight times through the day, as soon as a heat rash develops.

Urtica 6C: Take one tablet three times a day, for up to five days, when urticaria or hives occurs.

Sol 30C: Take one tablet three times a day for up to three weeks if you're in a hot and humid climate and prone to heat rash.

CALL YOUR DOCTOR

Heat rash will fade in cooler temperatures, but if you have hives and your rash persists or worsens, you should see your doctor.

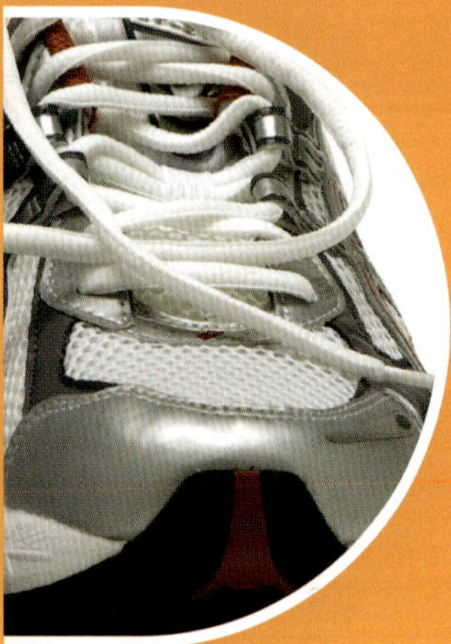

Athlete's Foot

This common skin condition, which affects the feet, is caused by a fungal infection. Anyone can get it (not just athletes), although it's more common among teenagers and men because they are more likely to wear airtight shoes. Known medically as *tinea pedis*, athlete's foot makes the skin on the foot, and between the toes, become red, itchy, dry, flaky, and scaly.

SYMPTOMS

- An itchy rash between your toes
- Dry, flaky, or scaly skin
- Redness
- Blisters
- Swelling
- Cracked skin
- A burning or stinging sensation

Did You Know?

Athlete's foot is usually mild and can be successfully treated at home, but, if left untreated, it can go on for prolonged periods.

PREVENTION

The athlete's foot fungus thrives in moist, warm, and dark environments, so some of your prevention strategies should focus on keeping your feet dry. It can also spread by walking bare foot in swimming pool changing rooms, showers, and saunas and from direct contact with someone who has it.

- Keep your feet clean and fresh by washing them every day.
- Dry your feet thoroughly, especially between the toes, before putting on clean socks or tights.
- Avoid sharing towels, especially with someone who has athlete's foot.
- Wash your towels and bedding regularly.
- Use talcum powder on your feet to help prevent them from sweating.
- Expose your feet to the air when you're at home by taking off shoes and socks.
- Wear different pairs of shoes regularly instead of always the same pair.
- In communal changing rooms, saunas, or showers, wear flip-flops or sandals.
- Don't share or borrow other people's shoes.

CONVENTIONAL TREATMENTS

Antifungal medications are commonly used to treat athlete's foot and come in the form of creams, lotions, sprays, or powder. These are applied to the affected area of the foot and the surrounding skin, and they are available over the counter in pharmacies. Oral antifungal pills are sometimes required and are prescribed by a doctor.

NATURAL REMEDIES

There are various natural remedies you can try for relieving athlete's foot.

AROMATHERAPY Tea tree essential oil can be effective for treating fungal infections. Try soaking your feet in a bowl of water with a drop of tea tree oil added. Alternatively, put one or two drops of oil onto a cotton ball and dab directly onto the affected area.

NUTRITIONAL REMEDIES Cutting out caffeine and sugar from your diet may help reduce the risk of fungal infection developing. Eat garlic, which is packed with antifungal and antibacterial properties.

Caution

Always wash your hands before and after treating your feet. If you don't, the fungal infection can spread to your hands, too, causing tinea manuum, a condition where your hands become dry, itchy, and red.

HERBAL REMEDIES

- Use some marigold or calendula cream to help soothe itching.
- Soak your feet in an infusion of goldenseal, which is known for its antifungal properties, and dust your dry feet with goldenseal powder.
- Help support your immune system by taking echinacea tablets or tincture during an athlete's foot outbreak.

HOMEOPATHIC REMEDIES

Homeopathic remedies can be useful in relieving some symptoms of athlete's foot:

Silica 6C: If you're prone to sweaty feet, this can help reduce the sweat and dampness that the infection loves. Take one tablet twice a day until the condition improves.

Sulfur 6C: To help aid the dry, cracked, and itchy skin of athlete's foot, take one tablet twice daily.

CALL YOUR DOCTOR

If none of the remedies work and athlete's foot persists, consult your doctor, because fungal infections can sometimes be an underlying sign of diabetes. In severe cases, it can spread to the toenails and, where the skin becomes very cracked, bacterial infections can develop, too.

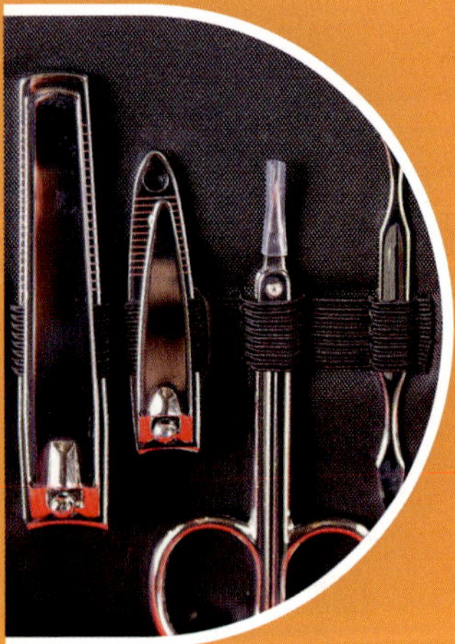

Nail Problems

Like other parts of your body, your nails can be subject to their own health complaints. Nail problems, such as fungal nail infections, ingrown toenails, and brittle nails, are all common. They can sometimes be a sign of nutritional deficiency or a hint of an underlying health condition, but most are easily treated once they are correctly diagnosed.

SYMPTOMS

FUNGAL NAIL INFECTIONS

- Thick, discolored, and crumbly nail
- Pain and inflamed skin under the nail
- Nail may fall off
- Discomfort when walking

INGROWN TOE NAILS

- Pain and discomfort
- A nail where the edge or corner grows into the skin
- Hard skin
- Swelling and pain
- Tenderness
- Bleeding
- Discharging pus

BRITTLE NAILS

- Nails that easily break, split, and chip
- Vertical splits

PREVENTION

- If you have, or suspect you could have, athlete's foot, then treat it, because if left, it can spread and cause fungal nail problems.
- Keep your feet clean and dry, because damp, hot, and sweaty feet encourage fungi to grow and cause nail fungal infections.
- To prevent reoccurrence of fungal nail problems, look after your nails properly.
- If you do a lot of dish washing or frequently have your hands in hot water, wear rubber gloves, because they can help prevent fingernail infections from occurring.
- Avoid biting your nails or using artificial nails to reduce the risk of fingernail infections.
- Avoid wearing tight shoes.
- Always cut your toenails straight across to help prevent ingrown toenails; however, avoid cutting them too short.
- To help avoid brittle nails and to prevent nail problems as a whole, always eat a healthy, balanced, and nutrition-filled diet.
- If you have nail problems or have difficulty cutting your toenails, you should visit a podiatrist regularly.

CONVENTIONAL TREATMENTS

FUNGAL NAIL INFECTIONS are treated with a paint-on, antifungal nail lacquer or through the use of prescribed antibiotics.

INGROWN TOENAILS can be softened by soaking your foot in warm water, three to four times a day. Painkillers can help alleviate the discomfort. The small part of the nail that's digging into the skin may have to be removed.

For bad cases, all or part of the nail may need to be surgically removed under local anaesthesic. This is usually done at a doctor's office or a surgery center.

BRITTLE NAILS, along with other symptoms, can sometimes be a sign of an underactive thyroid, so if your doctor suspects this, then blood tests may be required.

NATURAL REMEDIES

If you have regular nail problems, try the following alternative remedies.

HERBAL REMEDIES To help your nails become stronger, take evening primrose oil capsules daily or try the herb horsetail, which is rich in silica. Aloe vera gel or neem oil can be applied to nails that are affected by fungal infections.

HOMEOPATHIC REMEDIES Silica 6C can be taken to help fight fungal nail infections and also to aid brittle nails.

Aromatherapy

- Put a drop of tea tree oil on a cotton ball and dab onto nails affected by fungal infections, or soak your feet in warm water with two drops of tea tree oil.
- A foot soak with a few drops of soothing lavender oil can ease the discomfort of ingrown toenails.

NUTRITIONAL MEDICINE

Brittle nails can be a sign that you lack vitamins, such as the vitamin B group, and minerals, such as zinc and iron. Eat plenty of asparagus, broccoli, yeast extract, and meat for the B vitamins; a handful of pumpkin seeds for zinc; and some red meat, beans, or green leafy vegetables for iron. For an extra boost, you can take a multivitamin and mineral supplement. The overall effect of improved nutrition should be visible within three months or as the nails grow.

CALL YOUR DOCTOR

If you have a painful ingrown toenail that does not respond to self-treatment or visits to the podiatrist, call your doctor. You may need antibiotics to clear up any infection. If brittle nails or fungal infections persist and do not heal, you should also consult your doctor.

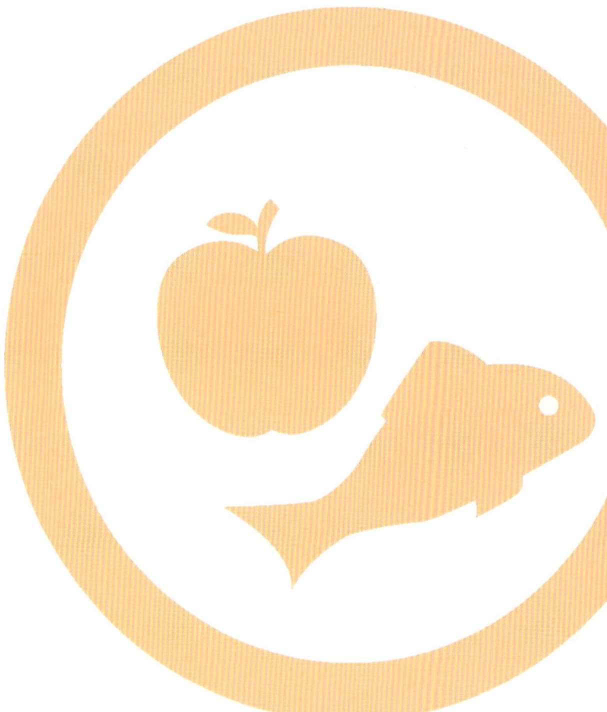

Corns and Calluses

Corns and calluses both involve skin that thickens and becomes painful on the feet. Corns appear on or between the toes, usually due to poorly fitting shoes; calluses appear on the soles, often caused by pressure when walking.

SYMPTOMS

CORNS

- Small, round hard area of skin
- A hard "plug" in the center
- Corns between the toes can be softer and are white and rubbery
- Pain
- Swelling

CALLUSES

- Hard, wide area of skin
- Undefined edge
- Pale or yellow color

PREVENTION

- Check your feet regularly and keep them in good condition.
- Soak your feet in warm water and gently remove hard skin with a foot file or pumice.
- Regularly moisturize with foot cream.
- Wear comfortable shoes that fit and don't put your toes or feet under pressure.
- Change your socks or tights every day.

CONVENTIONAL TREATMENTS

Corn bandages, padding, or insoles in shoes are the usual remedies for corns and calluses. A podiatrist may cut away the corn or callus to relieve the pressure. If soft corns become infected, antibiotics may be prescribed.

NATURAL REMEDIES

You can also try the following natural methods of dealing with these problems.

AROMATHERAPY Soften hard skin by soaking your feet in an aromatherapy footbath. Add a few drops of lavender, thyme, and rosemary essential oils to soothe and cleanse the skin. Once the skin is softened, gently rub it with a pumice stone or foot file.

HERBAL REMEDIES Moisturize your feet daily using herbal foot creams, such as calendula, to keep the skin soft and reduce the likelihood of painful cracking.

AYURVEDA Mix together one teaspoon of aloe vera gel with half a teaspoon of turmeric and apply nightly to your feet. Cover with cotton socks, and wash off in the morning.

FELDENKRAIS METHOD Learn awareness of how you walk and stand, because incorrect movements may increase pressure on your feet and toes.

Warts and Verrucas

Warts are small, rough benign lumps that appear on the skin; verrucas (plantar warts) occur on the feet. Although warts are normally painless, verrucas can be painful to walk on as they are pushed up into the foot.

SYMPTOMS

COMMON WARTS

- Firm, raised, and skin color
- Rough surface

VERRUCAS

- A white, hard area on the foot, with a black dot in the center

PREVENTION

Warts and verrucas are both caused by the human papilloma virus (HPV). They are contagious and skin-to-skin contact can easily pass them on, so preventive methods are important.

- Avoid sharing washcloths, towels, or shoes.
- Avoid touching someone's warts or verrucas.
- Wear flip-flops or sandals in communal changing rooms, saunas, or showers.

CONVENTIONAL TREATMENTS

Creams, gels, and medicated bandages are available over the counter. Most contain an ingredient called salicylic acid and, although it helps warts and verrucas, it can also damage healthy skin. Anyone with diabetes or circulation problems needs to be especially careful and should speak to a doctor before using salicylic acid remedies. Some warts are treated with cryotherapy, whereby a cold liquid is sprayed on to the affected area to freeze the wart and destroy it.

NATURAL REMEDIES

The following natural remedies may be helpful in treating warts and veruccas.

HERBAL REMEDIES Being susceptible to warts and verrucas can signify that your immune system is low, so you could try some immune-boosting remedies, such as echinacea. Thuja cream can be rubbed into the affected area daily.

AROMATHERAPY Oregano oil is packed with antiseptic properties and can help warts. Put a drop on a cotton ball and dab it on the wart daily until cleared.

HOMEOPATHIC REMEDIES

Homeopathic remedies that can help warts and verrucas include the following:

Causticum 30C: For getting rid of the infection, take one tablet daily

Thuja 30C: For hard, misshapen warts, take one tablet daily.

CALL YOUR DOCTOR

For severe and persistent cases of warts or verrucas that do not improve with over-the-counter or natural remedies, you should consult your doctor.

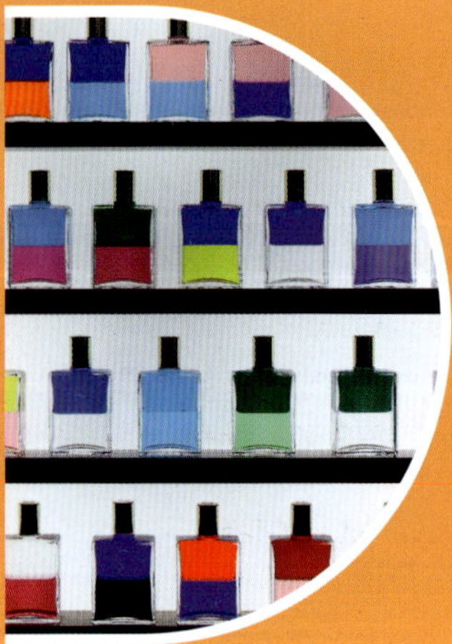

Body and Foot Odor

Everyone sweats, but some people have a tendency to sweat more than others, and men tend to sweat more than women. Body and foot odor occur when the bacteria living on your skin causes sweat to break down into acids, which create a strong or unpleasant odor. Body odor can be an embarrassing health problem, but there are natural and conventional remedies to help beat it.

SYMPTOMS

- Sweating
- An odor under the armpits
- Smelly feet

PREVENTION

- Body odor can be made worse if you are overweight or obese, so losing weight may help to prevent it.
- Dietary factors play a role in body odor—avoid eating spicy foods and you may be spared from body odor.
- Foot odor can be prevented by not wearing sneakers or any shoes that have a plastic lining, because it encourages your feet to sweat. Instead, opt for shoes that have a more foot-friendly leather lining.
- Make sure you change your socks every day and choose ones that are made from a mixture of wool and man-made fibers. These fibers will enable any sweat on your feet to evaporate.

Caution

Avoid using foot deodorants if you have a fungal foot infection—in this case, an antifungal foot spray or athlete's foot treatment is required.

CONVENTIONAL TREATMENTS

- Warm water helps kill the bacteria on your skin, so have regular showers or baths.
- Use antibacterial soap and a deodorant or antiperspirant. Deodorants are designed to make the skin acidic, which helps ward off bacteria, while antiperspirants help block sweat glands and reduce sweating. Foot deodorants and antiperspirants are also available to purchase.
- Wear clothing made of natural fibers, such as cotton, wool, or silk, because these let your skin breathe and sweat evaporate more easily.
- Using an extrastrong antiperspirant, such as aluminum chloride, may be recommended by your doctor.
- In severe cases, a cosmetic treatment with Botox injections may be recommended. These are injected near the armpit and help to destroy the nerves that are involved in sweating.

NATURAL REMEDIES

You can try some of the following natural remedies to combat body and foot odor.

HERBAL REMEDIES Use the herb marigold to help reduce sweating and body odor. Brew yourself a pot of marigold tea by adding one to two teaspoons of dried marigold to a teapot and pouring boiling water over it. Drink the tea twice a day.

NUTRITIONAL MEDICINE

Your diet can have an important effect on the smell of your sweat, so try adapting it as follows:

- Avoid eating garlic, spices, or meals such as hot Mexican or Indian dishes, because they could make your sweat smell stronger
- Try cutting back on eating red meat and dairy products—this may also help
- A zinc deficiency can contribute to sweating and body odor, so consider taking a daily zinc supplement.

CALL YOUR DOCTOR

Although they are usually harmless and fine to treat at home, sometimes a change in body odor, or suddenly having one, can be a sign of an underlying medical condition, such as diabetes, liver disease, or kidney disease. If you suddenly begin to sweat a lot, have cold sweats, start sweating at night, or notice that your body odor begins to smell fruity or like bleach, then call your doctor.

Aromatherapy

- Put a few drops of antibacterial tea tree essential oil into a bowl or bathtub of warm water and bathe your feet in it. After washing, dry your feet thoroughly.
- For body odor, add up to six drops of essential oil to a warm bath; choose lemon, clary sage, or lavender essential oils, or even a mix of all three, because they have deodorizing properties.

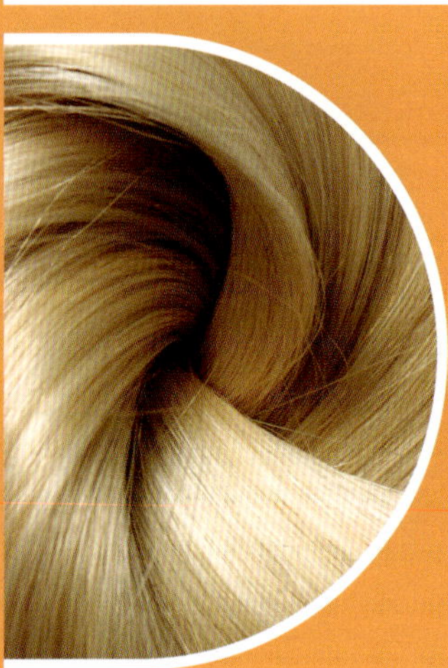

Dry hair

Silky, healthy-looking hair depends as much on good nutrition and how you feed it from the inside as the range of hair products you use and your hairdresser's skill. Indeed, your hair is an external barometer of your internal health, and its appearance and condition can be affected by many underlying medical problems as well as your lifestyle and environmental factors.

SYMPTOMS

- ▷ Dry, rough, and brittle hair
- ▷ Split, frayed ends
- ▷ Hair looks lackluster
- ▷ The texture feels harsh like string

PREVENTION

The good news is that there are a lot of effective remedies for dry hair and you don't have to worry anymore about bad hair days. Better still, try to keep your hair well-nourished and in good condition to prevent it from becoming dry and brittle. Here are some practical steps you can take to have healthy, shiny hair.

- Eat a healthy, balanced diet that contains all the essential nutrients. Make sure you get your five-a-day portions of fresh fruit and vegetables, and foods that are good sources of vitamins C (citrus fruits, bell peppers, strawberries, tomatoes, and leafy green vegetables) and E (avocados, whole-grain cereals, and leafy green vegetables).
- Don't expose your hair to excessive sun—always wear a sun hat in hot weather.
- Use a swimming cap in chlorinated swimming pools.

Did You Know?

Stress, hair colorants, heat from hair dryers and straighteners, sun and chlorine, and poor nutrition can all damage your hair and dry it out. You need to consider all these factors.

- If you color your hair yourself, always try to avoid chemical hair dyes and opt for natural colorants instead (see page 46).
- Visit the hairdresser for a trim at least once every six to eight weeks to keep the ends healthy and stop them from splitting (see box, below).
- Keep the use of heated hair appliances, such as hair dryers, hot rollers, curling tongs, and hair straighteners, to an absolute minimum.
- Try not to overdo applications of hairspray, mousse, or styling gel—bombarding your hair with chemicals weakens and dulls it.
- Do not wash your hair every day. In reality, too-frequent washing can strip out the natural oils.
- Always rinse your hair thoroughly in warm, not hot, water to get rid of all shampoo residues.
- Use a good-quality natural bristle brush, not a harsh nylon one, to prevent damage to your hair.
- Whenever possible, do let your hair dry naturally instead of using a hair dryer.

CONVENTIONAL TREATMENTS

- After shampooing in the usual way, always use a conditioner that is specially formulated for dry hair, and carefully comb it through from the roots to the ends of the hair. Let it sit for a few minutes or for the time specified on the container before rinsing it out thoroughly.
- To make an intensive-treatment conditioner more effective, apply it to your hair, then wrap your head in a hot, damp towel and let sit for 10 to 15 minutes before rinsing. Alternatively, you can use a stay-in conditioner with an in-built thermal protector—apply before blow-drying.

NATURAL REMEDIES

The natural remedies you select will depend on whether you want to treat the condition from the inside or outside.

AROMATHERAPY Mix together one drop each of geranium, patchouli, rosemary, and sandalwood essential oils with two teaspoons of jojoba oil. Massage into your scalp and hair with your fingertips and then wrap in a towel and let sit for at least 15 minutes before washing out.

YOGA Some devotees of yoga believe that practicing head and shoulder-stand asanas can help keep hair healthy by boosting blood flow and nutrients to the scalp.

HERBAL REMEDIES

- If your scalp is itchy, add a soothing chamomile infusion to the final rinse.
- Make a cleansing herbal tea by infusing one teaspoon of dried burdock or marshmallow in almost-boiling water. Steep for at least 5 minutes, then drain and drink.
- Make a preshampoo oil pack by heating some olive, almond, or jojoba oil in a heatproof bowl set over a saucepan of boiling water. Massage the warm oil into your dry hair and scalp and wrap in a towel or aluminum foil. Sit in a steamy bath for 15 minutes before rinsing and shampooing.

Split Ends

To prevent split ends, you can try massaging a natural commercial brand of mayonnaise into clean, dry hair or make your own by whisking one teaspoon each of almond or vegetable oil and vinegar with an extra-large egg, until smooth and emulsified. Let sit for at least 1 hour before rinsing out.

NUTRITIONAL MEDICINE

- Make sure you include some foods that are rich in Vitamin E in your daily diet. Good sources are avocados, nuts, seeds, olive oil, and leafy green vegetables.
- The most important nutrients of all for healthy hair are the B-complex group of vitamins, because deficiencies can lead to lackluster, dry hair and dandruff (see opposite). Every day, try to eat some of the following foods: whole-grain cereals, meat, poultry, fish, eggs, cheese, bananas, brewer's yeast, nuts, and dark green leafy vegetables.
- Zinc and sulfur will also help to keep your hair glossy, silky, and smooth.

CALL YOUR DOCTOR

If none of the remedies seem to work and your hair remains stubbornly dry despite all your efforts, perhaps you should consult your doctor. In rare instances, dry hair can be a symptom of a more serious underlying medical condition, such as an underactive thyroid gland or even psoriasis if it is accompanied by a dry, scaly, itchy scalp. You may even be referred to a specialist or trichologist for treatment.

Did You Know?

Your hair is a nonliving tissue made of a protein called keratin. The hair shaft in every individual strand is coated with a layer of protective cells. Hair grows at a rate of ½ inch per month and has a lifespan of three to six years.

HOMEMADE REMEDIES

- Add one tablespoon of cider vinegar to the rinsing water to add shine and soothe an itchy, dry scalp, which often accompanies dry hair.
- To add moisture and a healthy shine to your hair, mash up a ripe avocado with an egg yolk and a spoonful of olive oil. Massage into your hair and scalp and let sit for 20 to 30 minutes before washing out and shampooing.
- If you have any overripe discolored avocados and black bananas, don't throw them away. Mash them up with a fork and smooth into your hair, rubbing the mixture into the roots. Rinse off after 15 minutes and wash in the usual way.
- Another kitchen remedy is to beat up an egg with a cup of yogurt and the juice of a lemon. Mix in one teaspoon of coconut or olive oil and then massage into your hair and cover with a hot towel. Let sit for at least 30 minutes before rinsing and shampooing.

Natural Hair Colorants

Instead of using drying chemical hair colorants, try a herbal rinse for a soft and subtle effect.

- Chamomile flowers add sheen to blonde hair. Add a handful to a saucepan of simmering water and let simmer for 20 minutes before straining and cooling. Use as a herbal rinse after shampooing and then rinse out thoroughly. Diluted lemon juice will make it shine.
- Elderberries will add a subtle, deep mahogany color to dark hair. Prepare a herbal rinse in the same way as for chamomile above. Rinse it with a vinegar solution for extra shine.

Dandruff

This common scalp problem can vary in severity. Your skin cells are continuously being renewed and the old ones are shed. When this process is faster, the dead skin is more noticeable and is referred to as dandruff.

SYMPTOMS

- ▷ Flaking scalp
- ▷ Small white flakes falling from hair onto shoulders
- ▷ In acute cases, may be yellowish waxy scales on scalp with large greasy flakes

PREVENTION

- Eat a healthy, varied diet.
- Regular exercise will stimulate circulation and maintain hair health.
- Brush your hair regularly with a natural bristle brush, working from the scalp outward.
- Wash your hair at least twice a week.
- Don't color your hair with harsh chemical dyes.

CONVENTIONAL TREATMENTS

Dandruff is usually treated with conventional dandruff shampoos or lotions, but some can be harsh and irritate sensitive scalps. Ideally, opt for a mild, nondetergent-base one. Ask your pharmacist for advice on antidandruff and antifungal shampoos.

NATURAL REMEDIES

For a more natural approach, wash and rinse your hair and then gently massage half a cup of warm olive oil into your scalp. Cover with a towel and let sit for 30 minutes before shampooing and rinsing.

NUTRITIONAL MEDICINE Include B vitamins and sulfur in your diet by eating whole-grain cereals, wheat germ, eggs, and plenty of dark green leafy vegetables, such as cabbage. Cutting down on dairy foods may help alleviate dandruff.

HERBAL REMEDIES

- Try a simple rosemary rinse: put a few sprigs of fresh rosemary in a saucepan, cover with water, and simmer gently to 15 minutes. Cool and strain, then add a few drops of olive oil. After shampooing, use the rosemary water as a rinse before rinsing again with tepid water.
- Make an infusion of stinging nettles and add it to the final rinse.

HOMEOPATHIC REMEDIES

Choose the appropriate remedy for your symptoms.

Oleander 6C, for an itchy, dry scalp with white flakes falling from the hair.

Kali sulphuricum 6C, for moist or sticky flaky dandruff.

CALL YOUR DOCTOR

You can usually treat dandruff yourself at home, but if it is persistent, excessively flaky, and becomes acute, you should consult your doctor for an accurate diagnosis. It could be a symptom of psoriasis, seborrheic dermatitis, or a fungal infection.

Greasy Hair

Healthy hair should be clean, manageable, and glossy with plenty of bounce and natural shine. However, it is exposed on a daily basis to environmental pollution, wind, cold, heat, humidity, and air-conditioning, and all these factors can affect your hair type and condition. If you have greasy hair, don't worry—there are many natural beauty remedies as well as conventional ones.

SYMPTOMS

- ▷ Hair looks and feels oily
- ▷ It needs frequent washing
- ▷ It looks dirty soon after it is washed
- ▷ It is limp, lank, and lacks body

Did You Know?

Greasy hair is caused by overactive sebaceous glands beneath your scalp producing too much sebum (oil). Your diet, genetic inheritance, hormones, stress levels, and general state of health may all contribute.

PREVENTION

If you have a natural tendency toward excessively oily hair, you can take preventive measures to stop the condition from getting worse.

- Eat a healthy diet with plenty of fresh fruit and vegetables, and cut down on greasy, fried, and high-fat, sugary foods.
- Exercise regularly to increase the oxygen supply to your scalp.
- Do not use too much conditioner, or even try cutting it out altogether—some conditioners can leave an oily residue on the hair, making the problem worse.
- Taking oral contraceptive pills can worsen the condition for some people—if you suspect that this may be the case, discuss it with your doctor, who may suggest switching to another pill.
- Use mousse to style your hair—it does not contain oil and it will add volume.
- Don't use hair sprays—they attract dust and dirt from the air and will make your hair appear even more greasy.
- Wash your hair brushes and combs regularly in tepid, soapy water to avoid brushing grease back into your hair.

CONVENTIONAL TREATMENTS

Greasy hair is usually treated by washing it frequently with a specially formulated shampoo for oily hair types. It is advisable to shampoo and rinse it twice to thoroughly remove all traces of oil and leave it squeaky clean. You may not need to use a conditioner.

NATURAL REMEDIES

There are many natural treatments for the problem of oily hair, so why not try one of the following?

HERBAL REMEDIES Oily hair can benefit from lavender, peppermint, and white dead-nettle herbs, used fresh or dried, in herbal teas, infusions, and other preparations.

AROMATHERAPY Mix a massage oil by combining eight drops each rosemary, lavender, ylang ylang, and lime oils. Massage gently into your scalp at bedtime. Wash with a natural shampoo the following morning and then rinse out thoroughly.

HOMEMADE REMEDIES

- Add two beaten eggs and one tablespoon baking soda to two-and-a-half cups warm water. Pour over your hair and massage gently but firmly into your scalp. Let sit for 10 to 15 minutes before rinsing. Shampoo and then rinse again.
- Another effective old-fashioned kitchen remedy is to add some cider vinegar to the final rinse to degrease your hair.
- Like vinegar, lemon juice is acidic and can help control oil production. Try adding the freshly squeezed juice to a cup of warm water and pouring it over your hair after shampooing and rinsing. Let sit for 5 minutes and then rinse again with some tepid water.

CALL YOUR DOCTOR

Obviously, annoying as it may be, greasy hair is not a serious medical condition and there should be no need for you to consult a doctor. However, if it is persistent and affects your self-esteem, you may want to make an appointment with a dermatologist or trichologist to get expert advice.

Quick Fix

If you have an important meeting or a date and don't have time to wash your hair, just apply some dry shampoo or even gently shake a little fine talcum powder or baby powder onto the hair roots, wait a minute, and brush through thoroughly to absorb excess oil.

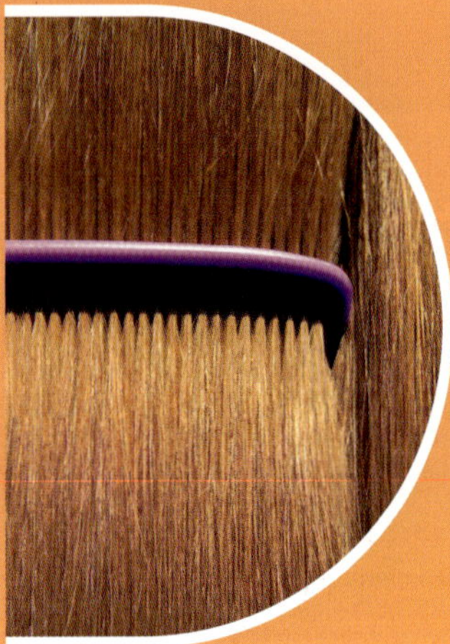

Head Lice

Head lice (or nits) are small, pinhead-size parasitic insects that live on the head, where they suck blood and lay their eggs. They can spread quickly, usually among young schoolchildren, and are then transmitted to other members of their family. Contrary to popular myth, dirty hair is not a cause—head lice always prefer clean, shiny hair, and healthy scalps.

SYMPTOMS

- Itching scalp—not usually an early symptom
- Lice look similar to dandruff in the host's hair
- The eggs are oval, yellowish white, and pearl-like in appearance

Did You Know?

Head lice cannot jump between heads; there has to be contact to enable them to crawl onto a new host. They lay their eggs on the sides of hair shafts close to the scalp. The eggs take 7 to 10 days to hatch, and the lice live for about 30 days, laying an average of 10 or so eggs per day.

PREVENTION

It is difficult to prevent head lice because they do not respect good hygiene and cleanliness, but if your child does come home with lice, you can try to stop other family members from becoming infested, too.

- Do not share hair brushes and combs.
- Avoid cross-infection by asking everyone to use only their own personal towels.
- Do not share a bed or bed linen.
- Check children's hair regularly by combing with a fine-tooth comb.
- Keep hair tied back and avoid head-to-head contact.

CONVENTIONAL TREATMENTS

The conventional treatment for head lice is to use a specially formulated, chemical insecticide shampoo or lotion. However, these are harsh and they should not be used too frequently, especially on young children or people who have asthma and allergies.

NATURAL REMEDIES

Because insecticides can have unwanted side effects, many people are seeking out more gentle natural remedies for treating head lice.

- Dampen your child's hair, adding conditioner, if desired, and comb through in sections with a special fine-tooth metal lice comb (available from pharmacies) to remove the eggs, wiping the comb clean on some tissue or paper towels between strokes. Repeat once every three days for two to three weeks until there are no signs of any lice or eggs.
- Try rinsing the hair in cider vinegar and rubbing some lemon juice into the scalp to destroy the eggs and combat oiliness.

HERBAL REMEDIES Make an infusion of bitterwood bark by adding the chips to freshly boiled water. Let sit and cool before straining into a bottle. Add witch hazel and spray onto the hair. You can also sprinkle wormwood in your linen cupboard and drawers of clothes to kill lice and fleas. Both these herbs are available from herbalists, some pharmacies, and health food stores.

AROMATHERAPY

- Put a few drops of undiluted thyme or tea tree essential oil on a fine metal comb and comb in sections, at least twice a day, preferably first thing in the morning and at bedtime.
- Alternatively, mix five tablespoons of a carrier oil, such as vegetable oil, with 20 drops tea tree oil, 15 drops each thyme and lavender oil, and 10 drops rosemary oil. Smooth onto the hair and massage gently into the scalp and hair. Cover for at least an hour and then rinse and shampoo as normal.
- Or you can make up a simple but effective homemade treatment by putting 10 drops of each of the following oils—eucalyptus, lavender, peppermint, rosemary, and tea tree—in a clean one-quarter cup bottle or container. Fill to the top with a carrier oil, such as almond, apricot kernel, or olive oil. Seal and then shake gently to mix well together. Use this mixture to rinse your hair twice daily.

CALL YOUR DOCTOR

Most cases of head lice can be treated quickly and effectively with natural remedies or over-the-counter products. However, if you do not respond to these treatments or have allergic reactions, you should consult your doctor.

Spring Clean

It is not enough to treat the infected person's head. You must wash all their towels and bedding and even, in some cases, treat the furniture, including couches and chairs where they recline and their heads may have rested.

Quick Fix

Before going to bed, smear some petroleum jelly over your scalp and hair and then cover with a shower cap. It will trap the lice. Shower off the following morning.

TOP 10
Skin-Care Recipes

If you care about what you put on your skin, and want to avoid harsh chemicals, then natural skin care is the way to go. As well as buying natural products, it's quick and easy to make your own. Here are 10 skin-care recipes to try at home—all need to be washed off after use.

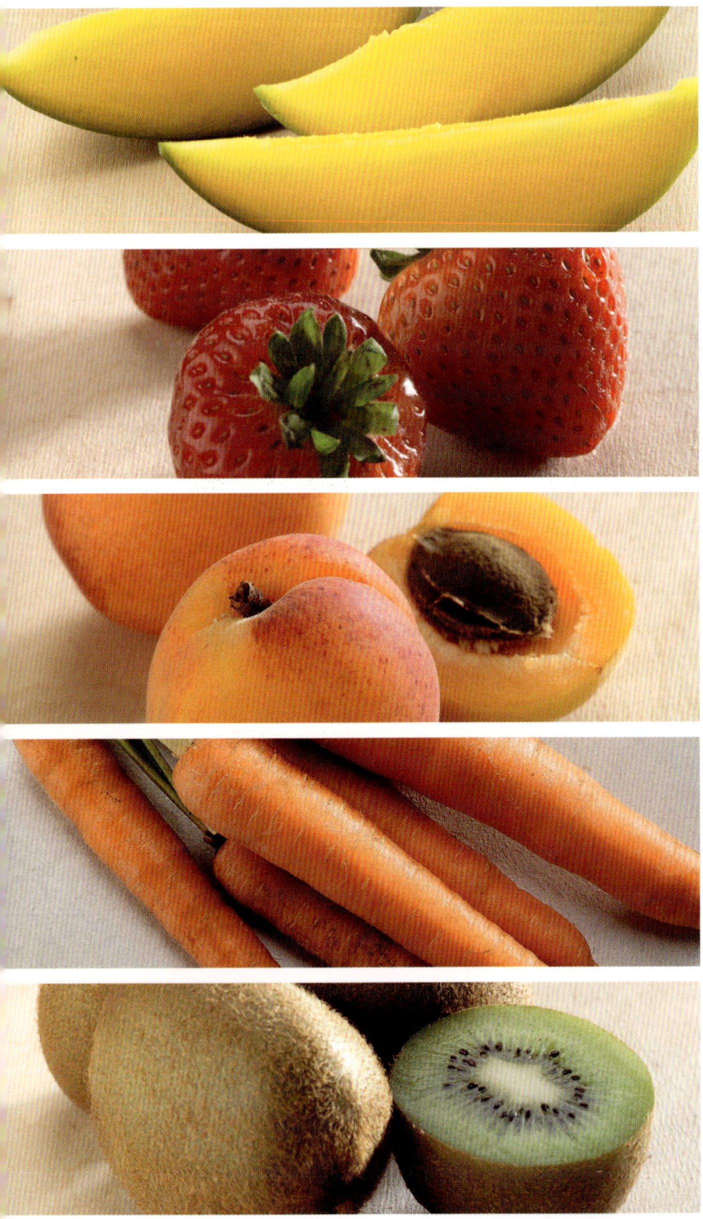

RETINOL-RICH MANGO SCRUB

BENEFITS

Mango contains retinol, or vitamin A, which helps regenerate collagen in skin.

INGREDIENTS

One ripe mango, one tablespoon of honey, two tablespoons of milk, and half a cup of sugar.

METHOD

Blend all the ingredients together, then apply to your face or body. Let sit for 10 minutes.

SUPER KIWI SKIN FIRMER

BENEFITS

Kiwi is rich in vitamin C and can rejuvenate tired looking skin.

INGREDIENTS

One ripe kiwi and one teaspoon of honey.

METHOD

Blend the ingredients, then drain off any excess liquid to leave a paste. Apply to your face for 15 minutes.

REFRESHING CUCUMBER TONER

BENEFITS

Cucumber is refreshing and witch hazel is cooling and astringent.

INGREDIENTS

Half a cucumber, three tablespoons of witch hazel.

METHOD

Chop and blend the cucumber, then strain off the juice. Mix the juice with the witch hazel. Dab onto your face with a cotton ball.

AVOCADO MOISTURIZER

BENEFITS

Avocados are packed with oily unsaturated fat, vitamins, and minerals. They nourish dehydrated or damaged skin.

INGREDIENTS

One avocado and one cup of warm olive or almond oil.

METHOD

Mash the ingredients together, then chill. Apply to the skin for 20 minutes.

APRICOT SHOWER SCRUB

BENEFITS

Apricot moisturizes the skin and sea salt exfoliates.

INGREDIENTS

Three fresh apricots, three tablespoons of apricot kernel oil, and two cups of sea salt.

METHOD

Blend the apricots and oil, then stir in the sea salt. Use as a scrub in the shower.

FINE LINE REDUCER

BENEFITS

Eggs contain the protein albumin and have amino acids that smooth fine lines.

INGREDIENTS

Two egg yolks and one teaspoon of sugar.

METHOD

Whisk the egg yolks until firm, then add the sugar and mix well. Apply to your face for 20 minutes.

STRAWBERRY FACE MASK

BENEFITS

Strawberries cleanse the skin and help remove excess oil.

INGREDIENTS

Half a cup of strawberries and one tablespoon heavy cream.

METHOD

Blend the strawberries and then add the cream. Apply this mixture to your face and neck for 10 minutes.

SIMPLE BANANA FACE MASK

BENEFITS

Banana nourishes the skin.

INGREDIENTS

Two ripe small bananas.

METHOD

Mash the bananas, then apply to your face for 20 minutes.

CREAMY CARROT FACE CREAM

BENEFITS

Carrots contain retinol, which is important for antiaging.

INGREDIENTS

One large, cooked carrot and two tablespoons of cream cheese.

METHOD

Mash the ingredients together. Apply to the face and neck for 15 minutes.

ZESTY WINTER SKIN MASK

BENEFITS

The Vitamin C in the fruit rejuvenates winter skin and the scent is uplifting.

INGREDIENTS

Juice of two lemons and one orange, one cup of instant milk, and a drop of water.

METHOD

Mix the ingredients together, adding enough water to make a thick, but spreadable, paste. Apply to your skin; let sit for 15 minutes.

Ear, Eye, and Mouth Problems

Your ears, eyes, and mouth are not only the sensory gateways to hearing, sight, and taste but are also distinctive characteristics that are individual to you and your appearance. They all have important functions in the body and mirror your general health.

Your ears enable you to hear and govern your sense of balance. They consist of an outer ear (outside the body up to your eardrum), middle ear (between your eardrum and the hearing nerve), and inner ear (containing the receptor hair cells, which convert sounds to nerve impulses). Common problems range from bacterial and viral infections to a buildup of wax.

Your eyes are your body's organs of vision, detecting light and sending messages to the brain via the optic nerve. Eye health is important and is affected by many factors, including your diet, your lifestyle, and state of health. Common problems include infections, inflammation (often due to allergies), visual disturbances, and focusing difficulties.

Your mouth is the entry point to your digestive and respiratory systems; you eat with it, and breathe through it when your nose is blocked. Inside are your teeth for chewing food, thousands of taste buds, and three pairs of salivary glands, which moisten the food. It is also where the vibrations produced by your vocal cords are converted into speech. Effective dental care is essential both for keeping your teeth and gums healthy and preventing problems elsewhere in the body. New research suggests that there may be a link between gum disease and the incidence of heart disease and stroke.

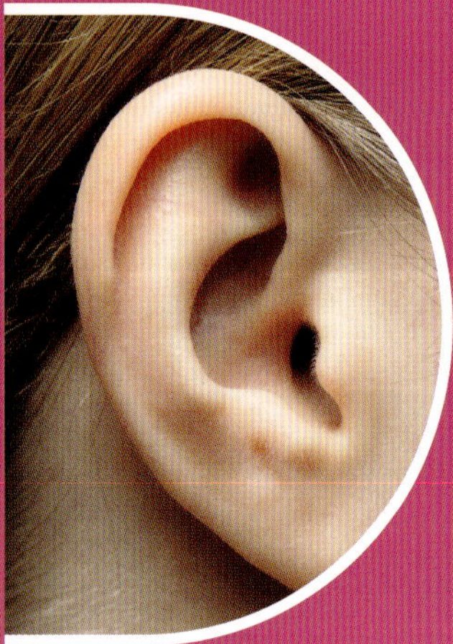

Ear Problems

Ears play an important role in helping you hear clearly and also maintaining your sense of balance. Common problems affecting the ears include a buildup of excessive ear wax, which blocks the ear and affects hearing; earache; and ear infections, where an infection develops in the middle ear.

SYMPTOMS

EARWAX BUILDUP

- ▷ Dulled hearing
- ▷ Ringing in the ear
- ▷ Mild dizziness or vertigo

EAR INFECTION

- ▷ Earache
- ▷ Dulled hearing
- ▷ Fever
- ▷ Feeling generally unwell
- ▷ Discharge from the ear

PREVENTION

- However tempted you may be to stick a cotton swab in your ear to clean and remove wax, don't do it! The cotton swab will push the wax back even more and will make it become compacted, which only increases the risk of blockage from a wax buildup.
- Earache can be brought on by exposure to icy cold winds, so wear a hat that covers your ears on cold winter days.
- Frequent swimmers are sometimes prone to ear infections. Wearing ear plugs can help to prevent water from getting into the ear and also reduce the risk of infection.

Did You Know?

One of the best ways of softening ear wax is olive oil. Use cooking olive oil, or buy special dropper medicinal bottles from pharmacies and insert a couple of drops in each ear. Often, this is the only treatment needed to clear ears from a wax buildup, although extremely blocked ears may take up to a week to clear.

CONVENTIONAL TREATMENTS

BLOCKED EARS AND EARWAX Over-the-counter eardrops can be purchased to apply to your ears for three to four days. Many drops contain an active ingredient called urea hydrogen peroxide, which creates a fizzing sensation in the ears. Sometimes drops can make the ears irritated or painful. For bad cases, and if ears are completely blocked, syringing may be required at your doctor's office (don't ever try to do this yourself).

EARACHE Painkillers are used to help relieve ear discomfort.

EAR INFECTION Antibiotics may be prescribed to relieve ear infections. For associated ear pain, painkillers may be required.

NATURAL REMEDIES

There are various natural remedies you can try to relieve ear problems.

HOMEOPATHIC REMEDIES Aconite 6C can be taken to aid earache that is brought on by being out in a cold wind. Belladonna 6C can help ear infections, especially when there is a lot of pain and fever. Take one tablet of each, twice daily.

NUTRITIONAL MEDICINE Take vitamin C tablets daily to boost your immune system, or eat foods that are rich in vitamin C, such as oranges, broccoli, kiwi, or strawberries.

Quick Fix

Hold a warm hot-water bottle or heat pad against your ear to relieve the distressing symptoms of earache.

HERBAL REMEDIES

- Garlic oil drops can be used to help the symptoms of ear infections. Add one or two drops into each ear, ideally with a different dropper to minimize the risk of spreading the infection.
- A liquid extract of St. John's Wort, which has antiseptic properties, can also be used for treating ear problems.
- Echinacea tablets or liquid can support your immune system during an infection.

HELPFUL THERAPIES

HOPI EAR CANDLING This unusual therapy uses special hollowed candles, which are lit at one end, while the other end is placed just inside the ear for short periods to help clear wax. This needs to be done by a qualified practitioner and may help to relieve ear problems without the need for other remedies.

CRANIAL OSTEOPATHY A buildup of fluid in the ear occurs with ear infections, but gentle manipulation of the skull by a cranial osteopath may help to drain this fluid. Only go to a properly qualified practitioner.

CALL YOUR DOCTOR

If you have severe and persistent earache, you should seek your doctor's advice—you may have an ear infection and need prescribed medication, such as antibiotics.

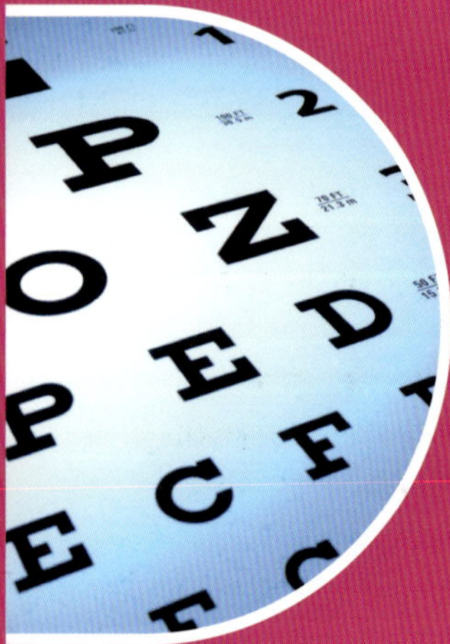

Eye Strain

You may experience eye strain after focusing on a visual task for a long time, such as when reading, driving, or using a computer. However, although your eyes will feel uncomfortable and tired, eye strain is unlikely to be anything serious and can be helped with a few simple measures. Eye strain is also known as asthenopia.

SYMPTOMS

- Tired, itchy, burning, stinging, or sore eyes
- Dry or watery eyes
- Headaches
- Blurred or double vision
- Sensitivity to light
- Difficulty focusing
- Problems concentrating
- Fatigue

PREVENTION

You can help to prevent eye strain by making a few adjustments when you are doing close-up work. Here are some practical examples.

- Use good lighting—dim light can cause your eyes to strain in order to see what you are doing. Make sure sunlight or artificial light is not shining directly at you or on your computer screen.
- Check that the contrast and brightness, text size, and resolution of your computer screen are all set at comfortable viewing levels for you.
- Sit at least one arm's length away from your computer screen.
- Occasionally look up from what you are doing and glance out of the window, or at things farther away from you in the room. This will relax your eye muscles.
- Take frequent breaks. Get up and move around, stretch out your arms, shoulders, neck, and back.
- When driving for a long time, glance at the speedometer or fuel gauge every now and again to shift your focus. If it's sunny, wear sunglasses to avoid squinting.

CONVENTIONAL TREATMENTS

Taking frequent breaks to rest your eyes should be enough to relieve eye strain. Use over-the-counter eye drops several times daily if eye strain is causing dryness. Glasses may be prescribed for driving, reading, or computer use.

NATURAL REMEDIES

The following natural remedies may help to prevent and soothe tired eyes.

HERBAL MEDICINE To relieve eye strain, take one to two 470-milligram eyebright capsules daily, or drink as a herbal tea.

AROMATHERAPY Soak a clean washcloth in a bowl of cold water in which two drops of lavender essential oil have been added. Place over your eyes for 10 minutes.

NUTRITIONAL MEDICINE Kale, spinach, peas, zucchini, Brussels sprouts, and broccoli are all good sources of lutein, a nutrient that is beneficial for eye health.

HOMEOPATHIC REMEDIES

These remedies may help to ease symptoms:

Ruta graveolens 6C: Take two tablets four times daily to relieve aching eye muscles

Apis mellifica 6C: Take two tablets four times daily for stinging or burning eyes.

EXERCISE

The following simple exercises may help to relieve eye strain and tension:

- Hold your thumb up six inches away from your nose and focus on it. Then focus on an object in the distance. Bring your focus back to your thumb. Repeat 15 times
- Keeping your neck and shoulders relaxed, drop your chin to your chest. Lift your head up, and then drop your head backward. Return to the starting position. Repeat six times
- Turn your head to the left, then back to the center. Turn your head to the right, and then back to the center. Repeat six times both sides.

CALL YOUR DOCTOR

If your eye strain symptoms do not resolve themselves with any preventive or self-help measures, consult your doctor or optician. You may have a vision problem or another condition that needs correcting. You should also seek medical advice if you experience pain in your eyes or loss of vision.

IMMEDIATE RELIEF

Close your eyes, and use your fingers to massage your temples in a circular motion for 60 seconds.

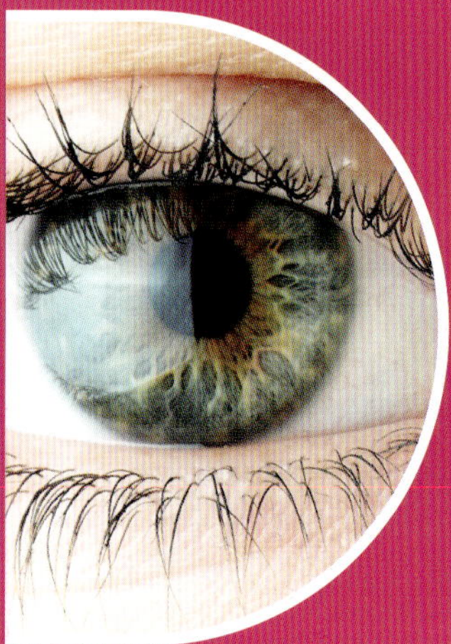

Eye Irritation

Eye irritation is uncomfortable and can be caused by dust, smoke, or other airborne irritants, eye makeup, tiredness, dry eyes, or infection. Equally irritating is a foreign body in the eye, such as grit, sand, dust, or fragments of wood, plastic, paint, or metal.

SYMPTOMS

- Watery or dry eyes
- Itching, burning, or stinging eyes
- Red eyes
- A sensation of something being stuck in your eye
- A rust stain in your eye if the foreign body is metal
- Eye pain
- Sensitivity to light
- Blurred vision

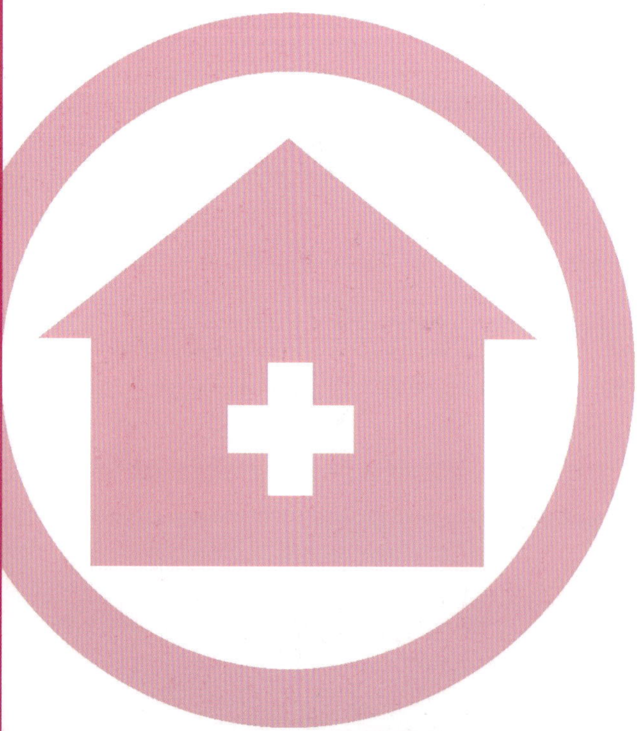

PREVENTION

Here are some simple, practical measures that you can take to avoid eye irritation and foreign bodies in your eyes.

- Wear sunglasses on windy days to protect them from airborne particles.
- Avoid smoky places.
- Replace your eye makeup regularly; if you keep it too long it will harbor bacteria.
- Spray household cleaning products and other eye irritants well away from your face, and always use only in a well-ventilated area.
- Don't rub your eyes, especially if you have been handling irritants.
- Wear safety goggles where there is a risk of stray objects or fluids going into the eye, such as: when doing home improvement work, strimming the lawn, hammering, mixing chemicals, sawing, sanding, drilling, or welding.

Did You Know?

In order to examine your eye, a doctor may use a special dye that is called fluorescein. This will stain the damaged areas of your eye bright green for easy identification.

CONVENTIONAL TREATMENTS

Eye drops or eye baths are used to soothe irritated eyes, but if the irritation is persistent or due to infection, anti-inflammatory medications or antibiotics may be necessary. If there is a foreign body trapped in your eye, it will need to be washed out with clean water to dislodge it. If the object won't budge, it will need removal by a doctor, who may also prescribe eye drops to prevent infection. Painkillers, such as ibuprofen or acetaminophin, can be taken to ease pain.

NATURAL REMEDIES

The following remedies may make your eyes feel more comfortable but do them under sterile conditions.

HERBAL REMEDIES Mix one teaspoon of dried eyebright with two cups boiling water. Let steep for 30 minutes, then strain. Soak a clean washcloth in the solution and place over closed eyes for 10 minutes. (Do not use if you wear contact lens or eye surgery.)

NUTRITIONAL MEDICINE For dry eyes, take 1,000 milligrams of flaxseed oil twice daily. This helps to encourage tear production and moisturize eyes.

AROMATHERAPY Add one drop of chamomile essential oil to a cup of warm water. Soak two cotton balls in the solution, squeeze them out, and then apply to your closed eyes for 10 minutes.

HOMEOPATHIC REMEDIES

Symphytum 6C: Take one or two tablets three times daily to relieve pain after injury to the eye.

Aconitum napellus 30C: Take four tablets four times daily to soothe irritation from a foreign body in the eye.

Sulfur 30C: Take two tablets four times daily to reduce redness, inflammation, and itching.

CALL YOUR DOCTOR

You should see your doctor if:

- You have an object in your eye and you can't remove it
- Your eye hurts continuously
- You have distorted vision
- You can see spots or other random shapes in your field of vision
- You have cut your eye
- There is redness in your eye
- Bright light is painful
- A foreign body entered your eye when traveling at high speed.

Caution

Do not attempt to dislodge an embedded foreign body by poking it with cotton swabs or other objects. You risk doing more harm than good.

Styes

A stye is a boil-like infection at the bottom of an eyelash on the upper or lower eyelid. Fortunately, most styes, although painful and annoying, do not warrant special treatment and they will usually burst or dry up within a week.

SYMPTOMS

- ▷ Irritation of the eyelid
- ▷ Redness and swelling
- ▷ Throbbing pain
- ▷ Small inflamed bump appears on the eyelid
- ▷ Feels as though you have something in your eye
- ▷ May discharge pus

PREVENTION

Styes may be a sign of general poor health and a low resistance to infection. Eating a healthy diet, regular exercise, and staying relaxed and stress-free will all help to prevent them from occurring.

- Take vitamin C and zinc supplements or eat foods that contain these nutrients. They will help boost your immune system.
- Eat foods that contain beta-carotene and vitamin A, such as oily fish, liver, dairy produce, eggs, dried apricots, carrots, and dark green leafy and yellow vegetables.
- If you already have a stye, always wash your hands after touching it.
- Don't rub the stye or you may spread the infection to other follicles on your eyelid.
- Use separate towels and washcloths from other family members, and change them often.

Did You Know?

If a stye bursts, wipe away the pus with some moistened cotton balls. Use a clean ball each time to avoid spreading the infection.

CONVENTIONAL TREATMENTS

Pain relievers may be taken for painful styes. If they do not clear up, however, they may require taking antibiotics.

NATURAL REMEDIES

The time-honored natural remedy for styes is to place a warm, used tea bag on your closed eye for 10 minutes. This is soothing and helps the stye to come to a head or point.

HERBAL REMEDIES Make a herbal tea (see page 142) of marigold and, after straining and cooling, use to bathe the affected area. Take echinacea capsules to boost your immune system.

HOMEOPATHIC REMEDIES Take Pulsatilla 6C for styes on the upper lid; and Staphysagria 6C for recurrent styes.

CALL YOUR DOCTOR

If your stye fails to heal within a week, consult your doctor, because the infection can spread to your eye.

Conjunctivitis

Also known as pink eye, conjunctivitis is the inflammation of the membrane that lines the inner eyelids and covers the eye itself. It may be caused by infection, an irritant, or an allergic reaction, and it is highly contagious.

SYMPTOMS

- ▷ Eye looks red, swollen, and inflamed
- ▷ Eye may be itchy
- ▷ Feels gritty, like sand in the eye
- ▷ Burning sensation in eye
- ▷ Sensitivity to light
- ▷ Sticky or watery discharge
- ▷ Eyelids may stick together after sleeping

PREVENTION

Although you cannot prevent conjunctivitis, you can stop it from spreading to your other eye.

- Try not to rub your eye, however itchy, because this will make the condition worse.
- Always wash your hands after touching the affected eye. Dry them with disposable paper towels or a hot hand dryer.
- When wiping away discharge from the affected eye, use a different tissue or cotton ball for each wipe and dispose of them.
- Use separate towels and washcloths from other family members, and change them often.
- Don't wear contact lenses or eye makeup until the infection clears up.
- Eat foods that contain beta-carotene and vitamin A, such as oily fish, liver, dairy produce, eggs, dried apricots, carrots, and dark green leafy and yellow vegetables.

CONVENTIONAL TREATMENTS

Conjunctivitis is usually treated with antibiotic eyedrops or ointment. Taking antihistamines may relieve the symptoms of allergic conjunctivitis.

NATURAL REMEDIES

You can soothe the itching and relieve inflammation by bathing the eye(s) with boiled, cooled water (salty, if preferred), or placing a used tea bag or thin slice of cucumber over the closed affected eye.

HERBAL REMEDIES Use a herbal eye bath of marigold or chamomile. Take echinacea capsules every day to fight the infection and boost your immune system.

CALL YOUR DOCTOR

Conjunctivitis can be potentially serious and unless the symptoms are very mild and disappear within a few days, you must consult your doctor—do not try to treat it yourself. Seek immediate medical help if you experience blurred vision.

Did You Know?

Allergic conjunctivitis can be triggered by a reaction to pollen, eye makeup, or even the cleaning solution used by contact lens wearers.

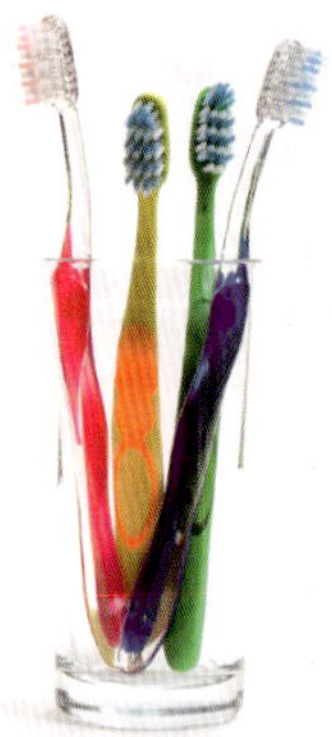

Gum Problems

Gum disease is a major cause of tooth decay and there are two main types: gingivitis and periodontal disease. Both conditions are caused by poor dental hygiene and, if left untreated, they can lead to painful abscesses and even loose teeth, which will fall out eventually.

SYMPTOMS

- Gums are inflamed, red, and swollen
- They bleed easily when brushing, flossing, or even eating
- Your breath may smell unpleasant
- Your teeth may become loose and wobbly
- You may develop a painful abscess

Did You Know?

Gum disease is caused by plaque, a film of food and bacteria on your gums and teeth. Most can be removed by brushing and flossing; if not, it builds up around the gum line, tartar forms on the surface of teeth, your gums shrink, and the resulting pockets cause abscesses and loose teeth.

PREVENTION

You may not even realize that you have gum disease because it may not be painful or evident in the early stages. However, most of us are affected, and if you visit your dentist regularly, brush and floss your teeth every day, and don't consume a lot of sugar, you can slow down the rate at which the disease develops and you will not lose your teeth.

- Brush your teeth with toothpaste twice daily, especially around the gum line.
- Use an electric toothbrush for more effective brushing around the gum line.
- After brushing, always floss.
- Quit smoking now—it produces more plaque and can make gum disease worse.
- Eat a healthy diet with plenty of crunchy, fibrous vegetables and daily vitamin C, found especially in citrus fruits.
- Sugar is your gums' worst enemy, so cut out sugary soft drinks and high-sugar foods.
- Always brush your teeth after high-sugar food and drink.
- Visit your dentist regularly for checkups.
- Get the hygienist to show you how to clean your teeth properly to remove all the plaque.

CONVENTIONAL TREATMENTS

You can buy specially formulated over-the-counter gels and mouthwashes in most pharmacies and supermarkets to bring instant relief to sore gums.

NATURAL REMEDIES

If your gums are sore, painful, and swollen, try these natural remedies.

- Gargle with saltwater to reduce germs in your mouth–dissolve one teaspoon of salt in a glass of hot water. Let cool before using.
- Make a paste of baking soda and water and apply sparingly to the gums.
- Gently massage your gums to boost circulation and blood flow.
- If your gums are swollen and painful or you have an abscess, you can apply an ice pack to your cheek over the painful area.

AROMATHERAPY Cypress, myrrh, rose, thyme, and tea tree oils can all be helpful in treating gum disease. Use them in mouthwashes.

HERBAL REMEDIES

- Make up some chamomile or thyme tea, then strain and cool. Use as a soothing mouthwash.
- Apply a little aloe vera gel to soothe inflamed gums.
- Add a few drops of echinacea liquid extract to a glass of warm water and rinse your mouth out three times a day.
- Rub a little calendula tincture onto sore gums to reduce inflammation.

HOMEOPATHIC REMEDIES

The remedy used will depend on the symptoms presented.

Merc sol 6C: Take one tablet three times a day to relieve inflamed, bleeding gums with bad breath.

Kreosotum 6C: Take one tablet three times a day for swollen gums that bleed easily and painful teeth.

Call Your Dentist

If your gums are sore, bleeding, or receding and you notice a buildup of yellowish tartar around your teeth, you must visit your dentist. The scale can be removed and you will be given advice on how to take care of your teeth and keep your gums healthy. Make an appointment if you have a loose tooth or painful gums with a fever or swollen glands in your neck—these may be symptoms of an abscess that requires urgent treatment.

Quick Fix

There is no quick fix for gum disease—you have to be eternally vigilant—but if your gums are painful, you can rub in some soothing babies' teething gel.

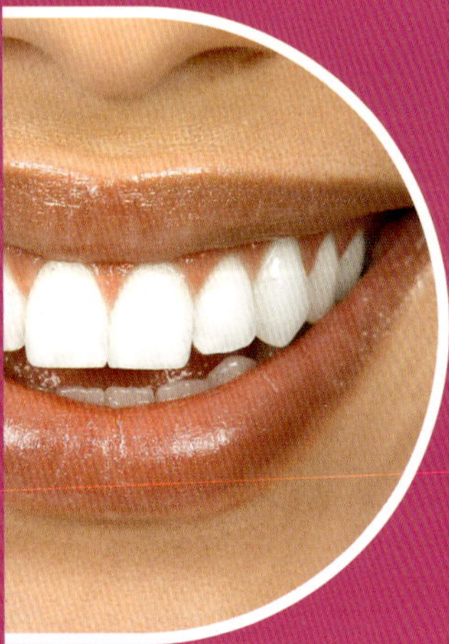

Toothache

Most toothache is caused by dental decay, gingivitis (gum disease), or an abscess, often due to poor dental hygiene. If your gums become inflamed and infected, they can recede, exposing the root of the tooth. The affected tooth can be sensitive to hot and cold food or liquids and may start throbbing.

SYMPTOMS

- Pain around a tooth—throbbing or severe
- Sensitivity to extremes of temperature
- Red, swollen gums
- Bleeding when brushing or flossing

PREVENTION

Good oral hygiene, regular visits to the dentist, and eating a healthy diet that is low in sugar are the best ways to keep your teeth and gums healthy and prevent toothache, gum disease, and dental problems.

- Brush your teeth with toothpaste twice daily, especially before going to bed.
- Brush in a circular motion.
- After brushing, floss carefully around each tooth—gum disease is the major cause of tooth decay and loss, and flossing can help prevent it.
- Eat a healthy diet with plenty of foods containing vitamin C, especially citrus fruits and leafy green vegetables.
- Cut out sugary soft drinks—check the labels carefully to be sure no sugars have been added to fruit juices.
- Reduce your sugar intake and always brush your teeth after consuming high-sugar foods.
- Visit your dentist regularly for dental checkups.
- Make regular appointments with an oral hygienist.

Did You Know?

If you have an abscess, with sensitive swollen gums, intense pain, and even a fever, your dentist may prescribe antibiotics to fight the infection before treating it.

CONVENTIONAL TREATMENTS

The conventional treatment for toothache is to take painkillers and make an appointment to visit your dentist. However, do read the instructions carefully to be sure that you do not exceed the recommended dose.

NATURAL REMEDIES

Conventional painkillers are not always effective and may have side effects, so you may prefer to try natural remedies instead to deal with the nagging pain of tooth and gum disease while you wait to visit your dentist.

- The traditional way to ease the pain is to dab the painful tooth and the gum surrounding it with some cotton balls soaked in clove oil.
- Alternatively, you can chew on a clove with the affected tooth—biting into it will release the oil.
- Chewing a peeled garlic clove may also bring some relief.
- A soothing warm saltwater mouthwash can be repeated several times a day to fight infection—use one teaspoon salt to a cup of hot water.

HERBAL REMEDIES Add five drops tincture of myrrh (available from herbalists) to a small glass of warm water and then use as a mouthwash. You can apply a tincture of calendula to swollen gums to ease the pain and swelling.

AROMATHERAPY Rub a little clove or chamomile oil around the affected tooth.

ACUPRESSURE Try applying pressure to the area between your thumb and index finger (point 4) for up to a minute.

HOMEOPATHIC REMEDIES

The remedy used will depend on the symptoms presented.

Chamomilla 30C: Take one tablet every two hours to relieve pain aggravated by coffee and warm drinks.

Magnesia carbonica 30C: Take one tablet every two hours for pain that is worse at night and aggravated by cold.

Staphysagria 30C: Take one tablet every two hours for pain that is aggravated by cold and by eating.

Quick Fix

If you don't have any oil of cloves, you could try rubbing a little brandy around the affected tooth to deaden the pain.

Call Your Dentist

Even if the remedies you try are effective at relieving the pain of toothache, you must make a dental appointment without delay to deal with the root of the problem and try to save the affected tooth.

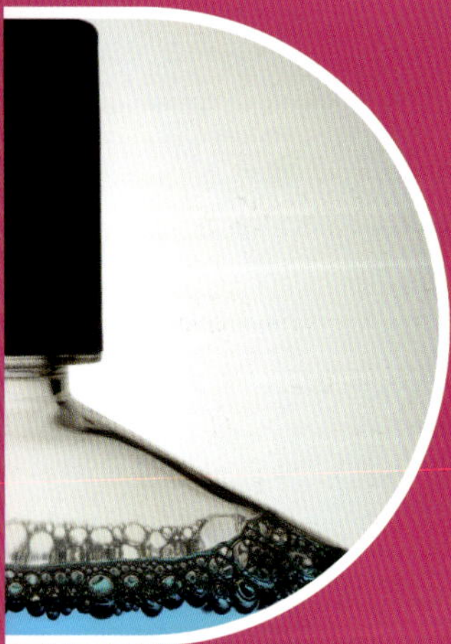

Canker Sores

Although canker sores look small and insignificant, they are sore, painful, and irritating. They may occur inside the lips and cheeks, on the roof of the mouth, the tongue, and gums. They are usually nothing to worry about and are the result of injuries, such as biting your lips, ill-fitting dentures, or a jagged, sharp-edged tooth.

SYMPTOMS

- Small white or yellowish craters
- They may have a red border
- Appear singly or in clusters

Did You Know?

Canker sores can be caused by some medicines, toothpastes, smoking, alcohol, and heavily spiced and salted foods. If you suspect that one of these is the culprit, try avoiding or eliminating them, or talk to your doctor about it.

PREVENTION

Recurrent canker sores may signal stress, poor diet, or underlying health problems. You can help prevent them by doing the following.

- Eating a healthy diet containing the B vitamins and vitamin C: meat, poultry, whole-grain cereals, beans, wheat germ, leafy green vegetables, citrus fruits, tomatoes, and bell peppers.
- Taking a daily vitamin supplement.
- Putting aside some time every day to relax if you have a hectic, stressful lifestyle or taking up yoga or meditation.
- Eating some yogurt with live cultures every day to replace friendly bacteria in your mouth.
- Avoiding salty, hot, spicy, and acidic foods.
- Checking that your toothpaste does not contain sodium lauryl sulfate, a substances that may cause canker sores in some individuals.
- Taking garlic capsules every day.
- Check your diet because some foods can trigger outbreaks of canker sores, notably wheat and other cereals, shellfish, citrus, fruits, strawberries, and chocolate.

CONVENTIONAL TREATMENTS

Most canker sores clear up quickly on their own accord but you can apply a soothing teething gel (sold for babies) or try sucking pain-relieving lozenges that contain local anaesthetic.

NATURAL REMEDIES

There are many traditional remedies that you can make yourself for treating canker sores.

- Peel a clove of garlic, then cut in half and dab the cut surface on to the sore. Repeat three or times a day.
- Cut the top off a vitamin E capsule and squeeze out the contents onto the sore.

AROMATHERAPY Dab a drop of tea tree oil on to the canker sore, or make a mouthwash by adding two drops myrrh oil or myrrh tincture to a glass of warm water.

HERBAL REMEDIES

- Cover some fresh or dried sage with boiling water, stand for 10 minutes, and then strain and use as a mouthwash when cool. Alternatively, you can make a mouthwash with some raspberry leaves, marigold, rosemary, myrrh, or chamomile.
- Dab the sore with a goldenseal tincture or add a few drops to a glass of warm water and use as a mouthwash.
- Use a little aloe vera gel on the canker sore—apply frequently to soothe and heal it.

HOMEOPATHIC REMEDIES

Do not use the following remedies if you have anemia. Take them for a maximum of five days and stop as soon as the condition improves.

Borax 6C: Take one tablet twice a day for painful sores that bleed on touch or when eating.

Mercurius sol 6C: Take one tablet twice a day for sores on the tongue, mouth, and throat with a metallic taste in the mouth.

Nitric acid 6C: Take one tablet twice a day for sores on the tongue and soft palate that bleed easily.

CALL YOUR DOCTOR

If you have painful and recurrent canker sores, it is worth consulting your doctor because there may be an underlying medical disorder that merits investigation.

Quick Fix

Chewing licorice is thought to be beneficial; you can buy special DGL licorice tablets in some health food stores.

Bad Breath

If you have bad breath (halitosis), you will probably be the last to know, and many friends may be too polite to tell you. It is rarely a sign of more serious medical conditions, but it can be difficult identifying the cause.

SYMPTOMS

▷ Breath smells unpleasant

PREVENTION

Bad breath is usually caused by poor dental hygiene or an unhealthy diet. Luckily, there are plenty of things you can do to prevent it.

- Brush and floss your teeth twice a day, preferably after every meal, and brush or scrape your tongue—gum disease is the most common cause of bad breath.
- Change your toothbrush every two to three months and keep it clean.
- Avoid sugary soft drinks as well as sugar-free carbonated ones.
- A dry mouth can contribute to bad breath, so drink eight glasses of water a day.
- Avoid using minty mouthwashes, which can dry up breath-freshening saliva.
- Visit your dentist regularly.
- Eat plenty of fiber to improve digestion and avoid constipation, which may contribute to bad breath.
- Onions, garlic, alcohol, smelly cheeses, and spicy food may be the cause, so try eliminating them.
- Quit smoking and you will notice an immediate improvement in breath freshness.

CONVENTIONAL TREATMENTS

Choose from a wide range of over-the-counter breath fresheners and antiseptic mouthwashes.

NATURAL REMEDIES

- Chew on some mint leaves, fennel, dill, or caraway seeds, or even a coffee bean.
- Change to a tea tree oil toothpaste.
- For a quick breath deodorizer, chew a sprig of parsley or sugar-free gum after meals, or eat an orange to stimulate the production of saliva.

HERBAL REMEDIES Make a cup of thyme tea with fresh or dried herbs and boiling water. Stand for 10 minutes, then strain.

AROMATHERAPY Use lemon, peppermint, or tea tree oil in a mouthwash or gargle.

CALL YOUR DOCTOR

There should be no need to visit your doctor if you improve your dental hygiene and eat healthily. However, make an appointment if your breath smells sweet because this could indicate diabetes.

Did You Know?

Bad breath is caused by bacteria in your mouth on your gums, teeth, and tongue. The best way to combat it is to develop a good oral hygiene routine.

Dry Mouth

If you have a dry mouth, which is caused by a lack of saliva, you can make it feel moist and more comfortable by trying the remedies below. You need saliva to lubricate your mouth, break down food, and help you swallow.

SYMPTOMS

- Mouth feels parched, dry, and lacks saliva
- Frequent thirst
- May be bad breath, canker sores, and cold sores
- Difficulty in tasting, chewing, and swallowing food
- Prickly or burning sensation in the mouth

PREVENTION

There are many possible causes, but the most probable one is that your dry mouth is a side effect of a medication you are taking. Check the label or any accompanying instructions to see if dry mouth is listed and consult your doctor.

- Drink plenty of water—carry a bottle around with you and sip some whenever you feel parched.
- To stimulate saliva production, suck sugar-free boiled candies or chew on sugar-free gum.
- To prevent dehydration, cut down on caffeine-containing drinks, such as coffee, alcohol, and carbonated drinks.
- Visit your dentist regularly to prevent increased risk of gum disease.
- Quit smoking now—saliva is reduced by cigarette smoke.
- Try not to breathe with your mouth open.
- Put a humidifier in your bedroom and don't sleep in air-conditioning, which can be very drying.

Quick Fix

You can try sucking an ice cube or a frozen chunk of melon for instant relief.

CONVENTIONAL TREATMENTS

These include over-the-counter and prescription oral rinses and artificial saliva substitutes.

NATURAL REMEDIES

- Munching celery stimulates the saliva glands and makes your mouth feel moist.
- Suck on a small piece of peeled fresh ginger root to boost saliva production.
- Switch from regular tea and coffee to Chinese green tea or chamomile tea.

CALL YOUR DOCTOR

Dry mouth can be a side effect of certain diseases, infections, medical treatments, and medication, so discuss it with your doctor.

Chiropractic Care and Osteopathy

These two complementary therapies involve touch and movement to treat disorders of the spine, joints, and muscles, as well as a variety of other conditions, but each has its own characteristics and healing approach. Here are the key facts about chiropractic care and osteopathy.

CHIROPRACTIC CARE

The term "chiropractic" comes from the ancient Greek words *cheiro*, which means hand, and *prakitikos*, which means "done by hand" or manipulation. Various forms of spinal manipulation have been practiced for centuries, but chiropractic care itself was developed in 1895 by Canadian Daniel D. Palmer. He claimed to have managed to restore the hearing of his office caretaker, who had been deaf for 17 years due to a back and neck injury. After manipulating his back, there was a noticeable "click" and the man's hearing was restored.

Key Ideas

Chiropractors view the spine as the main structure of the body. The spinal cord carries essential nerves around the body and links the brain as well. When any problems with the spine occur, it has an effect on other parts of the body, too, including internal organs and blood vessels. When the spine is properly aligned and in its natural position, the rest of the body's systems can work in harmony, which helps the body's self-healing ability to work effectively.

Which Conditions Can Chiropractic Care Help?

Chiropractors can help a range of conditions, as well as back problems:

- Spine problems
- Neck and shoulder problems
- Leg pain
- Sciatica
- Sports injuries
- Muscle, joint, and postural disorders
- Repetitive strain injury (RSI)
- Headaches and migraines
- Menstrual problems
- Asthma

Chiropractic Treatment

Chiropractic treatment is individually tailored to your needs, but involves special adjustments–controlled techniques that slowly, and sometimes rapidly, move joints. Sometimes a "click" can be heard when the joint change occurs.

OSTEOPATHY

The word osteopathy also stems from Greek origins and is formed from the words *osteon*, which means "bone," and *pathos*, which means "suffering." This therapy was developed in the late nineteenth century by Dr. Andrew Taylor Still, an American doctor. His wife and three children died from meningitis and he developed osteopathy while seeking a way to encourage the body's self-healing abilities.

Key Ideas

At the heart of osteopathy is the holistic idea that, if your musculoskeletal system is in good working order and structurally balanced, then the rest of your body will work well, too. The musculoskeletal system supports and protects the main organs of the body, and any physical or emotional stress, injuries, or incorrect posture puts strain on the system.

Not only are osteopaths concerned with treating health problems, but they are also eager to find out what caused them in the first place.

Which Conditions Can Osteopathy Help?

An osteopath can help treat a variety of health conditions:

- Spine and neck problems
- Muscle, joint, and posture problems
- Sports injuries
- Sciatica
- Headaches and migraines
- Repetitive strain injury (RSI)
- Tinnitus
- Vertigo
- Menstrual problems

Osteopathy Treatment

Osteopathy treatment is also tailored to your own unique needs but may involve stretching techniques, manipulation of the joints, muscle energy techniques, or massage.

Musculoskeletal Problems

The musculoskeletal system consists of bones, joints, and muscles, which, in turn, are linked by ligaments, tendons, and cartilage. While the skeleton supports the body and protects the vital organs, the joints and muscles (the locomotor system) provide our ability to move.

The skeleton consists of 206 bones, supplemented by cartilage. The bones have several functions: some act as levers, operated by muscles, to aid movement (the limbs); some protect internal organs; and others contain bone marrow, where red blood cells are made. The spine is made up of 33 bones (vertebrae), and it provides a protective casing for the spinal cord, which connects with the brain. To keep your bones healthy and strong, you need to exercise regularly and eat a healthy diet that contains protein, calcium, and Vitamin D.

A joint is the area where two bones meet. Joints may be fixed to promote stability (as in the skull); cartilaginous, allowing for some flexibility (as in the spine); or synovial, providing greater mobility and flexibility (as in the shoulders, elbows, or knees). Ligaments hold together the ends of the bones.

Muscles, which enable the body and its internal organs to move, are arranged in overlapping layers. They work in pairs, contracting and relaxing in opposition to one another. Voluntary muscles (which control body movement) are connected to the bones via bands of fibrous tissue called tendons. Involuntary muscles (within the major organs, arteries, and veins) control functions within the body, such as digestion. To build and maintain strong muscles, you need to use them regularly—exercise is the key.

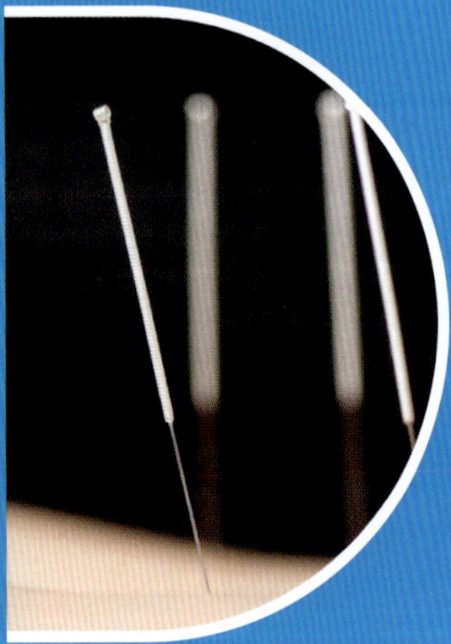

Back Pain

Most of us experience back pain at some time in our lives; it affects four out of five people and is the largest single cause of sickness absence from work. However, precise diagnosis is difficult and there is no simple universal treatment. The pain may occur along any part of the spine, with the lower back being most common.

SYMPTOMS

- A sharp pain in a localized area
- Stiffness in part of the back
- A general aching in the lower back
- Difficulty in bending
- Pain is often worse after standing or sitting for long periods

Did You Know?

Extending down the back from your head to your coccyx, the spine is designed to keep your head and body upright. Its 33 bones (vertebrae) are supported by muscles and ligaments and separated by disks (cartilage). The spine also protects the spinal cord.

PREVENTION

Prevention is always the best treatment, and if you have ever experienced back pain, you will become more aware of your body, your posture, and your habits. Problems may occur from sitting or standing in an unnatural or uncomfortable position, straining the back muscles when lifting heavy objects, twisting awkwardly in the process, or simply from being overweight. Luckily, there are some lifestyle changes and positive measures that you can take to prevent this painful and debilitating condition.

CHECK YOUR POSTURE Is your posture putting your back at risk? You should maintain good posture at work, at home, when driving your car, and in your leisure interests.

CHECK YOUR FURNITURE Do your chairs and couches have firm seats and good upright back support? Try using a lumbar support or foam wedge behind your lower back. Is your desk or work station the correct height? Are you hunched over your computer? Do you have a firm mattress on your bed that supports your spine?

CHECK YOUR HABITS Don't wear high heels or carry a shoulder bag on one side—split the load evenly between two lighter bags. Do not twist as you bend, and make sure you keep your back straight and bend your knees when reaching down to lift anything heavy.

CHECK YOUR FITNESS If you are fit and supple, you will be less likely to get low back pain and you will reduce the chances of it recurring. Cycling and swimming are both beneficial, but do not overexercise because doing so can lead to pulled and torn muscles.

VARY YOUR MOVEMENTS When you are performing household chores, cleaning, or gardening, do not make the same repetitive movements for a long time. Stop and do something else and then go back to the original task later. Do everything in moderation.

CONVENTIONAL TREATMENTS

You can ease the pain and discomfort by taking painkillers, such as ibuprofen, as soon as the pain occurs and then regularly thereafter. It is best to remain as active as possible—going about your normal daily routines can help recovery, but your doctor will advise you about this. In addition, you can apply hot and cold compresses to the affected area or take a prescribed muscle relaxant or nonsteroidal anti-inflammatory drugs (NSAIDs).

NATURAL REMEDIES

These fall into two main types: remedies that ease the symptoms; and natural therapies that improve posture, stabilize, and strengthen the spine, and that help prevent the pain from recurring.

ALEXANDER TECHNIQUE This therapy can improve posture and balance to prevent putting pressure on the spine, joints, and musculature system. It teaches you a more balanced and efficient way of using your body. Consult a qualified practitioner.

REFLEXOLOGY Work on the medial longitudinal arches of the feet, where the spinal reflexes are located. Use firm pressure along the bony ridges.

CHIROPRACTIC CARE This can help some people with chronic back pain. The joints of the spine are manipulated by the practitioner to ease pain and facilitate movement. Your doctor may refer you to a chiropractor.

ACUPUNCTURE This is another form of treatment for relieving back pain.

Caution

Always read the small print and instructions regarding recommended dosages on any over-the-counter or prescription pain relief packaging. Never exceed the stated dose.

Quick Fix

Try rubbing some deep heat ointment (available in tubes from most pharmacies) into the area for instant pain relief, or use a custom-made heating pad or heat spray.

HOMEOPATHIC REMEDIES

The remedy you use will depend on the type of pain you experience and its location. Here are some common symptoms and remedies for back pain.

Aesculus hippocastanum 12C: Take one tablet three times a day until the pain subsides for continuous, severe, dull pain in the lower back and hips.

Bryonia alba 12C: Take one tablet three times a day until the pain subsides for stiffness and pain in the small of the back.

Pulsatilla 12C: Take one tablet three times a day until the pain subsides for lower back pain with tiredness.

Kali carbonicum 12C: Take one tablet three times a day until the pain subsides for severe back pain shooting down into the buttocks; a back that feels weak and stiff; back pain when feeling cold or lying on the affected side.

Rhus toxicodendron 12C: Take one tablet three times a day until the pain subsides for back stiffness, pain deep in the back muscles, which feel bruised and hurt on movement, and pain that feels worse in bed but is better for warmth.

HERBAL REMEDIES

To ease back pain and sciatica, you can try taking one of the following herbal remedies.

- Gently massage some St. John's Wort oil into the affected area for temporary relief.
- Apply a warm paste to the painful area made by blending two teaspoons ginger with one teaspoon turmeric.
- Drink some willow bark, nettle, or chamomile tea.
- Take one 200-milligram capsule devil's claw (an anti-inflammatory) six times a day.
- Take one 250-milligram capsule valerian four times a day.
- Add a cup of rosemary, chamomile, or peppermint tea to a warm bath.

AROMATHERAPY

Use warming, soothing oils for muscular problems; and calming, soothing oils for painful disk problems.

- For muscular pain, use lavender, marjoram, or ginger essential oils in a carrier oil to massage the affected area, or add a few drops to a hot bath and then lie back and relax your aching muscles.
- For disk pain and to relieve inflammation, you can use chamomile, marjoram, or lavender, either in a compress or in a bath.

Did You Know?

For many people, back pain can become a chronic, long-lasting problem with at least 50 percent of people with back pain experiencing some recurring pain.

Posture Checklist

1 Stand up straight and pull your stomach muscles in to help straighten your spine.

2 Make sure your weight is distributed equally between both feet.

3 When seated, don't slouch—keep your back straight and sit equally on both buttocks. Do not cross your legs.

IMMEDIATE RELIEF

Ice and heat will bring immediate relief when you experience a twinge of back pain.

ICE Apply an ice pack or a bag of frozen peas that has been wrapped in a towel to the affected area, and let sit for 15 to 20 minutes. Repeat several times during the first couple of days until the swelling subsides and the pain goes.

HEAT If the pain persists, however, you should use heat instead of ice. You can apply a heat pack (available from pharmacies) or immerse a small towel in hot water, then wring it out and use to cover the painful area. Let it sit there until it loses its heat.

CALL YOUR DOCTOR

You should see your doctor if you experience any of the following symptoms:

- The back pain persists and it does not respond to any of the remedies you try
- You experience numbness in a limb
- You have difficulty in controlling your bowel or bladder functions
- The pain is associated with extreme weight loss
- If you also have fever, chest pain, labored breathing, or stomach cramps.

If you experience any of the above, there may be a serious underlying cause and you must consult your doctor immediately.

Old-Fashioned Remedies

The time-honored way of relieving back pain is to rub in a liniment. You can choose from old favorites like mustard poultices to modern versions, such as capsaicin cream. To make a mustard poultice, blend one-third mustard powder with two-thirds flour and a little water to a paste. Put it on a clean cotton cloth and fold the ends over, so the filling is completely enclosed before placing it on the affected area for a short period—no more than 30 minutes' maximum. The paste must never be applied directly to the skin as it can burn and cause painful blisters.

Yoga

This ancient holistic system of exercises, postures, relaxation, and breathing will help to relieve back pain, improve posture, and make your back more flexible and supple.

- For instant relief, lie flat on your back on a mat on the floor with your arms at your sides, knees bent and shoulder-width apart, and feet flat on the floor.
- Breathe in deeply and slowly, then exhale and repeat 20 times.

Sciatica

Sciatica is any compression or irritation of the sciatic nerve, which runs from your pelvis through your buttocks down the back of each leg to your feet. Sciatica is usually due to a prolapsed disk, putting pressure on the nerves.

SYMPTOMS

- ▷ Pain along the sciatic nerve
- ▷ Sharp pain radiates down the back of the leg to the foot
- ▷ May be numbness or tingling
- ▷ Pain can range from mild to severe
- ▷ May be due to a slipped disk

PREVENTION

The fitter and healthier you are, the less probable it will be that you experience sciatica.

- Exercise regularly—at least three times a week. Swimming, cycling, and walking briskly are all beneficial.
- Improve your posture with yoga, Pilates, or the Alexander Technique.
- Eat a healthy varied diet that contains all the essential nutrients you need for good health. Poor diet can contribute to blood and lymph stagnation and accumulation in the tissues of the lower back.

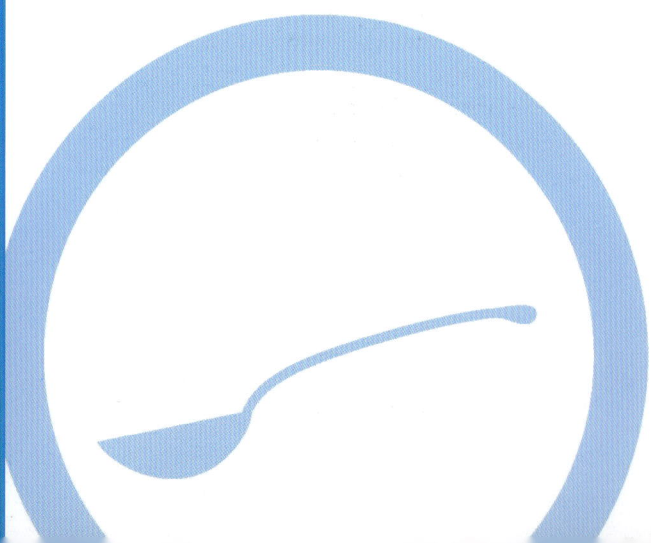

CONVENTIONAL TREATMENTS

Acute sciatica can last for up to six weeks and may not need medical attention. If over-the-counter painkillers do not work, you may need prescription painkillers, physical therapy, or even surgery.

NATURAL REMEDIES

Applying alternate hot and cold compresses to the painful area may be helpful in relieving the pain temporarily.

HERBAL REMEDIES Drink willow bark, nettle, or chamomile tea to relieve sciatic pain. Evening primrose oil can be an effective anti-inflammatory. To relax the nerves, try rubbing St. John's wort oil, mixed with olive oil, into painful areas at bedtime.

AROMATHERAPY Massage the lower back with a carrier oil to which is added three of the following essential oils: chamomile, lavender, rosemary, eucalyptus, peppermint, and wintergreen.

CALL YOUR DOCTOR

If the pain persists for several weeks, consult your doctor. You may be prescribed stronger painkillers, advised on the best types of exercise, or referred to a physical therapist or back specialist. Acupuncture, chiropractic care, or osteopathy may be suggested.

Trapped Nerve

This term refers to a nerve that is pinched or compressed. It is most commonly felt in the neck and mid- and lower back areas, and it may also cause pain in the parts of the body to which the nerve leads, such as arms, hands, legs, and feet.

SYMPTOMS

- Intense pain in a localized area
- Numbness or tingling in other areas
- Most commonly occurs in lower back

PREVENTION

You cannot prevent having a trapped nerve at some time in your life, but you can improve your posture and lifestyle to reduce the likelihood of this painful condition happening.

- Don't wear particularly high heels or always carry a purse or shoulder bag on only one side. Always bend your knees when lifting heavy weights.
- Practice good posture when you are standing, sitting, or lying down—don't slouch and support your back. Yoga, Pilates, and the Alexander Technique can also be helpful.
- A healthy diet with the B vitamins is essential for nerve tissue health. Good sources are poultry, fish, eggs, nuts, seeds, whole-grain cereals, beans, brown rice, dried fruit, and green vegetables.

CONVENTIONAL TREATMENTS

Ice packs, anti-inflammatories, muscle relaxants, and painkillers are the usual conventional treatments for a trapped nerve.

NATURAL REMEDIES

Although exercise may be painful, try to stay mobile and walk a little each day. Apply heat packs to the affected area and relax in a warm bath.

HERBAL REMEDIES St. John's wort oil is often used for spinal nerve pain. Apply to the affected area in a carrier oil.

CHIROPRACTIC CARE This therapy, which involves manipulating the joints in the spine, can be useful in treating a trapped nerve.

CALL YOUR DOCTOR

If the pain lasts for several weeks and over-the-counter pain relievers are not helpful, consult your doctor. Likewise if you experience chest pain, numbness in your legs, or the pain is getting progressively worse, not better, call your doctor.

Caution

Always read the directions on over-the-counter and prescription painkiller packages carefully and never exceed the stated dose.

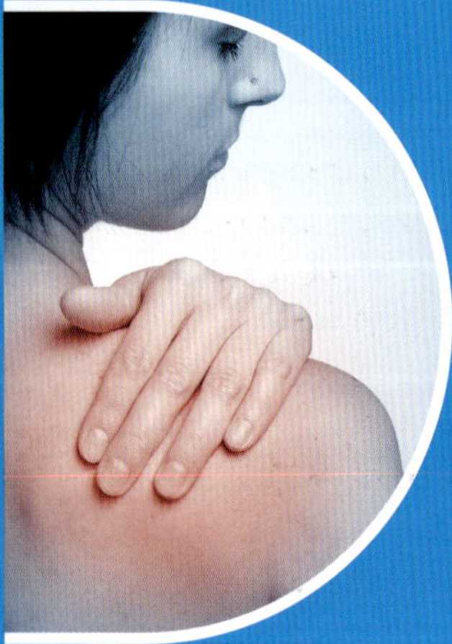

Neck and Shoulder Pain

There are many possible causes of this pain, including injury, arthritis, wear and tear in spinal bones and disks, tendinitis, and bursitis. Even just sitting in an awkward position for too long can cause problems.

SYMPTOMS

- Pain in the neck and when moving your head
- Stiffness and pain in the shoulder
- You cannot lift your arms above your head
- Difficulty in performing simple, everyday tasks

Did You Know?

Neck ache may be one of the first symptoms of a migraine coming on or, indeed, it can be caused by tension headaches.

PREVENTION

As with all other back problems, adopting good posture is the best means of preventing neck and shoulder pain.

- When standing or seated, your ears, shoulders, and hips should all be in a straight line—don't slouch.
- Keep your weight anchored evenly on both legs and feet—don't favor one leg over the other.
- Make sure that the chairs you use (including your car seat) support your back and neck. If necessary, fit a lumbar support or use a small pillow or cushion.
- Don't sit for too long in one position, especially at a computer. Get up, have a stretch, and walk around occasionally.
- Don't hold the phone in the crook of your neck with your head on one side.
- Wrap a scarf around your neck in cold, damp weather.
- Don't wear high heels that tilt you forward out of line.
- Split heavy weights or groceries between two bags, one in each hand, to spread the load more evenly.
- Don't wear a heavy shoulder bag—a backpack is a better option.

- Don't sleep in a draft under an open window, and always make sure that your head and neck are supported properly by a firm pillow.
- Keep your neck and shoulder muscles flexible and strong by performing regular, gentle stretches and rotations.

CONVENTIONAL TREATMENTS

Painkillers, heat pads, and gels containing ibuprofen are the usual over-the-counter remedies for neck or shoulder pain. Nonsteroidal anti-inflammatories, such as ibuprofen, can also be helpful.

NATURAL REMEDIES

For quick and effective pain relief, nothing beats heat. It helps relieve stiffness, relaxes muscles, and promotes healing. You can hold a hot water bottle, a heat pad, or even a towel soaked in hot water and then wrung out against the affected area. Or just treat yourself to a relaxing warm bath or an invigorating shower with the jets of water trained on your neck and shoulders.

HERBAL REMEDIES Make a hot compress to boost blood circulation, or massage the area with a soothing massage oil to which you have added a few drops of lavender oil. You could try taking devil's claw (available from health food stores in capsule form) for its anti-inflammatory properties.

OTHER THERAPIES Acupuncture, chiropractic care, or osteopathy may also bring relief to many neck and shoulder problems. Manipulation can alleviate pain in the area, especially after injury.

HOMEOPATHIC REMEDIES

The remedy used will depend on the exact symptoms, but shoulder pain may improve if it is treated with Sanguinaria (right shoulder) or Sulfur (left shoulder). Cimicifuga is sometimes used for muscular neuralgic pain affecting the neck, while Rhus toxicodendron is helpful for general neck pain and stiffness.

CALL YOUR DOCTOR

Neck and shoulder pain are common and at least half of us will be affected at some time or another in our lives. Although it is seldom a long-term or serious problem, it can make you feel miserable and affect every aspect of your daily routine. If the pain persists in your neck and/or shoulders for several days and does not improve after treatment with painkillers, anti-inflammatories, heat, and massage, consult your doctor. If you also have a fever, headache, sensitivity to light, or cannot lift your arms above your head, you must seek medical advice.

Quick Fix

For instant relief for stiffness and soreness in your neck, try using a hair dryer to blow warm air directly onto your neck.

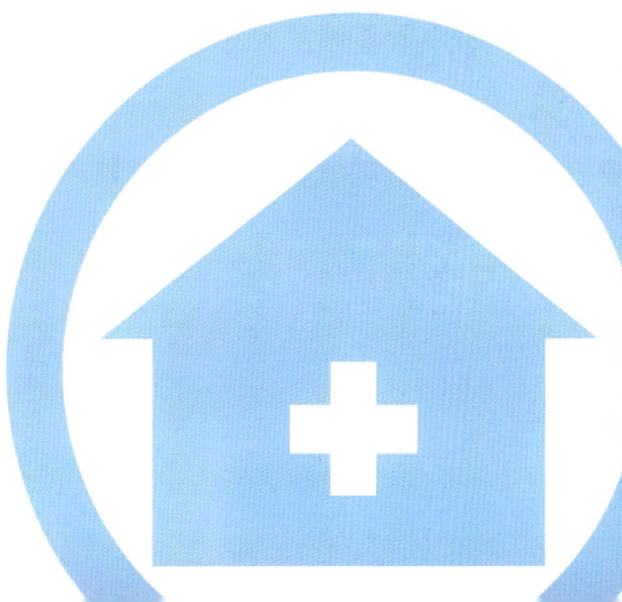

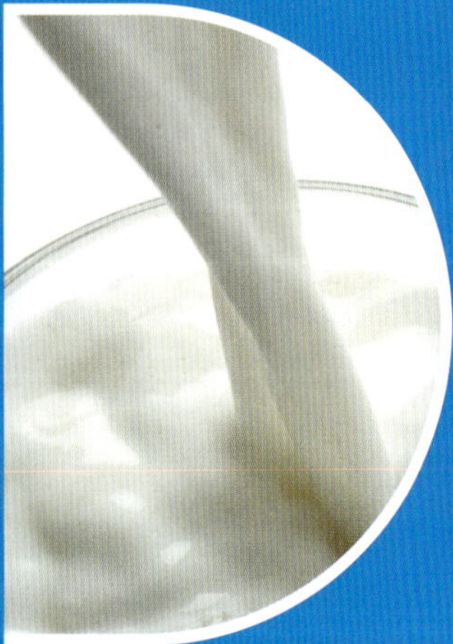

Osteoporosis

Osteoporosis occurs when the bones become less dense, more fragile, and increasingly susceptible to a break if a person falls down. This happens because the bone cells begin to break down faster than they are being replaced. Osteoporosis is a common problem, usually seen in people 50 years old and over, but you are unlikely to know if you have it until you experience a bone fracture.

SYMPTOMS

- Joint pain
- Bone fractures, particularly of the wrists, hips, or spine
- Problems standing or sitting upright
- Curvature of the spine
- Loss of height

Did You Know?

Bone growth happens during our early life, but from our mid-thirties onward we begin to lose bone mass. Therefore, the more bone we can build when we are young, the better.

PREVENTION

Following a healthy lifestyle from a young age is key to keeping your bones strong and preventing osteoporosis in later life.

- Eat a well-balanced diet containing plenty of fruit and vegetables and high-quality protein. This will ensure you get enough vitamins, minerals, and amino acids to build healthy bones.
- Make sure you get enough calcium, which is found in dairy products, green leafy vegetables, nuts, beans, small-boned fish, such as sardines, and fortified foods.
- Get a few minutes of sunlight exposure each day (without getting sunburned). Sunlight allows us to make vitamin D, which is necessary for the absorption of calcium. Vitamin D is also found in oily fish, fortified foods, and supplements.
- Exercise regularly. Weight-bearing and resistance exercises, such as walking, running, aerobics, and weight lifting, stimulate bone growth.
- Avoid excess alcohol, coffee, and sodium consumption. These substances cause calcium to be lost from the body.
- Don't smoke. Smoking encourages calcium loss and slows bone growth.
- Maintain a sensible body weight. Extreme dieting or exercising excessively can increase your risk of osteoporosis.

CONVENTIONAL TREATMENTS

Treatment for osteoporosis focuses on strengthening your bones and on decreasing the risk of additional fractures. Dietary changes may be necessary to increase calcium and vitamin D levels, or high-dose supplements may be recommended. You may be offered medications, such as bisphosphonates or calcitonin, to slow down the rate of bone loss. Some people may need to wear hip protectors in case they fall down.

NATURAL REMEDIES

Here are some natural therapies that may help to prevent osteoporosis.

NUTRITIONAL MEDICINE Omega-3 fatty acids, found in cold-water fish and flaxseeds, may increase calcium absorption and reduce calcium loss and help to maintain bone mass.

HERBAL REMEDIES Black cohosh contains phytoestrogens, which may have an effect that is similar to estrogen and help protect against bone loss. Try taking 80 milligrams twice daily.

ACUPUNCTURE A practitioner will stimulate points that restore the flow of energy from the kidneys, which may help prevent bone loss.

Exercise

Although some rest may be necessary after a fracture, resting for a long time will contribute to additional reduced bone strength. Stay as mobile as possible, starting with a little gentle exercise at first and working up gradually to a greater intensity. For example, just going for a gentle stroll for a few minutes each day will make a difference until you are able to go for longer walks.

HEALING FOODS

- Onions contain a compound that, according to research, may inhibit bone loss and help to prevent osteoporosis.
- Green leafy vegetables contain vitamin K, which is also needed for strong bones.

CALL YOUR DOCTOR

The long-term use of corticosteroids, thyroid, or blood-thinning medications can increase the risk of osteoporosis. Consult your doctor if this applies to you.

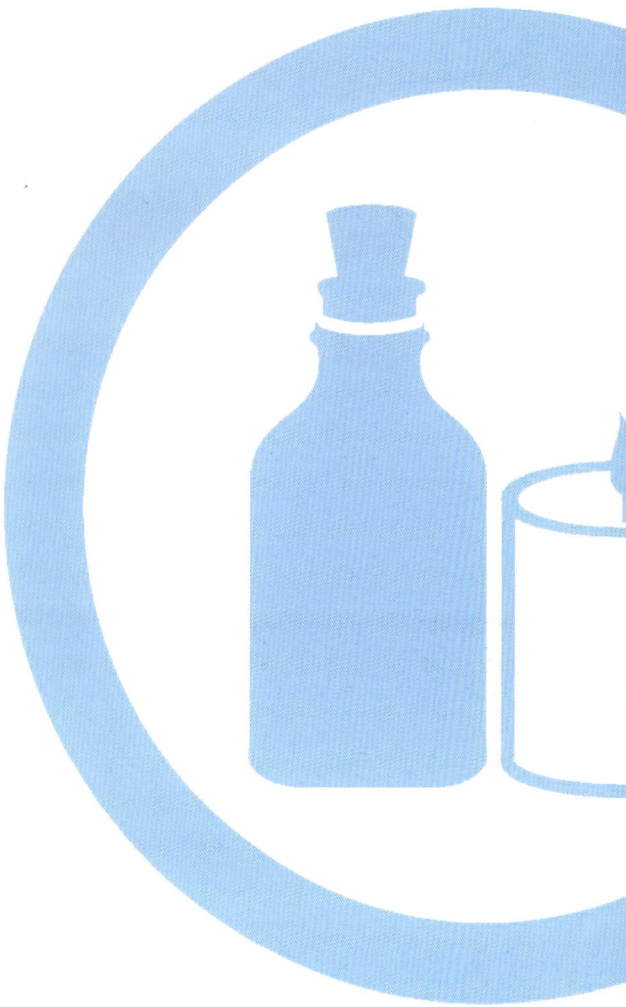

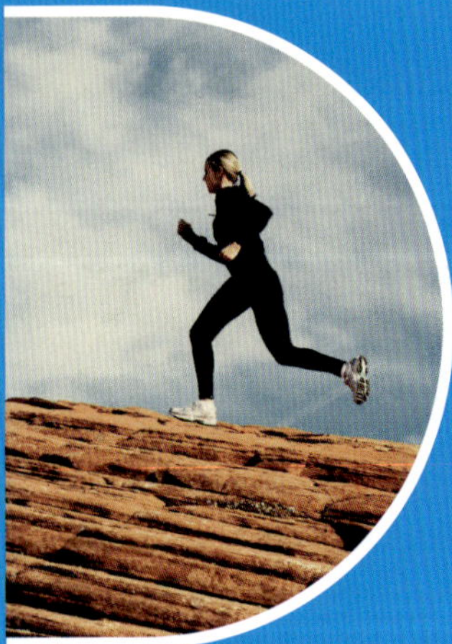

Shin Splints

As an increasing number of people are taking up jogging and running, shin splints are becoming more common, especially among new, inexperienced runners. This painful condition is an overuse injury, arising from constant strain on the muscles along the front of the lower leg. People who are training for marathons may get shin splints if they increase their weekly mileage too rapidly.

SYMPTOMS

- ▷ Shooting pains in the shins while out running
- ▷ May get worse with pain when walking

Did You Know?

Shin splints can affect sports people, ballet dancers, and people who engage regularly in any form of strenuous exercise that puts pressure on the muscles of the lower legs.

PREVENTION

You don't have to experience the pain of shin splints—they are preventable. Your running style, the surface you run on, and the shoes you wear can all make a difference and help to keep you fit.

- Make sure that your running shoes have adequate cushioning to provide essential shock absorption. Discard old shoes that make the problem worse and buy new ones.
- Put padded insoles in your running shoes.
- Always purchase good-quality shoes in a store the specializes in running equipment and get the assistant to check that you do not overpronate, because this can make shin splints worse. The shoes you choose can compensate for this tendency.
- Run on grass—not hard roads and sidewalks—to protect your shins from the impact. Grass is softer and you will be less likely to injure yourself.
- Don't overdo it by trying to run too far, too fast, or too soon. Progress gradually and build days of rest into your schedule.
- Listen to your body and alternate days of running with cross training, gymwork, or whatever exercise you enjoy.

CONVENTIONAL TREATMENTS

Aspirin and ibuprofen will help ease the pain of shin splints, and you can aid and speed up recovery with anti-inflammatory drugs. If the condition persists, you should consult a sports physical therapist.

NATURAL REMEDIES

For quick, effective pain relief, try the time-honored sports medicine remedy known as RICE:

REST As soon as you feel any pain in your shins, rest. Take a rest from running or the sport activity while the condition improves and heals

ICE Apply an ice pack to reduce pain and swelling. Use every four or five hours for no longer than 15 to 20 minutes.

COMPRESSION Wrap a bandage or towel around the ice pack to secure it in place. You can also wear an elastic compression bandage after removing the ice pack.

ELEVATION Raise your legs above your heart whenever possible. Lie on the floor or bed with your legs resting on the wall above.

Stretching

A few minutes stretching can be helpful in preventing and relieving shin splints. Always make time to stretch and ease out your calf muscles after running. To stretch the muscles in your shins, lie on your back and wrap a towel or belt around the ball of your right foot. Raise your leg, holding onto the ends of the towel or belt, and then pull it down with your left hand, so your foot and leg are pulled down over your body to the left. Feel the stretch in your lower leg and hold for a count of five. Repeat three times, change legs, and repeat on the right.

HERBAL REMEDIES

Make a hot compress with some comfrey tea (see page 142) and apply to the affected area.

HOMEOPATHIC REMEDIES

Ruby Arnica montana ointment or gel gently into the shins to help speed up your recovery.

CALL YOUR DOCTOR

If you rest and abstain from running, shin splints will usually heal up of their own accord. However, if rest and ice do not do the trick and the condition persists for more than a couple of weeks, ask your doctor for advice—you may have a stress fracture, which will get worse if it is not treated.

Quick Fix

Ease shin pain and bring instant relief by kneeling with your toes flat on the ground, heels together. As you slowly sit back on your feet, you will feel a soothing stretch in your shins.

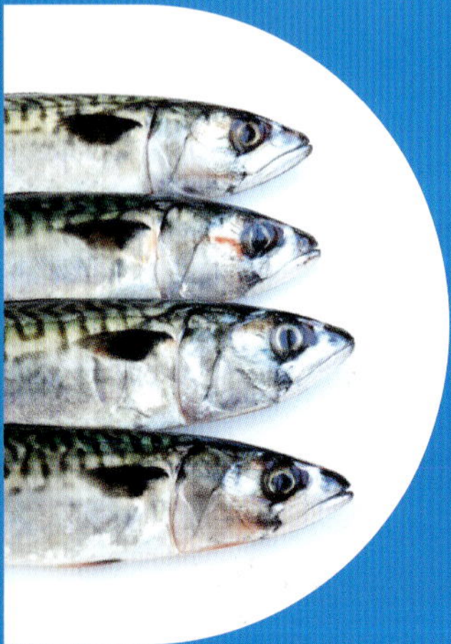

Arthritis

Arthritis is the collective term for more than 200 conditions that affect the joints and bones. In osteoarthritis, the most common form, cartilage degenerates as a result of wear and tear on joints, causing pain and stiffness. Rheumatoid arthritis is a more serious, long-term disease in which the body's immune system attacks and destroys joints, causing pain and inflammation.

SYMPTOMS

- General fatigue
- Pain in the joints, especially the knuckles of the hand
- Joints are swollen, red, stiff, and sore
- Inflammation and pain are worse early in the morning
- Periods of improvement are followed by a relapse
- Joints may look abnormal in shape
- Hands and feet may feel cold

Did You Know?

Gout is another form of arthritis, and it is caused by uric acid crystals accumulating in the joints, especially the big toe, and creating swelling, pain, heat, and tenderness.

PREVENTION

You can help to protect yourself against osteoarthritis as you get older. However, we do not know for sure what causes rheumatoid arthritis and it cannot be prevented. It may be triggered by a virus or an infection, but this cannot be proven.

- Being overweight puts additional stress on weight-bearing joints, especially the knees, hips, ankles, and feet. If you are significantly overweight, go on a weight-reducing diet or join a dieting club.
- Whatever weight you are, eat a healthy diet with plenty of calcium (dairy foods, preferably low-fat ones) and omega-3 fatty acids (found in oily fish). These help build strong bones and healthy joints.
- If you like to pound the streets while running, wear good-quality sneakers with shock-absorbing features and run on grass and soft surfaces. This reduces the impact on weight-bearing joints. Overuse of joints in sport and old sports injuries often cause arthritis in later life.
- Engage in sports that are more gentle on your body, such as swimming or cycling, where your joints are supported.
- Regular exercise will keep you active, mobile, and make your muscles stronger to help support your joints. If possible, exercise four or five times a week.
- Wear comfortable shoes that fit properly with plenty of room for your feet—avoid high heels and pointed toes, which can lead to bunions (arthritis in the big toe).

CONVENTIONAL TREATMENTS

Arthritis cannot be cured but you can relieve the symptoms with many over-the-counter analgesics and nonsteroidal anti-inflammatory drugs (NSAIDs), taken orally or as creams and gels. Your doctor may prescribe stronger painkillers or capsaicin cream, which blocks the nerves that send pain messages. In serious cases, physical therapy with TENS, intra-articular injections, or even surgery may be offered. Rheumatoid arthritis will require special care and treatment.

NATURAL REMEDIES

Severe arthritis is difficult to treat yourself with home remedies, but you can ease the symptoms. Heat can be helpful—keep your joints warm and use heat pads or a hot-water bottle.

ACUPRESSURE AND ACUPUNCTURE Both these therapies can help control pain levels. Go to only a qualified therapist.

AROMATHERAPY Some essential oils can soothe localized pain. Massage lavender, chamomile, eucalyptus, rosemary, ginger, or wintergreen oils into inflamed joints.

YOGA This aids suppleness and mobility, but only move or stretch as far as the affected joint will permit without pain.

Supplements

Many people believe that a daily supplement of chondroitin or glucosamine is helpful in alleviating stiffness and keeping joints mobile.

HERBAL REMEDIES

The traditional remedy for arthritis is devil's claw. Teas made with anti-inflammatory herbs, such as meadowsweet, birch, and willow, can be taken, as can ginger tea.

HOMEOPATHIC REMEDIES

It is wise to consult a qualified homeopath before treating your symptoms yourself. The usual remedies are Rhododendron (smaller joints susceptible to cold), Rhus toxicodendron (damp weather aggravates the condition), and Ruta (wrists and ankles). Take one 6C tablet twice a day until you notice an improvement.

HEALING FOODS

Diet may play a role in relieving arthritis and you can try eating healthy, anti-inflammatory foods to see if they make a difference.

- Eat a variety of fresh vegetables an fruit.
- Eat foods that contain omega-3 fatty acids, such as oily fish and flaxseeds.
- Eat less processed, high-refined, and sugary foods.
- Eat less polyunsaturated vegetable oils and partly hydrogenated oils.

You may also find that cutting out red meat, caffeine, and acidic fruits and tomatoes is helpful.

CALL YOUR DOCTOR

It is important to get a correct diagnosis, and if you suspect that you have arthritis, you must see your doctor as soon as possible.

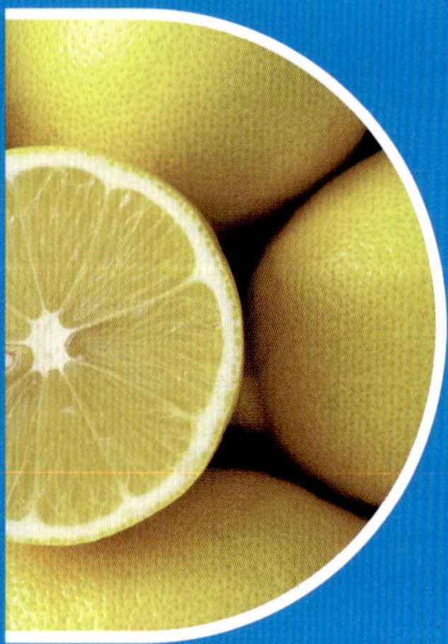

Rheumatism

Rheumatism is not a specific disease but a vague collective term we use to cover a wide range of aches and pains affecting joints, muscles, tendons, and connective tissues. It does not include arthritis (see page 88). When no arthritis or specific disease can be diagnosed, the problem is often referred to as "rheumatism."

SYMPTOMS

- ▷ Swollen, stiff joints
- ▷ Aching joints that look red and inflamed
- ▷ Joints are swollen, red, stiff, and sore
- ▷ Recurring or constant joint pain
- ▷ Pain is worse in cold or damp weather

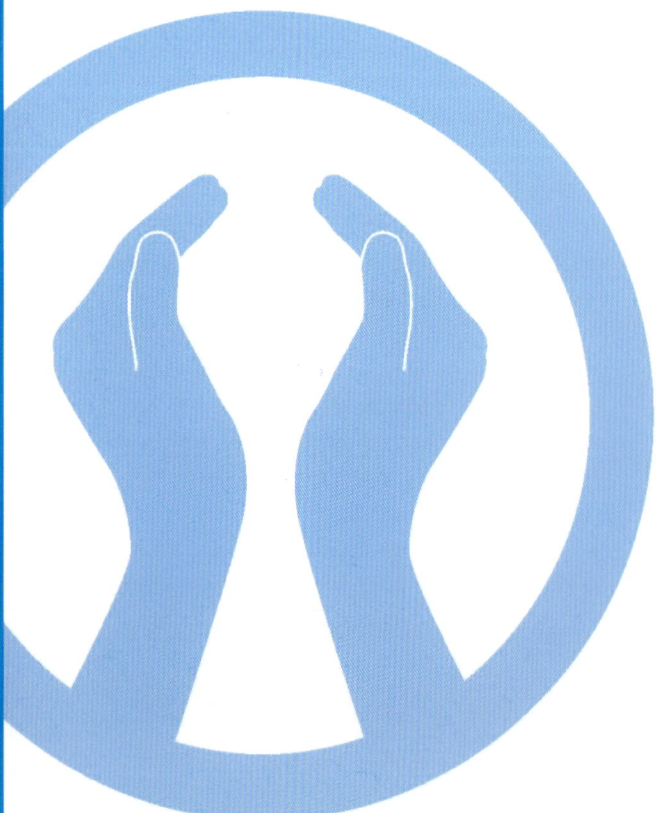

PREVENTION

Rheumatism tends to affect people as they get older and their joints age. It is more common among women and people who have experienced sports injuries. As with arthritis, eating a healthy diet and exercising regularly can help to minimize your risk of developing rheumatism and alleviate painful symptoms.

- Eat a varied diet that contains all the essential nutrients, especially vitamins A, C, and E, as well as selenium and zinc.
- Abstain from foods that may raise levels of uric acid: yeast, yeast extracts, liver, and kidney.
- Cut down your alcohol intake and choose white wine instead of red.
- Switch to herbal or green tea and reduce your coffee consumption.
- Eat oily fish (salmon, tuna, sardines, herring, mackerel) containing omega-3 fatty acids at least twice a week.
- Eat less red meat or cut it out altogether.
- Exercise regularly to boost circulation and build strong muscles to support your joints. Choose a nonweight-bearing activity that is appropriate for you.
- Lemon juice may be beneficial. Try drinking the squeezed juice of half a lemon added to a glass of warm water three times a day.
- Wrap up warmly in cold weather and avoid air-conditioning.

CONVENTIONAL TREATMENTS

The usual advice is to rest until the symptoms clear up or improve, and to take pain relief or anti-inflammatories as required to alleviate the pain.

NATURAL REMEDIES

There are many self-help treatments you can try. The following natural remedies may bring effective relief from rheumatic aches and pains.

HERBAL REMEDIES Anti-inflammatory massages, cleansing teas, and warm compresses can all be helpful. The herbs you choose depend on your symptoms; consult a herbalist. Add rosemary or two handfuls of Epsom salts to a warm bath.

AROMATHERAPY Experiment with different essential oils, using them in a carrier oil for a massage or adding a few drops to a warm bath. Choose from chamomile, ginger, lavender, and rosemary.

CALL YOUR DOCTOR

To avoid any doubt and to obtain a precise diagnosis of your particular problem, you should consult your doctor, especially if the symptoms last for longer than three weeks.

Yoga

Many stretches and postures can be beneficial if you have aching, stiff joints. You will develop better body awareness and increased suppleness and mobility. Find a local yoga class and tell the instructor that you have rheumatism. They will be able to devise a custom-made program for you.

HOMEOPATHIC REMEDIES

Rheumatism affects people in so many ways and the homeopathic remedy selected must be applicable to the symptoms. To be on the safe side, you should seek advice from a qualified homeopath.

Bryonia alba 6C: Take one tablet three times daily for acute pain with hot, red joints that are aggravated by movement or relieved by external heat.

Colchicum 6C: Take one tablet three times daily for severe pain that is worse in the evening or at night.

Ranunculus bulbosus 6C: Take one tablet three times daily for rheumatism that is worse in cold and damp conditions.

Caution

Always follow the package instructions for taking pain relievers carefully, and never exceed the recommended dose in any 24-hour period.

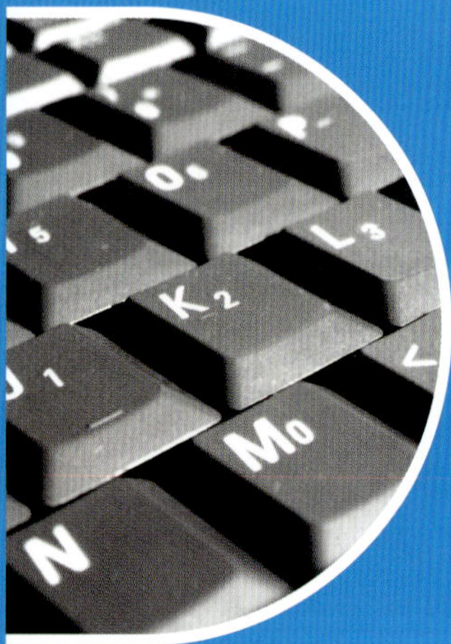

Repetitive Strain Injury

Repetitive strain injury (RSI) is an extremely debilitating musculoskeletal condition that commonly affects the arms, wrists, elbows, hands, neck, shoulders, and upper back and involves chronic pain.

SYMPTOMS

- Sudden onset of bad pain
- Painful spasms
- Stiffness
- Numbness
- Tingling
- Weakness
- Cramp
- Some swelling

PREVENTION

- If you have a desk-base job, particularly typing, working at a computer, or data entry, then be sure to take regular breaks.
- Changing your job and doing different work is a good way of eliminating the problem, but if you can't do that, take time to stretch your arms.
- Make sure your working environment lets you work with an upright body, so that you don't have to twist or stretch too much.
- Learn to touch type, because using all your fingers to press the right keys and looking straight ahead at the computer screen can help to prevent RSI.
- Work at reducing stress in your life, because stress can increase the risk of RSI pain.
- Regular massage can help to relieve any tension and stress in your upper body, neck, shoulders, and arms.

Did You Know?

RSI is caused by overuse of a particular area of the body, often due to repetitive work, such as using a computer for long periods of time in the same position, or working in a factory and repeating movements again and again.

CONVENTIONAL TREATMENTS

Over-the-counter painkillers can help, and your doctor may prescribe nonsteroidal anti-inflammatory drugs (NSAIDs). Bandages or splints, for example, worn on the wrists to ensure they remain straight, can offer support and relieve symptoms. For severe RSI, steroid injections may be recommended. If the pain and discomfort of RSI is interrupting your sleep, then medication to help you sleep may be prescribed for a short time. You may be referred to a physical therapist, who will suggest exercises you can do to build up your strength in the muscle affected by RSI.

NATURAL REMEDIES

The following natural remedies may help to relieve pain and other symptoms.

NUTRITIONAL MEDICINE Shiitake mushrooms are often used as a herbal remedy for RSI, becaue they are good for easing inflammation and helping the body to cope with stress. You can make a nutritional soup from three ounces of fresh shiitake mushrooms and eat for lunch.

AROMATHERAPY Mix together two drops of black pepper and two drops of rosemary essential oils, with two tablespoons of a carrier oil, such as sweet almond, to create an anti-inflammatory RSI blend. Very gently rub it into the affected area—don't initially try to massage your wrist, neck, shoulder, arm, or hand much at all, because it may well be painful.

HELPFUL THERAPIES Body and movement therapies, such as yoga, Pilates, and the Alexander Technique, can help bring relief from stress, develop better posture, and ease strain from your muscles. See a qualified practitioner for individual guidance.

RELAXATION AND MEDITATION

If stress could be at the heart of your RSI, then try out relaxation and meditation techniques to fully relax your body.

1 Use a guided meditation or relaxation CD to help you relax, or try a do-it-yourself meditation.

2 Sit quietly with your back supported and let all your muscles relax.

3 Breathe slowly and deeply and forget about any stress in your life.

NOTE It may help to visualize a blackboard with your stresses written on it—and then imagine you are wiping them away.

HERBAL REMEDIES

- Take a tincture of the herb meadowsweet. It contains salicylates, which help to reduce inflammation and pain. Add one teaspoon of tincture to a glass of water and take three times a day until your symptoms improve.
- Make a compress from yarrow, because it helps reduce inflammation in joints and muscles and reduces pain. Soak a piece of cheesecloth in 10 drops of yarrow oil and apply to the affected area.

CALL YOUR DOCTOR

If changing your lifestyle and rest do not ease the symptoms of RSI, see your doctor. You may be referred to a specialist or physiotherapist.

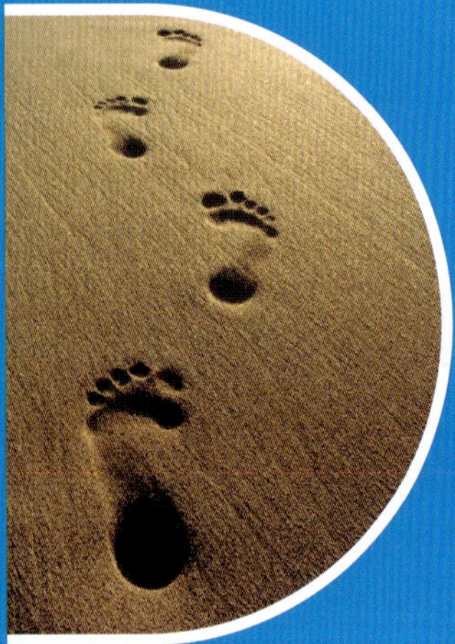

Foot Pain

Feet can easily be taken for granted, but they need as much care and attention as the rest of your body. You rely on them being healthy and fine for walking and moving around, but when foot pain occurs, everything goes out of kilter. Pain is usually due to injury, disease, or a health condition, or how the foot is interacting with external factors, such as the shoes you wear.

SYMPTOMS

- Pain or discomfort in the foot
- Rubbing, blisters, or bleeding
- Painful to put your foot on the floor
- Swelling

PREVENTION

There are plenty of steps you can take to keep your feet in tip-top condition. Here are some suggestions.

- Wear shoes that fit well and don't rub your feet. High heels are a big culprit for causing foot problems. If you can't resist wearing them, choose a thicker heel, because this can give more stability and more evenly distribute the weight on your feet. It also helps to choose shoes without such a steep "slope," and open toes can relieve the pressure on your toes.
- Wear in new shoes before wearing them for long periods of time, because this can help prevent them from rubbing and causing sores, blisters, or bleeding.
- Add orthotics or insoles to your shoes to aid comfort and prevent foot pain.
- Wear the right type of recommended shoe or boot for walking, running, playing baseball, or other sports activities. If you are running, avoid surfaces that are too soft (sand), too hard (concrete), or uneven, because all these can put unwanted pressure on your feet. Also, remember to warm up properly before exercising.

CONVENTIONAL TREATMENTS

The RICE method—Rest, Ice, Compression, and Elevation—is commonly recommended for foot pain caused by injuries. Never apply ice directly to the foot; put it in a plastic bag and wrap in a cloth before applying to your foot for 20 minutes at a time.

Large blisters on the foot, filled with pus, which are caused by rubbing, can be drained by a doctor. Covering them with a large bandage or blister pad can prevent additional rubbing. Over-the-counter painkillers can help ease pain and discomfort in the foot.

NATURAL REMEDIES

Among the most common natural remedies for foot pain are the following.

HERBAL REMEDIES If your feet are bruised or tender, apply arnica ointment to help aid healing. Rub it in well, but don't use on broken skin. Take five drops of cayenne tincture in a glass of water to help ease foot pain caused by nerve damage.

ACUPUNCTURE This can help to relieve foot pain. Depending on the location of the pain, an acupuncturist can work on areas of the foot and lower leg, helping to relieve pain and discomfort. Book an appointment with a qualified practitioner.

ALEXANDER TECHNIQUE Sometimes poor posture can put increased pressure on your feet, causing pain and discomfort. An Alexander Technique practitioner can work with you to identify old habits that are harming your health and develop new ones that relieve pain.

AROMATHERAPY

- Relieve tired, painful, or aching feet by adding a few drops of aromatherapy oils to a bath or foot bath and soaking your feet. Try using anti-inflammatory peppermint, soothing lavender, refreshing lemon, or antibacterial eucalyptus.
- If your foot pain is related to rheumatic aches and pain, try rosemary, which is a mild stimulant.

HELPFUL THERAPIES

Try practicing exercises, such as yoga or Pilates. They'll work by increasing the strength and stability in your foot, improve muscle strength, and aid flexibility. When your muscles are stronger and more flexible, you will reduce the risk of additional foot injuries.

CALL YOUR DOCTOR

If your feet are particulary painful and none of the remedies you try seem to work, you should either consult your doctor or visit a podiatrist.

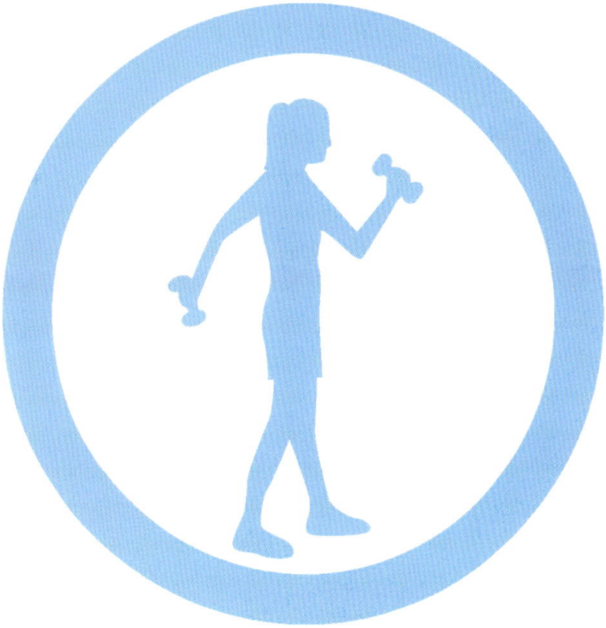

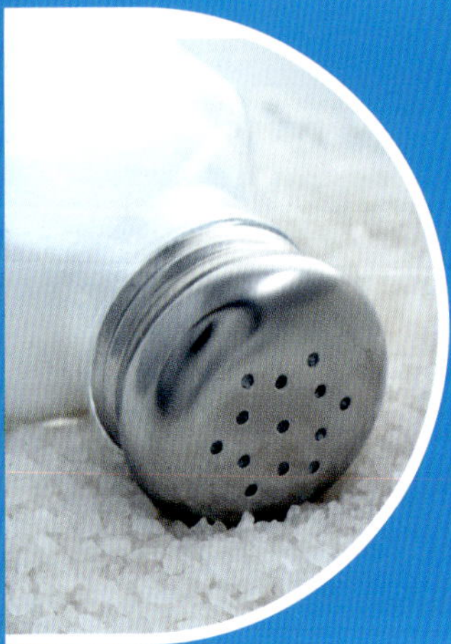

Muscle Cramps

Muscle cramps can come on suddenly, usually lasting from a few seconds to several minutes, and they are caused by a spasm of a muscle. A cramp commonly occurs in the calf muscles of the legs, or in the feet, and can happen when you're sitting still, standing up, exercising, or lying in bed. The amount of pain felt varies, but the affected muscle can remain uncomfortable for up to 24 hours.

SYMPTOMS

- ▷ A sharp or sudden pain in your leg or foot
- ▷ The muscle affected by a cramp feels rigid and hard to move
- ▷ The muscle is tender for some time afterward

PREVENTION

To prevent muscle cramp from occurring, it helps to do the following.

- Drink plenty of fluids each day, including eight glasses of water.
- If you're exercising, always warm up properly beforehand and avoid doing excessive exercise involving a lot of repetitive movements, because this can trigger a muscle cramp.
- Avoid drinking too much alcohol, because this can cause a cramp.
- Sometimes a cramp can be linked to stress or exhaustion, so make sure you get plenty of sleep and try to avoid stressful situations.
- Drinking some tonic water, which contains quinine, before going to bed may help to prevent nighttime muscle cramps.

Did You Know?

A cramp can sometimes be caused by losing salt through sweating, such as when you're exercising. Drinking a glass of water with a little added salt can help rebalance the loss of salt and relieve a muscle cramp.

CONVENTIONAL TREATMENTS

To relieve the after effects of a cramp, such as a tender calf muscle, you can take painkillers. In instances of a severe, recurring cramp, quinine sulfate tablets may be prescribed.

NATURAL REMEDIES

There are several natural remedies that help to ease the symptoms of a cramp.

NUTRITIONAL MEDICINE Muscle cramps can sometimes be caused by a lack, or imbalance, of minerals in your diet. Zinc and magnesium are two key culprits. Eat foods such as shellfish, corned beef, whole grains, or nuts to increase your levels of zinc. To boost levels of magnesium, eat foods such as dark leafy vegetables, shellfish, nuts, seeds, lentils, or whole-grain cereals.

HOMEOPATHIC REMEDIES The homeopathic remedy Magnesia Phosphorica 8C can provide relief for a cramp. For instant relief, take four tablets every 30 minutes until the effects wear off. If you have regular cramps, take three doses daily.

HERBAL REMEDIES

- Take cramp bark tincture to help relieve the discomfort of muscle cramps. Add one teaspoon to a glass of water and take three times a day during a bad bout of a cramp. Cramp bark lotion can also be rubbed into the affected muscle.
- Mexican wild yam has muscle relaxant properties. Take a one-milliliter tincture when a cramp occurs. In bad cases of a persistent cramp, repeat the dose every 15 minutes until the cramp eases.
- Guelder rose has anti-inflammatory and relaxant properties. Add two tablespoons of tincture to five tablespoons of rose water, or to an unscented skin cream, and gently massage it onto the affected muscle.

CALL YOUR DOCTOR

If you have a recurring cramp or it does not ease up, you should seek medical advice. It could be a sign of an underlying or serious condition, such as a blood clot or underactive thyroid, and tests and investigations will be carried out. In some cases, medications that have been prescribed for other conditions, such as diuretics or water tablets, can result in a cramp. If this is the case, your doctor may need to review your medication.

IMMEDIATE RELIEF

- For a cramp in your foot, put your bare foot on a cold floor.
- For a cramp in a calf muscle, stand an arm's width away from a wall, put your feet flat on the floor and lean toward the wall, stretching your calf muscle.
- If you're prone to a cramp in bed, sleep on your back and prop your feet up on a pillow—this helps prevent your toes from pointing downward when sleeping, which is a position linked to cramps.

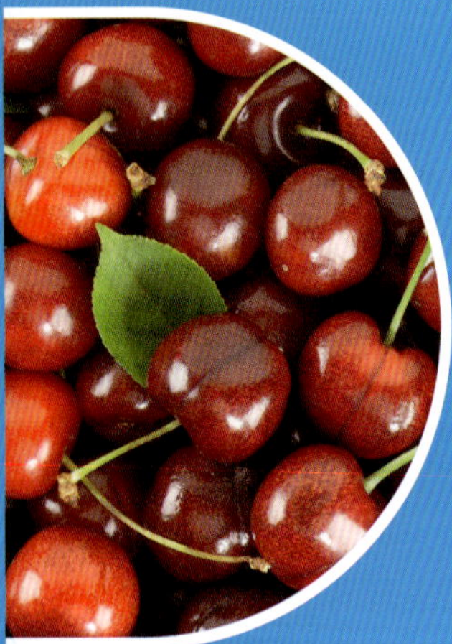

Gout

Gout is an extremely painful form of arthritis, and while it can occur in any joint, it most often affects the big toe. The condition is caused by a buildup of uric acid in the blood, which leads to crystals forming in the joints, but, fortunately, there are many things that you can do to help yourself if you have gout.

SYMPTOMS

- Inflammation and swelling of joints
- Extreme pain in your joints that comes on suddenly
- Red, shiny, hot, itchy skin around the joints
- Visible lumps underneath the skin
- Difficulty walking or moving about
- Fever

PREVENTION

You can help prevent gout by leading a healthy lifestyle. In particular, you should avoid foods that are high in purines, because these increase uric acid. Here are some things you can do to prevent gout.

- Limit your consumption of red meat, liver, kidney, oily fish, such as mackerel and sardines, shellfish, and some vegetables, including beans, asparagus, mushrooms, and spinach.
- Reduce your alcohol intake, especially beer, stout, fortified wines, and port.
- Keep conditions, such as high blood pressure, diabetes, psoriasis, high cholesterol, obesity, kidney disease, and vascular disease, under control, because these can increase uric acid.

Did You Know?

Although gout is more common in men over forty, anyone can experience gout at any age. Some people will experience gout only once in their lifetime.

CONVENTIONAL TREATMENTS

Treatment for gout focuses on reducing pain and inflammation in your affected joints, and controlling blood uric acid levels to prevent additional attacks. It is important to elevate and rest the affected joint, and you may like to keep it cool with an ice pack. Don't apply ice directly to your skin, because this can cause damage. You can also take nonsteroidal anti-inflammatory drugs (NSAIDs), such as ibuprofen, to reduce inflammation and pain. In some cases, medications, such as colchicine or steroids, may be prescribed to reduce uric acid. Sometimes a medication known as allopurinol may be given to reduce uric acid in the blood and prevent any additional attacks of gout.

Change Your Lifestyle

Focusing on a healthy lifestyle will reduce the likelihood of developing gout.

- Cut down on the amount of alcohol you drink or, better still, eliminate it altogether. Avoid binge drinking.
- Stay well hydrated by drinking plenty of water and herbal teas. Try to avoid sugary soft drinks.
- Exercise regularly (but never with an inflamed and painful joint) to improve your circulation and overall health.
- Eat a healthy, balanced, diet (not one that is high in protein), and minimize your consumption of processed, refined foods.
- Lose weight sensibly and gradually if you are overweight.

NATURAL REMEDIES

Here are some natural remedies you might consider for treating gout.

NUTRITIONAL MEDICINE Try to eat a handful of tart cherries each day. They contain anthocyanins that have anti-inflammatory properties. You can also try taking cherry concentrate, capsules, or teas.

HERBAL MEDICINE Take devil's claw extract three times daily to help reduce the pain and inflammation. You may also like to try extracts of green tea or turmeric.

AROMATHERAPY Add five drops of juniper oil to a massage oil, and massage it into painful joints several times daily. Or try adding juniper, rosemary, lavender, or eucalyptus oils to a foot bath.

CALL YOUR DOCTOR

Although gout is relatively common, you should see your doctor if:

- You have frequent attacks of gout, because this may increase the risk of permanent joint damage
- You develop lumps in your joints that are particularly bothersome or painful
- You have difficulty getting about and gout is severely affecting your day-to-day life
- Your gout symptoms are making you depressed.

Alexander Technique and Pilates

The Alexander Technique and Pilates are two popular body and movement therapies. The two approaches share similarities, as they both aim to help you improve your posture, correct muscle imbalances, help specific health concerns, and generally aid overall health and vitality.

ALEXANDER TECHNIQUE

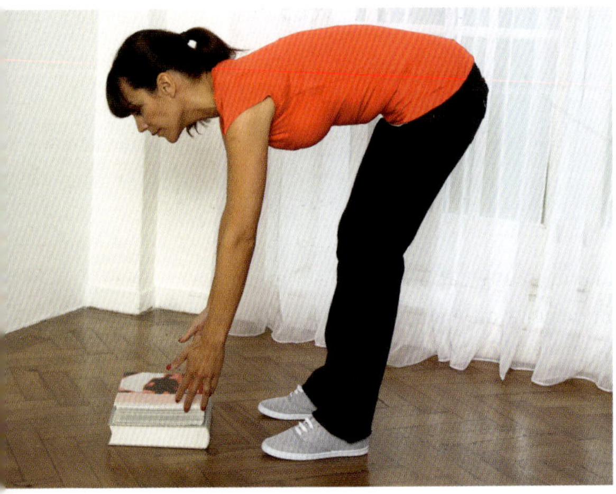

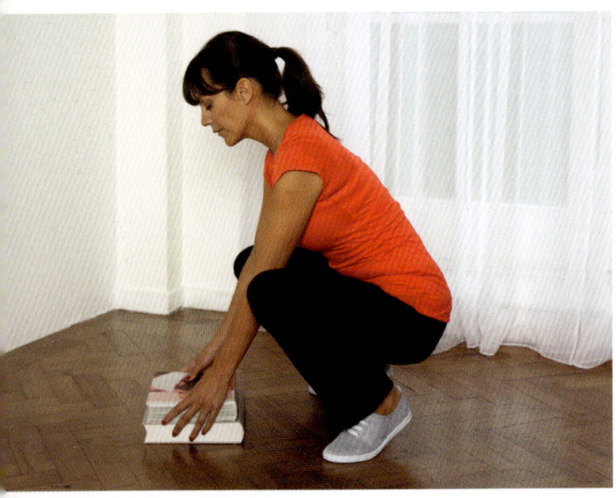

Top The incorrect technique for picking up heavy objects; this should be avoided

Bottom The correct technique for picking up heavy objects that will protect your back

The Alexander Technique was developed by the Australian actor Frederick Matthias Alexander. He made the discovery that he could stop his voice from becoming strained by improving his posture and relaxing his throat muscles. He subsequently moved to London in 1904 and worked on developing his technique.

Key Ideas

One of the key ideas behind the Alexander Technique is the idea that, as we go through life, we develop poor postural habits and they are difficult to break. Alexander believed that bad posture affects the body and mind, resulting in health problems, such as back pain, headaches, muscle strain, or stress.

By relearning a series of basic movements, such as the movements needed to go from a sitting position to a standing position, or standing up straight, it is possible to become more aware of the bad habits and realign the body in such a way that movement becomes more natural and harmonious.

Learning the Alexander Technique

To gain proper insight and expertise into the Alexander Technique and how it can help you, book a series of sessions with an experienced practitioner. One-to-one sessions are ideal for helping you discover your bad postural habits and how they could be affecting your health. An Alexander Technique practitioner will help you to become aware of these habits when you're active and resting and will provide you with a series of exercises to practice to help you change your posture. It can be hard to recognize that your lifetime habits are not healthy and learn to change them, but the benefits are worth it.

PILATES

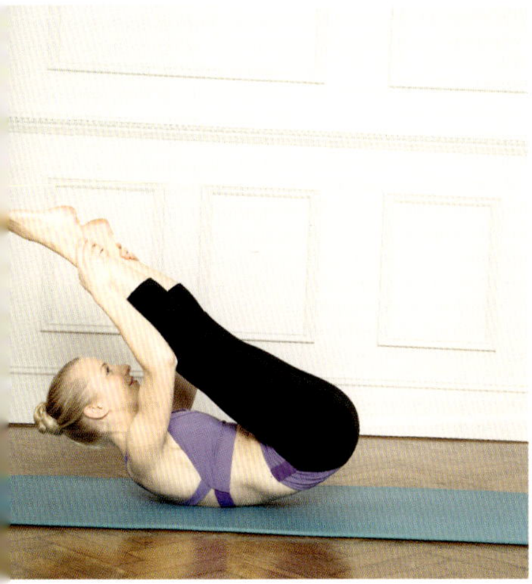

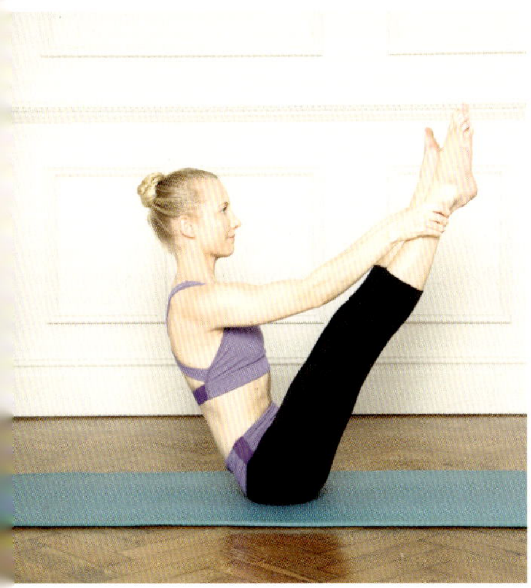

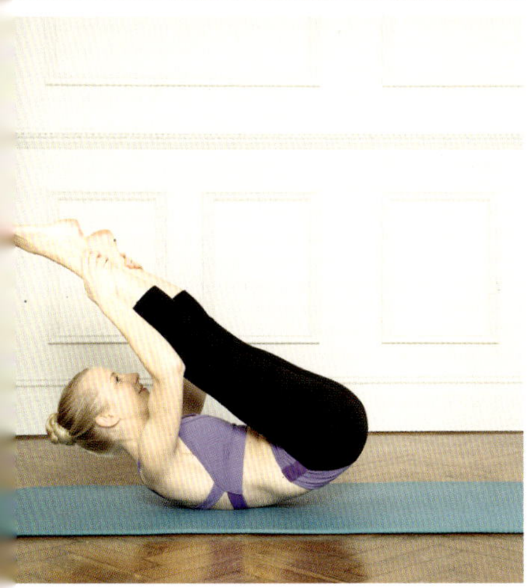

Pilates was created by Joseph Pilates, a German fitness trainer. During his childhood, Joseph was often ill and started practicing gymnastics to try to improve his health. He studied yoga and tai chi before inventing his own form of exercise, which became known as pilates, in the early 1900s.

Key Ideas

Joseph Pilates noticed that other exercises paid attention to the outer muscles, but he believed that it was important to focus on the deeper, inner muscles because they hold the key to all movements.

Pilates focuses on the core muscles in the center of the torso, such as the lower back, abdomen, buttocks, and hips. Precise movements help you to gain control over muscles while breathing exercises help circulate oxygen and improve your energy levels.

Learning Pilates

If you would like to try out this holistic approach to movement and posture, go along to a session with a qualified pilates teacher. Sessions are available on a one-to-one basis, or in small groups. Some simply involve mat work, while others use special apparatus to help you with the exercises. Regularly practicing pilates can help alleviate many health conditions, such as back problems, arthritis, and pain. It also results in longer and leaner muscles and more stability, strength, and flexibility.

Heart and Circulation Problems

A healthy heart and circulatory system are essential for our well-being. Eating a varied, nutritionally balanced diet, not smoking, and getting regular exercise will help to keep them strong and healthy and prevent relatively minor problems, such as chilblains, restless legs, and varicose veins, as well as more serious ailments, including high or low blood pressure, palpitations, and angina. And even if you have heart problems, there are positive steps you can take to embrace a healthy lifestyle, and useful home remedies to prevent any additional damage and help repair the system.

A properly functioning heart muscle and efficient blood circulation are vital for the health of every organ. Your blood transports oxygen and nutrients around your body and carries away waste products. The pressure of the circulating blood must not be too high or too low, and the blood vessels must remain free from obstructions, including clots and fatty deposits.

Cardiovascular disease is increasing but you can minimize the risk of developing it by making simple lifestyle choices and changes, as outlined in the following pages. Many natural therapies, such as herbal remedies, aromatherapy, homeopathy, reflexology, and yoga, can be used to complement conventional medicine in this area. If you are unsure about their safety or are receiving medical treatment, always first check with your doctor.

Learn how to recognize the early warning symptoms of heart and circulation problems and you may be able to take some simple steps to relieve them now and prevent them from becoming more serious in the future.

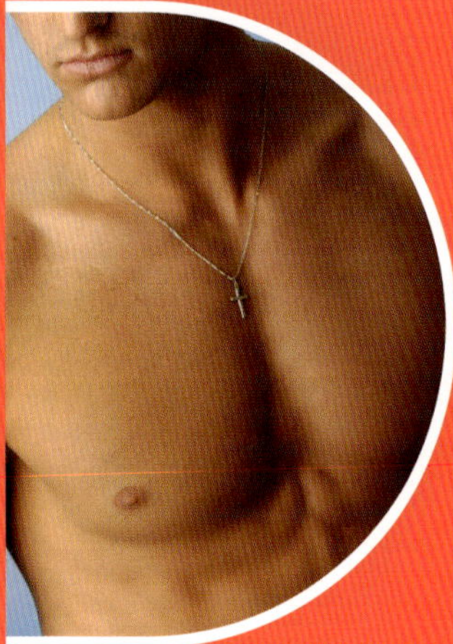

Angina

Angina is a sudden, acute pain in the chest and is due to restricted oxygen-rich blood flow to the heart. This is usually caused by hardening and narrowing of the arteries that supply the heart with oxygenated blood. Fatty deposits can gather inside these arteries and block them, a condition that is known as atherosclerosis. Angina increases the risk of having a heart attack or stroke.

SYMPTOMS

- ▷ Sudden pain, squeezing, or pressure in the chest
- ▷ Pain in the jaw, neck, left arm, or back
- ▷ Breathlessness
- ▷ Tiredness
- ▷ Feeling sick
- ▷ Dizziness
- ▷ Burping

PREVENTION

There are some lifestyle factors you need to address in order to prevent angina and reduce your risk of having a heart attack or stroke.

- Obesity, stress, high blood pressure, and diabetes cause damage to the artery walls, so these conditions need to be managed properly.
- Exercising five times per week for 30 minutes at a time can strengthen your heart, lower blood pressure, reduce cholesterol, and improve blood circulation.
- Excessive alcohol consumption increases cholesterol levels and raises blood pressure, so drink only in moderation.
- Don't smoke. Smoking increases blood pressure, damages artery walls, and also increases the risk of blood clots.
- Try to reduce the amount of saturated fat in your daily diet, because it increases blood cholesterol and blocks the arteries.

Did You Know?

There are two main types of angina: stable and unstable. Stable angina is caused by triggers, such as strenuous exercise and stress, and lasts for only a few minutes. Unstable angina happens even when resting, and needs immediate medical attention.

CONVENTIONAL TREATMENTS

Healthy lifestyle changes are important for treating angina, including eating less saturated fat, limiting alcohol consumption, exercising regularly, and giving up smoking. Your doctor may prescribe nitroglycerin to relieve the pain during an angina attack. Other medications that slow the heart rate, increase blood flow to the heart, lower blood pressure, or lower cholesterol may also be recommended. Antiplatelet medicines, such as aspirin, help to prevent blood clots. If your angina does not improve as a result of these measures, surgery may be required.

NATURAL REMEDIES

Here are some suggestions for how you can treat your angina naturally.

HERBAL REMEDIES Hawthorn may help to increase blood circulation and benefit your heart. Try taking 150 milligrams three times daily.

NUTRITIONAL MEDICINE Increase the amount of "good" cholesterol in your diet. This is found in avocados, oily fish, nuts and seeds, olive oil, and sunflower oil.

YOGA Practicing yoga may help to lower your blood pressure, improve blood circulation, and help you to cope with stress and anxiety.

CALL YOUR DOCTOR

Do not attempt to treat your angina on your own without medical supervision; it could lead to serious health consequences. Only take supplements and herbal remedies to treat your angina after discussing it with your doctor. You should also see your doctor if you feel particularly anxious, stressed, or depressed because of your angina.

Lifestyle Changes

You should make the following changes to your lifestyle if you have angina.

- Your diet should contain plenty of fresh fruits, vegetables, and whole-grain cereals. Keep saturated fats to a minimum.
- Reduce your salt intake because it raises blood pressure. Aim for a maximum of 1,500 milligrams—about two-thirds of a teaspoon—per day. Remember that processed food often has added salt.
- Drink alcohol in moderation. Men should consume no more than two drinks a day, and women no more than one drink a day.
- Exercise regularly. If you have angina, you will need to avoid vigorous exercise, so, to begin with, stick with gentler forms of exercise, such as swimming and walking.
- Lose weight if necessary. You should be able to accomplish this with regular exercise and eating a healthy low-fat diet.
- Quit smoking.

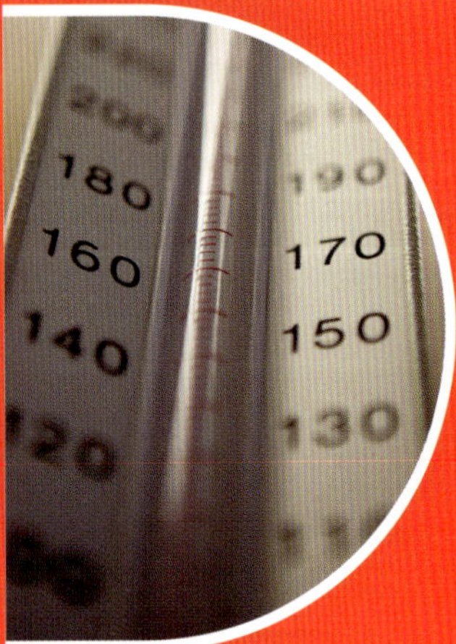

Blood Pressure

High blood pressure (hypertension) is when the force of the blood being pumped around your body is greater than considered normal. Although it rarely has symptoms, if this condition is left unchecked, prolonged high blood pressure can damage the blood vessels and increase the risk of developing serious health conditions, such as kidney disease, heart disease, and stroke.

SYMPTOMS

- Vision disturbances
- Nosebleeds
- Breathlessness
- Headaches
- Blackouts
- Seizures

Did You Know?

High blood pressure is defined as 140/90mmHg. The first figure represents systolic blood pressure (when the heart beats), and the second represents diastolic blood pressure (when the heart is at rest in between beats); 120/80mmHg is normal.

PREVENTION

Diet, exercise, and general lifestyle factors all play a major part in preventing high blood pressure.

- Get regular exercise: 30 minutes of moderate to vigorous intensity exercise five times per week will strengthen your heart, improve your blood circulation, and help you to manage stress.
- Avoid becoming overweight or obese; concentrate on maintaining a healthy weight for your height.
- Make sure you have a healthy, balanced diet consisting of plenty of fruit, vegetables, and whole-grain cereals. Minimize your intake of processed foods and foods high in sugar.
- Watch your cholesterol levels. Foods high in saturated fat increase blood cholesterol, causing narrowing of the arteries and contributing to high blood pressure.
- Drink alcohol in moderation. High alcohol consumption increases blood pressure, especially binge drinking. Men should consume no more than two alcoholic drinks a day, and women no more than one a day.
- Pay attention to your stress levels—large amounts of stress increase blood pressure.
- Reduce your salt intake to under 1,500 milligrams, or two-thirds of a teaspoon, per day.
- Reduce your daily caffeine intake to no more than five cups of coffee; go easy on caffeinated drinks.
- Avoid smoking.

CONVENTIONAL TREATMENTS

A few simple lifestyle changes can have a huge effect on your blood pressure levels. Exercise regularly, eat healthily, watch your salt and caffeine intake, drink sensibly, quit smoking, and lose weight if necessary. Your doctor may prescribe medications that widen your arteries or slow down your heart rate in order to lower your blood pressure. They may also treat any underlying medical conditions that are contributing to your high blood pressure.

NATURAL REMEDIES

Here are some natural remedies you could try for high blood pressure.

NUTRITIONAL MEDICINE Add more fish to your diet, such as salmon and halibut. These contain omega-3 fatty acids, which help to reduce blood cholesterol levels. Alternatively, you could take a fish oil supplement.

HERBAL REMEDIES Try taking ginkgo biloba daily to improve blood circulation and reduce blood pressure.

RELAXATION TECHNIQUES Transcendental meditation may be helpful to reduce stress, relax your mind, and lower your blood pressure.

CALL YOUR DOCTOR

If you are 40 years of age or older, you should have your blood pressure checked regularly, especially if you have a family history of high blood pressure, or other factors that increase your risk of hypertension.

Low Blood Pressure

If you have low blood pressure (hypotension), which is classified as 90/60mmHg or less, you are unlikely to need treatment. To a degree, low blood pressure protects you against some of the things that cause high blood pressure, such as too much salt in your diet and weight gain. Low blood pressure can simply be a result of being particularly relaxed or physically fit. However, it can sometimes cause dizziness, light-headedness, fainting, and weakness. Beta-blockers, diabetes mellitus, adrenal gland problems, dehydration, injury, or shock can cause low blood pressure, but it is often nothing to worry about.

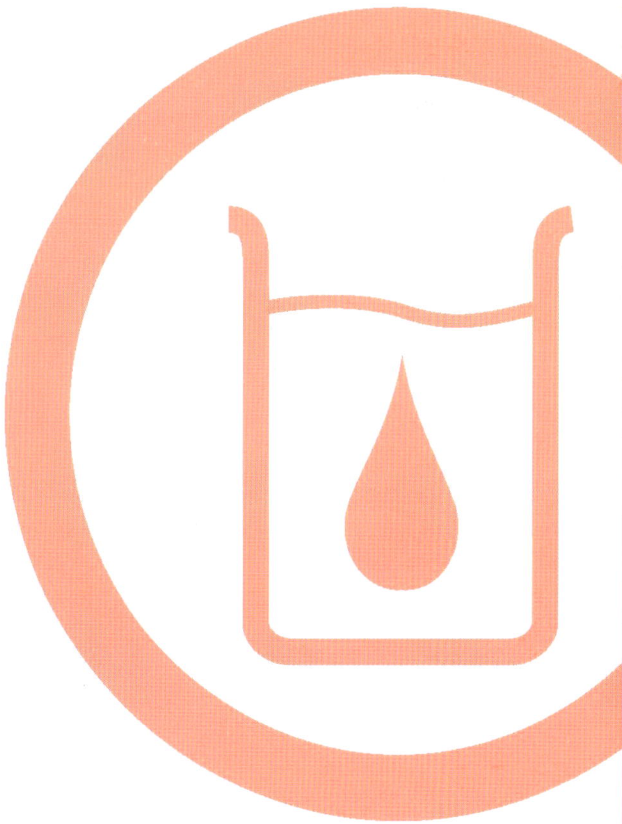

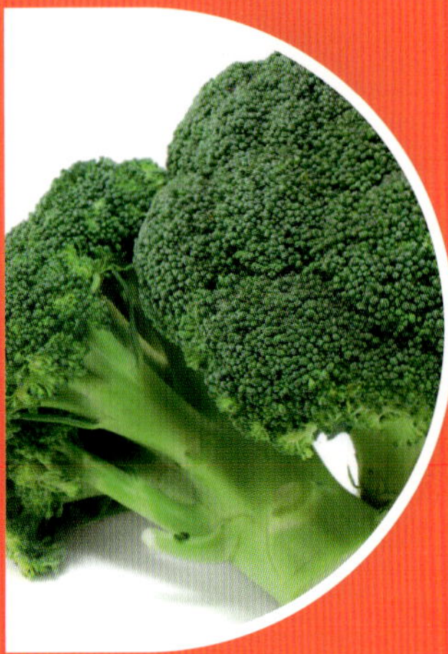

High Cholesterol

Cholesterol is a type of fat, which is important for cell membranes and other functions within the body. However, high levels of blood cholesterol can cause health problems. Excess cholesterol builds up inside the walls of the arteries, restricting blood flow and increasing the risk of developing heart disease and stroke.

SYMPTOMS

- Yellow deposits around your eyes or on your skin
- White rings around the eyes
- Blood cholesterol of more than 5mmol/L
- Angina or leg pain (caused by narrowed arteries)

Did You Know?

Low-density lipoprotein (LDL) is "bad cholesterol" because it builds up in your arteries. High-density lipoprotein (HDL) is "good cholesterol" because it helps to get rid of excess LDL cholesterol.

PREVENTION

There are several lifestyle factors that affect your risk of developing high blood cholesterol. In particular, you should do the following.

- Eat a healthy balanced diet with plenty of fruit and vegetables.
- Restrict your intake of saturated fat. This is found in red meat, meat pies, cream, hard cheese, butter, and pastries.
- Exercise regularly, because lack of exercise increases LDL cholesterol levels and decreases HDL cholesterol. Aim for 30 minutes of moderate-intensity exercise five times a week.
- Lose weight if you are overweight. Obesity increases the risk of high LDL cholesterol and low HDL cholesterol.
- Avoid excessive alcohol consumption; men should have no more than two drinks a day and women no more than one drink a day.
- Don't smoke. Smoking reduces your level of HDL cholesterol.

CONVENTIONAL TREATMENTS

Treatment for high cholesterol begins with making some important lifestyle changes: eat less saturated fat, lose weight, exercise more, and quit smoking. You may also be offered medication, such as statins, niacin, or ezetimibe, to lower your cholesterol, or aspirin to help prevent blood clots.

NATURAL REMEDIES

You may like to try the following natural remedies to lower your cholesterol.

NUTRITIONAL MEDICINE Eating foods high in vitamin C may help to lower cholesterol. Add bell peppers, broccoli, kale, parsley, Brussels sprouts, kiwi, strawberries, and oranges to your diet.

ACUPUNCTURE This treatment focuses on rebalancing your body and improving blood flow in order to lower your cholesterol levels.

YOGA Yoga helps to reduce stress, which has been associated with high cholesterol. Deep breathing exercises, postures, and meditation increase blood circulation, improve digestion, and aid relaxation.

HEALING FOODS

Some foods will have a positive effect on your blood cholesterol levels.

- Increase your level of HDL cholesterol by replacing saturated fat with healthier, unsaturated fat. This is found in oily fish, olive oil, avocados, nuts, and seeds.
- Soluble fiber helps to remove cholesterol from the body. Good sources include psyllium, oat bran, beans, peas, potatoes, and apples.
- Substituting some animal meat with soy protein, such as tofu, miso, and tempeh, may help to lower blood cholesterol levels.

HERBAL REMEDIES

The following remedies are helpful for protecting against high cholesterol.

HAWTHORN Take 150 milligrams three times daily.

GARLIC Eat it fresh, or take an odorless supplement one to four times a day.

OLIVE LEAF EXTRACT Take 500 milligrams one to two times daily.

PSYLLIUM HUSK Take 1,000 milligrams three times a day.

CALL YOUR DOCTOR

In addition to lifestyle factors, there are other things that can put you at greater risk of high cholesterol. You should consult your doctor and get your cholesterol checked if:

- You have high blood pressure or diabetes
- You have heart disease or have had a stroke
- You have a family history of heart disease or stroke
- A member of your immediate family has familial hypercholesterolemia (high cholesterol that runs in the family)
- You have kidney or liver disease or an underactive thyroid gland.

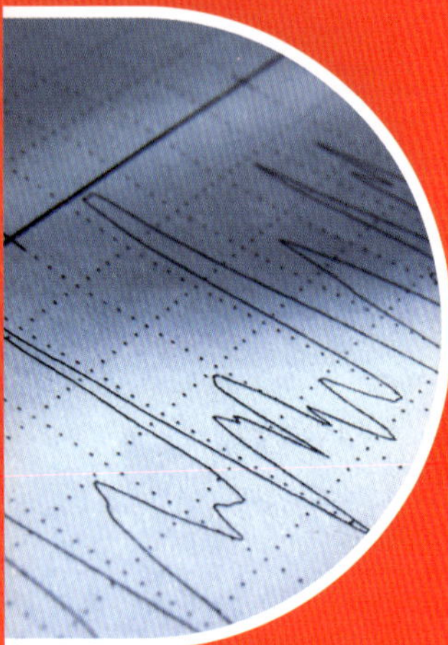

Palpitations

Palpitations (also known as arrhythmias) are variations in normal heartbeat rhythm, caused by a disruption of the electrical impulses that make the heart muscles contract. A normal heart rate is between 60 and 100 beats per minute when you are at rest, but sometimes your heart may beat faster or slower than usual or you may feel as though your heart skips a beat.

SYMPTOMS

- Rapid heartbeat
- Slow heartbeat
- Your heart feels as though it skips a beat, or thumps suddenly
- Irregular heartbeat
- A fluttering sensation in your chest
- Sudden awareness of your heartbeat

Did You Know?

Most people experience extra heartbeats (ectopic beats) daily. An ectopic beat sometimes feels like a sudden thump in the chest, or as though your heart has missed a beat, but it is usually nothing to worry about.

PREVENTION

Depending on the type of palpitations you experience, they may be prevented easily with some simple lifestyle changes.

- Some medications can cause palpitations, such as beta-blockers, calcium channel blockers, and asthma and thyroid medications. You may need to discuss your medication with your doctor.
- Over-the-counter cold remedies can cause palpitations, but this is only probable if you have had heart problems in the past.
- Some substances, such as caffeine, tobacco, alcohol, and recreational drugs, including cocaine, amphetamines, and marijuana, can stimulate the heart and cause palpitations, so avoid them.
- Manage your stress levels. Stress increases adrenaline, which can cause a rapid heartbeat and palpitations.
- Reduce your risk of heart disease by exercising regularly and eating a healthy diet.

CONVENTIONAL TREATMENTS

Treatment for palpitations may be as simple as avoiding particular substances or situations that trigger them. Depending on the type of palpitations you have, your doctor may prescribe medicines for controlling your heart rhythm, such as beta-blockers to slow your heart rate, or antiarrhythmic medicines. An injection of adenosine can also be given to normalize the heart rate. In some cases, surgery may be necessary to control the heart's rhythm, and a pacemaker may need to be fitted.

NATURAL REMEDIES

Here are some natural ways of controlling your palpitations.

HERBAL REMEDIES Hawthorn contains flavonoids, which may help control an irregular heartbeat. Try 150 milligrams three times daily.

AROMATHERAPY Try adding a few drops of neroli, ylang ylang, or lavender essential oils to bathwater to help calm palpitations.

NUTRITIONAL MEDICINE Include foods rich in magnesium in your diet, such as fish, spinach, nuts, and dairy products. Magnesium is a mineral that helps to regulate the heart's rhythm.

Caution

Seek immediate medical attention if you:

- Have pain or pressure in your chest
- Feel extremely weak
- Feel dizzy or faint
- Have shortness of breath
- Feel nauseous while having palpitations.

HELPFUL THERAPIES

Regularly practicing yoga, tai chi, or meditation will help you to relax and reduce the frequency of palpitations caused by anxiety or stress. Try the following deep breathing exercise when you feel anxious or stressed:

1 Relax your shoulders and breathe in deeply through your nose for the count of two.

2 Then breathe out through your mouth for the count of four. As you breathe, you should be able to feel your diaphragm (the muscle just below your breastbone) moving in and out.

CALL YOUR DOCTOR

Although palpitations are common and often harmless, sometimes they can be signs of an underlying medical condition that is more serious. For example, they can be caused by an overactive thyroid gland, anemia, high blood pressure, or heart problems. Call your doctor if your palpitations seem to last a long time and are worrying you.

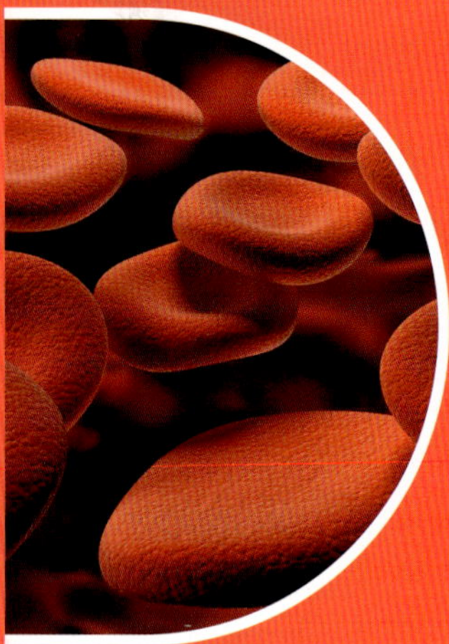

Anemia

You have anemia when you have too few red blood cells or too little hemoglobin (an oxygen-carrying protein) in your blood. This is most likely caused by an iron deficiency, but can also be due to a deficiency in vitamin B12 or folate. Anemia is most likely to occur in premenopausal women, especially during pregnancy.

SYMPTOMS

- Tiredness and lack of energy
- Palpitations (rapid or irregular heartbeat)
- Light-headedness
- Pale skin
- Shortness of breath
- Feeling cold
- Headaches
- Changes in taste
- A sore or smooth tongue
- Sore corners of the mouth
- Itching
- Dry, peeling, or spoon-shape nails

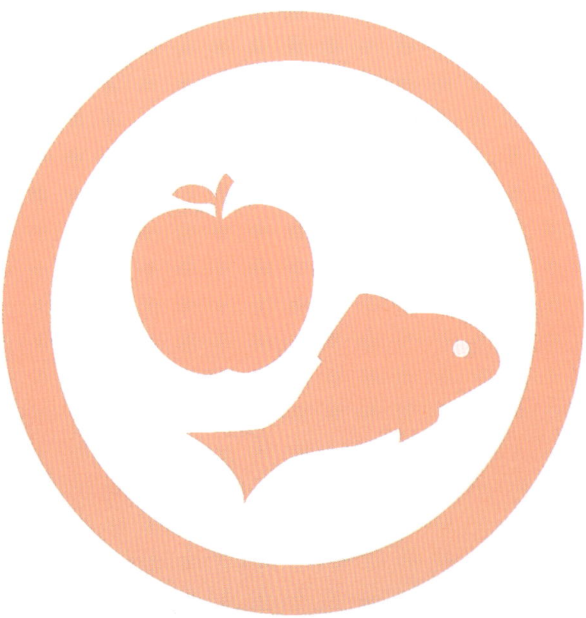

PREVENTION

Prevention involves making sure you eat a healthy balanced diet to get the nutrients you need, as well as addressing any other medical conditions that may be causing the anemia.

- Be sure you get an adequate supply of iron, vitamin B12, and folate in your diet, especially if you are pregnant.
- Women who experience heavy menstruation may need treatment to prevent anemia.
- Nonsteroidal anti-inflammatory drugs (NSAIDs), such as ibuprofen and aspirin, can cause gastrointestinal bleeding, which can lead to anemia. It may be necessary to change medicines.
- Some people have underlying medical conditions that need attention. For example, stomach ulcers and Crohn's disease may cause blood loss, and celiac disease can interfere with iron absorption.

CONVENTIONAL TREATMENTS

As well as treating any underlying problems that may be making you anemic, your doctor may prescribe iron supplements to address an iron deficiency and bring your iron levels back to normal. Your red blood cell count and hemoglobin levels will be monitored carefully to make sure you are responding well to treatment. It may also be necessary to make dietary changes and take vitamin B12 or folate supplements.

NATURAL REMEDIES

Here are some natural treatments you might consider.

HERBAL REMEDIES Spirulina is a type of blue-green algae that may help to treat anemia. Try taking one heaping teaspoon per day.

NUTRITIONAL MEDICINE Vitamin C helps your body to absorb iron from food. Good sources include broccoli, bell peppers, tomatoes, berries, and citrus fruits.

HOMEOPATHIC REMEDIES Ferrum phosphoricum is a tissue salt that is used to treat iron deficiency. Try taking four tablets of Ferrum phosphoricum 6C twice daily until relief is obtained.

HEALING FOODS

The following foods contain iron, vitamin B12, and folate, and they will help your body make enough red blood cells and hemoglobin.

IRON Found in dried fruits, such as apricots, raisins, and prunes, green leafy vegetables, meat (especially liver), nuts, beans, and molasses. Some foods are fortified with iron, such as bread and breakfast cereals.

VITAMIN B12 Occurs naturally in meat, dairy products, eggs, and fortified foods. If you follow a vegan diet, take a vitamin B12 supplement or eat fortified foods, because this vitamin is not found naturally in nonanimal products.

FOLATE Found in many fruits and vegetables. Good sources include green leafy vegetables, beans, peas, oranges, bananas, yeast extract, liver, and fortified foods.

Caution

If you are taking medications, supplements, or if you are pregnant, consult your doctor before trying alternative remedies.

CALL YOUR DOCTOR

It is important that anemia is investigated by your doctor, because failure to do so may have other health consequences, such as an impaired immune system or heart and lung problems. Iron deficiency in pregnancy may increase the risk of low birth weight, premature birth, and postnatal depression if it is left unchecked, whereas a folate deficiency can cause neural-tube defects, such as spina bifida, in a developing baby. If you have the classic symptoms of anemia (see opposite), consult your doctor without delay.

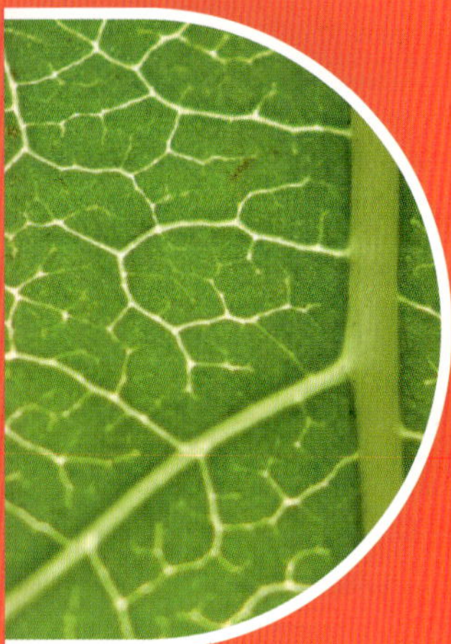

Varicose Veins

Varicose veins are a common problem, most often occurring in the legs. Veins contain tiny valves that control the direction of blood flow, making sure it flows upward toward the heart. However, sometimes the valves become weaker, letting blood flow backward and pool in the veins, causing swelling. While varicose veins don't usually cause health problems, they can become bothersome and unsightly.

SYMPTOMS

- ▷ Lumpy, swollen, twisted blue or purple veins
- ▷ Aching, painful, heavy legs
- ▷ A throbbing or burning sensation
- ▷ Cramp in the legs
- ▷ Skin discoloration
- ▷ Ulceration
- ▷ Eczema-like rash (varicose eczema)

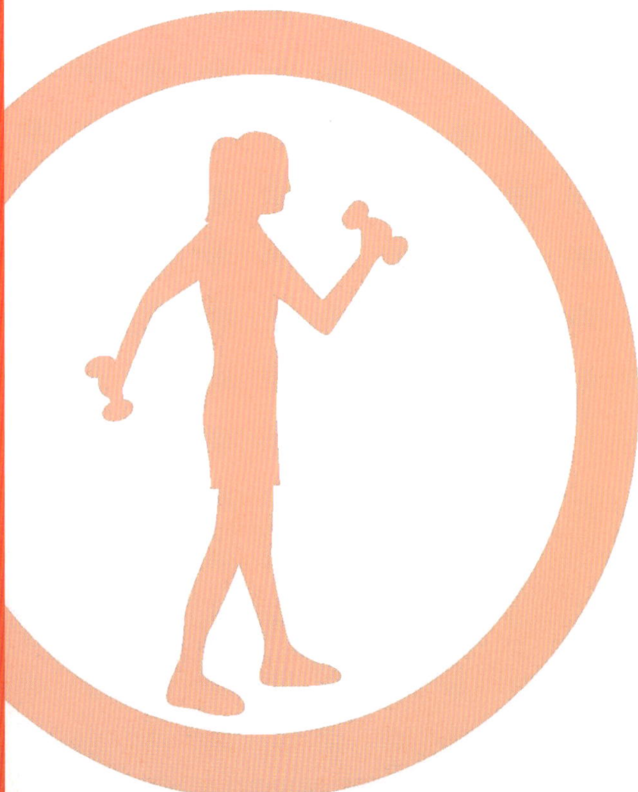

PREVENTION

A healthy lifestyle and good blood circulation may help to prevent varicose veins.

- Maintain a sensible weight. Obesity seems to increase the risk of varicose veins, because the extra weight puts pressure on the veins.
- Get regular exercise to keep your legs moving and improve blood circulation.
- Try to avoid standing or sitting for long periods of time because this can affect blood flow and make your varicose veins worse. Change your position often, and try to move about at least every 30 minutes.
- Don't smoke; it disrupts your body's circulation.

Did You Know?

Applied several times daily, witch hazel ointment may help soothe the swelling and bruising that are associated with varicose veins. This is due to its astringent properties.

CONVENTIONAL TREATMENTS

Varicose veins don't usually require treatment and can be left alone if they are not giving you trouble. However, sometimes they can become uncomfortable or painful and require medical attention. Compression stockings can ease pain and discomfort; these apply pressure to the legs and encourage blood flow up toward the heart. Varicose veins can also be treated with sclerotherapy, which involves injecting the veins with a chemical to close them off. In some cases, varicose veins may need to be removed with surgery.

NATURAL REMEDIES

There are a number of things you can try to help relieve symptoms of varicose veins.

HERBAL REMEDIES Horse chestnut (*Aesculus hippocastanum*) is helpful for treating chronic venous insufficiency. Take two 300 milligram tablets of horse chestnut extract (standardized to contain 20 percent aescin) daily.

NUTRITIONAL MEDICINE Rutin is a bioflavonoid that may help to improve vein function and the symptoms associated with varicose veins. Try taking one 500 mg rutin tablet daily.

YOGA Yoga postures will help improve circulation and encourage blood flow back to the heart. Try the shoulder stand for a few minutes each day to drain blood from your legs or, for a simpler option, lie with your body flat on the floor and your legs resting up against the wall.

HOMEOPATHIC REMEDIES

You can buy specially prepared homeopathic remedies for varicose veins and circulatory disorders, or try the following.

Arnica montana 6C: Take one tablet three times daily for bruised, swollen legs that are very sore and feel better when you are lying down.

Hamamelis 6C: Take one tablet three times daily for large, sore, stinging, purple, and bruised veins, and a tendency to experience bleeding hemorrhoids.

Pulsatilla 6C: Take one tablet three times daily for swollen, painful veins and heavy legs, which feel worse during warm temperatures.

CALL YOUR DOCTOR

If your varicose veins bother you, cause pain, or keep you awake at night, call your doctor. This is especially important if:

- Your veins bleed
- You have excessive swelling
- Your skin changes color
- You notice a rash or you develop ulcers.

IMMEDIATE RELIEF

To ease pain and discomfort when you are lying down, place some pillows under your legs to raise them above the level of your heart. When sitting, sit with your legs raised to help improve blood circulation, and don't sit with your legs crossed.

Restless Legs

Restless legs is characterized by unpleasant sensations in the legs and the overwhelming urge to move them. Most people have mild symptoms, but they can be more severe, causing interrupted sleep and interfering with daily life.

SYMPTOMS

- The need to move your legs when resting
- Aching, tingling, itching, or pain in your legs
- Involuntary leg movements during the night
- Difficulty sleeping

PREVENTION

Lifestyle changes may help to prevent symptoms and aid restful sleep.

- Exercise regularly.
- Avoid alcohol, caffeine, and tobacco before going to bed.
- Do something relaxing before bed.
- Make sure your bed is comfortable and your bedroom is quiet and dark.
- Get up and go to bed at the same time each day.

Did You Know?

It is not clear what causes restless legs, but it is believed to be related to a low level of dopamine (a neurotransmitter) in the brain.

CONVENTIONAL TREATMENTS

If your symptoms are mild, simple lifestyle changes may be enough to provide relief. Dopamine agonists, such as ropinerol and pramipexole, which increase the level of dopamine in the brain, may be prescribed for more severe cases of restless legs.

NATURAL REMEDIES

The following natural therapies may help relieve the symptoms of restless legs.

HERBAL REMEDIES Take 20 to 30 drops of butcher's broom extract in a little water up to three times daily to improve circulation.

NUTRITIONAL MEDICINE Restless legs may be associated with low iron levels. Good sources of iron include beef, chicken, beans, lentils, and molasses.

CALL YOUR DOCTOR

If your symptoms are getting worse and disrupting your sleep and daily life, see your doctor. Restless legs can be due to an underlying health condition, such as kidney disease, diabetes, or anemia. It can also occur as a side effect of some medications, such as antidepressants.

Deep Vein Thrombosis

Deep vein thrombosis (DVT) is a blood clot in a deep vein, usually in the leg. The risk of developing this condition is increased by being immobile for a long time, such as during a long-haul flight or car journey, or a stay in hospital.

SYMPTOMS

- ▷ Pain and swelling in the leg
- ▷ Heavy, aching leg
- ▷ Leg feels hot
- ▷ Skin changes color

PREVENTION

Here are some simple measures to help prevent DVT.

- Walk regularly to boost circulation in your legs.
- Obesity increases the risk of DVT, so lose weight if necessary.
- Eat a healthy diet.
- Stay well hydrated by drinking plenty of water.
- Don't drink alcohol.
- Don't smoke.
- Don't use sleeping pills while traveling.
- Wear special flight socks on long flights.

CONVENTIONAL TREATMENTS

DVT is treated with the anticoagulant medicines heparin and warfarin. These stop the blood clot from getting bigger and help prevent additional blood clots from forming. Wear compression stockings relieve pain and swelling and encourage blood circulation in the legs. After DVT, it is important to keep mobile with gentle exercise.

NATURAL REMEDIES

The following may help to prevent additional clots.

NUTRITIONAL MEDICINE Vitamin E, vitamin K, and garlic have natural blood-thinning properties. (Seek medical advice if you are already taking anticoagulants.)

EXERCISE With your toes on the floor, raise and lower your heels 10 times. Then raise and lower your toes 10 times while keeping your heels on the floor. On long flights or car journeys, do these exercises at regular intervals to prevent blood from pooling in the lower legs.

CALL YOUR DOCTOR

If you think you may have DVT, call your doctor as soon as possible. If a blood clot is not treated, part of it may break off, travel to your lungs, and block a blood vessel. This is a potentially life-threatening condition known as a pulmonary embolism.

Did You Know?

If you have a family history of deep vein thrombosis, you have an increased risk of developing thrombosis yourself.

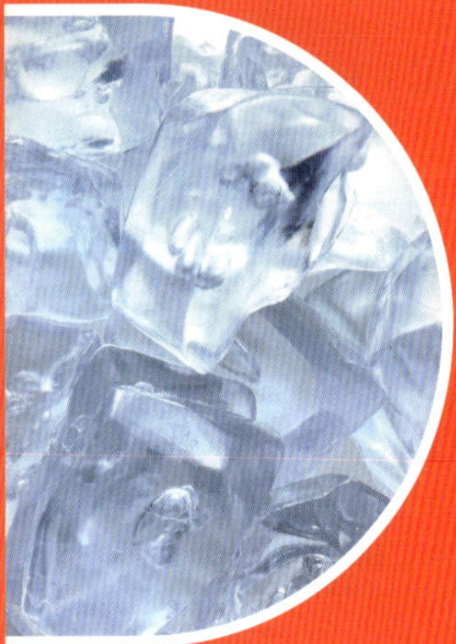

Chilblains

Chilblains are small, itchy lumps on the fingers, toes, ears, or nose that appear a few hours after prolonged exposure to cold. Although chilblains cause some discomfort, they usually go away on their own without other complications. Children, older people, and people with poor circulation are more likely to get chilblains.

SYMPTOMS

- Small swellings on the skin
- Itching, burning skin
- Red or purple skin
- Sore and broken skin
- Blistering or ulceration of the skin

Did You Know?

In cold weather, the blood vessels in your fingers, toes, and ears become narrower. When you go back into a warm environment, these blood vessels expand, which sometimes causes fluid to escape into nearby tissues. This leads to chilblains.

PREVENTION

Here are some simple things you can do to protect yourself from the cold and help prevent chilblains.

- Keep warm. Wear gloves, socks, a hat and scarf, and other insulating clothing when you are outside in the cold.
- Warm your shoes and gloves on the radiator before you go outside.
- Make sure your home is warm, and free of drafts and damp.
- Wear socks in bed if you get cold feet.
- Don't wear tight-fitting shoes; this puts pressure on your feet and increases the risk of chilblains.
- Keep your hands and feet moisturized to prevent your skin from drying out.
- Have at least one hot meal a day in cold weather to warm up your body.
- Keep as active as possible to maintain good circulation.
- Don't smoke—nicotine contributes to poor circulation.

CONVENTIONAL TREATMENTS

Always keep the parts of your body affected by chilblains warm. There are over-the-counter ointments that may relieve the symptoms of chilblains. Antiseptic cream can be used on areas of cracked skin. A medication known as nifedipine, which dilates blood vessels, is sometimes prescribed for people who repeatedly get chilblains.

NATURAL REMEDIES

The following remedies may help provide some relief from chilblains.

NUTRITIONAL MEDICINE Use plenty of ginger, garlic, chile, and turmeric to add flavor when you are cooking. These foods are good for enhancing circulation.

AROMATHERAPY Add a few drops of peppermint, lavender, rosemary, or eucalyptus essential oils to a carrier oil and massage into the affected areas.

ACUPUNCTURE This treatment may help to prevent chilblains by improving circulation to the hands and feet.

HERBAL REMEDIES

The following herbs are thought to be helpful in improving general circulation.

- Take 30 milligram ginkgo biloba three to four times daily.
- Take 20 to 30 drops of hawthorn berry extract with water two to three times daily.

HOMEOPATHIC REMEDIES

You might like to try one of these remedies, depending on your symptoms.

Sulfur 30C: Take two tablets four times daily for chilblains that are inflamed.

Pulsatilla 30C: For painful chilblains, take two tablets four times daily.

Nux vomica 30C: For throbbing or pulsating chilblains, take two tablets three times daily.

CALL YOUR DOCTOR

If you have cracked, broken, or sore skin, call your doctor. Your skin may have become septic and need treating with antibiotics. Also, narrowing of the blood vessels may be a side effect of some medications, such as beta-blockers. Speak to your doctor if you think your medication may be making you more susceptible to chilblains.

Caution

When you come in from the cold, never sit right next to a heater or place something hot directly on your skin. This increases the risk of chilblains. Warm yourself up slowly.

TOP 20 Conventional Treatments

In case of accidents, minor aches, pains, and common ailments, it's a good idea to keep some conventional medicines handy at home. Here are the top 20 remedies for your medicine cabinet with information on their uses. Always keep them in a safe place out of the way of children and pets.

1 SIMPLE ANALGESICS

- **Common names** Acetaminophen, Tylenol
- **Used for** Pain relief, headaches, fever

!!! **Caution** Do not use if you have liver problems

2 NONSTEROIDAL ANTI-INFLAMMATORY DRUGS (NSAIDS)

- **Common names** Ibuprofen, aspirin, naproxen
- **Used for** Pain relief, especially where there is inflammation, swollen joints, sprains, arthritis

!!! **Caution** Do not use if you have asthma, irritable bowel syndrome, or stomach ulcers; do not give aspirin to children under 16

3 ANTIHISTAMINES

- **Available as** Pills, creams
- **Used for** Hay fever, allergies, rashes, insect stings and bites, poison ivy, poison oak, stinging nettles

!!! **Caution** Some may cause drowsiness

4 ANTACIDS

- **Common names** Aluminum salts, Milk of Magnesia, Gaviscon, Alka-Seltzer
- **Used for** Heartburn, indigestion, and trapped gas

!!! **Caution** Consult your doctor before taking if you have a kidney disorder

5 ORAL REHYDRATION SALTS

- **Common names** Dioralyte
- **Available as** Powder sachets
- **Used for** Treating dehydration, diarrhea, loose bowel movements, vomiting, and restoring body's natural balance of minerals and fluids

6 ANTIFUNGAL TREATMENTS

- **Common names** Clotrimazole
- **Used for** Relieving yeast infections, and treating oral thrush and fungal skin infections

7 HYDROCORTISONE 1% CREAM

- **Common names** Hydrocortisone acetate
- **Used for** Mild skin irritation, itching, and mild eczema

8 CALAMINE

- **Available as** Lotion or cream
- **Used for** Itchy skin, rashes, sunburn

9 ANTIDIARRHEA PILLS

- **Common names** Imodium
- **Used for** Diarrhea, food poisoning, gastroenteritis

!!! **Caution** Do not give to children under 12

10 SUNSCREENS AND SUNBLOCKS

- **Available as** Lotions, creams, sprays
- **Used for** Protecting skin against the sun's burning rays and minimizing risk of skin cancer. Choose one that offers UVA protection with an SPF of at least 15

!!! **Caution** If sensitive to perfumes, opt for nonscented, hypoallergenic products

11 ANTISEPTIC

- **Common names** Dettol, Sudocream
- **Available as** Lotions, creams, sprays, wipes
- **Used for** Cleaning cuts, grazes, and wounds

12 THROAT LOZENGES AND SPRAYS

- **Common names** Benzocaine, Chloraseptic
- **Used for** Relieving sore throats

13 EMOLLIENTS

- **Common names** Aquaphor, Eucerin
- **Available as** Creams, gels
- **Used for** Relieving itching and moisturizing dry skin, eczema, dermatitis

14 BANDAGES

- **Used for** Covering cuts and wounds

15 EYEWASH SOLUTION

- **Used for** Washing grit and dirt out of eyes and treating eye injuries where tap water is not readily available

16 DECONGESTANTS

- **Available as** Pills or nasal sprays
- **Used for** Relieving cold symptoms, such as blocked nose, and easing hay fever symptoms

17 MUSCLE PAIN RELIEF

- **Common names** Biofreeze, Deep Heat
- **Available as** Sprays, gels, heat pads
- **Used for** Muscular pains, and sprained joint pain

18 INSECT REPELLENTS

- **Available as** Sprays, creams, gels, lotions, medicated towelettes
- **Used for** Preventing insect bites and stings

19 INFANT SUSPENSION

- **Available as** Flavored liquids and sachets
- **Used for** Relieving pain, teething pain, fever, cold symptoms in babies and young children

!!! **Caution** Contains acetaminophen

20 COUGH MEDICINES

- **Types** Suppressants for dry coughs; expectorants for chesty coughs with phlegm
- **Used for** Relieving painful and irritating coughs

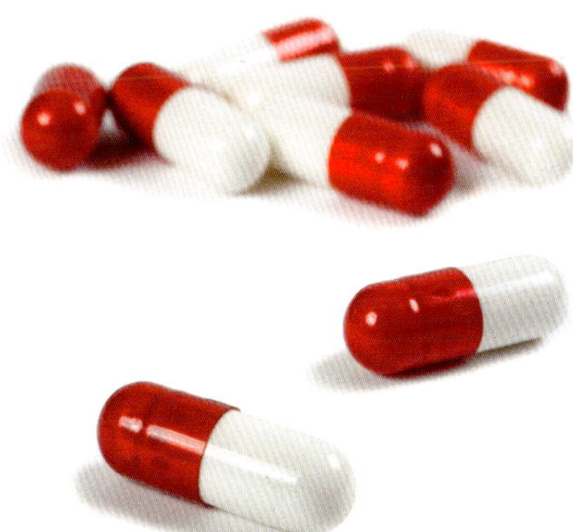

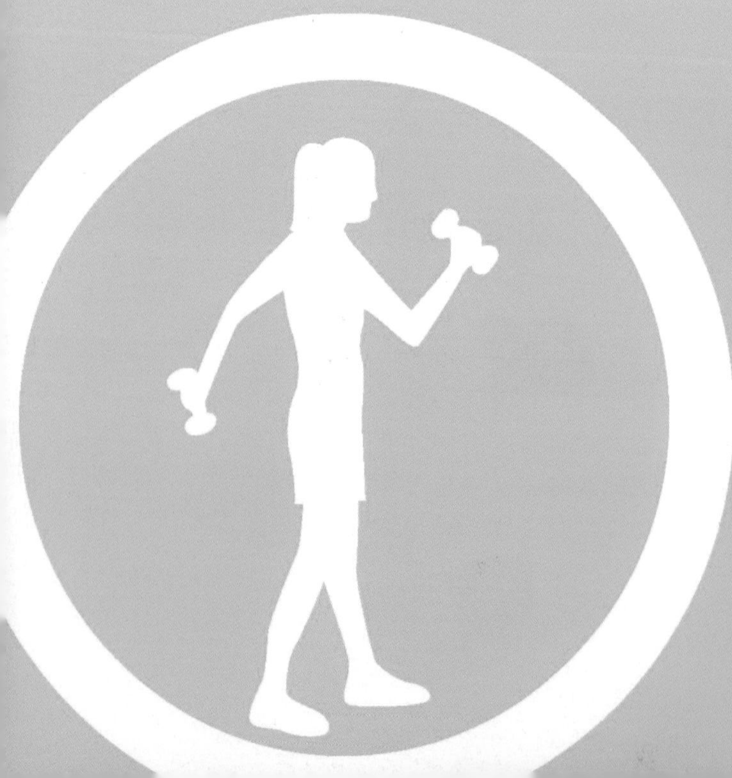

Respiratory Problems

The respiratory system comprises the airways, breathing muscles and lungs, together with the arteries and veins that carry oxygen to and from the lungs. Its function is to supply oxygen, which is essential for the healthy and efficient functioning of all the body's cells, and to take away waste products, such as carbon dioxide.

When you inhale, air is breathed in through your nose and mouth and passes down the windpipe through the bronchi into your lungs. Inside the lungs are millions of tiny air sacs called alveoli where an exchange of gases takes place. The oxygen is passed into the bloodstream for distribution to the heart and thence to the rest of the body, while carbon dioxide is exhaled.

A properly functioning respiratory system is essential for good health, but diseases are becoming increasingly common in industrialized countries due to pollutants in the atmosphere, tobacco smoke, and exhaust fumes. There is evidence that repeated exposure can increase the likelihood of developing respiratory problems, such as asthma, chronic bronchitis, emphysema, and even lung cancer. Many minor common respiratory problems and disorders, such as coughing, runny nose, and sore throat, are caused by infection, and these can be treated with conventional, traditional, and natural remedies.

Your lifestyle and diet play an important role in building and maintaining healthy lungs. Regular exercise will make them strong and expand their capacity, while eating healthily helps your body to fight infections. However, the best protection you can give your lungs is not to smoke; if you are already a smoker, quit now before it is too late. Even second-hand smoke and passive smoking can affect your respiratory health, so get your partner or friends to give up cigarettes.

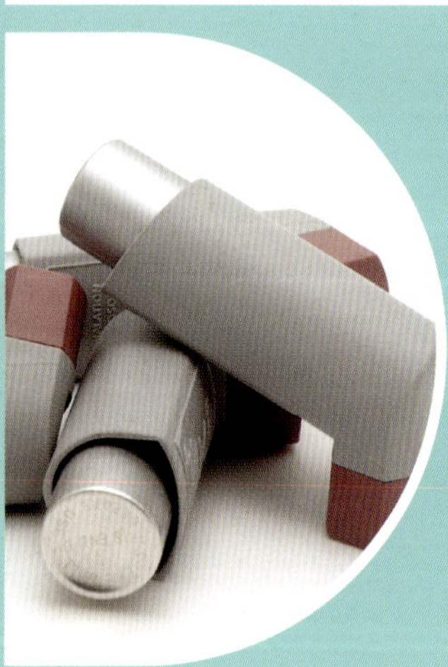

Asthma

The respiratory condition asthma affects around millions people around the world. It causes the bronchi—the airways of the lungs—to become irritated, inflamed, and swollen, which results in a narrowing of the airways. In many cases, asthma begins in childhood, but it can also develop at any point during life. Although there is no overall cure for this condition, there are many ways in which the symptoms can be managed and treated.

SYMPTOMS

- Coughing
- Shortness of breath
- Wheezing
- A tight feeling in the chest

PREVENTION

- Asthma can be triggered by common allergens, such as dust mites, pollen, smoke, animal fur, or feathers, so reducing contact with these can help reduce the risk of an asthma attack. For dust mites, regularly cleaning your home is beneficial.
- Dust, fumes, or chemical substances you come into contact with regularly (for instance, through your work environment) can also trigger asthma attacks. Being aware of this and trying to limit exposure wherever possible can help reduce the risk of an asthma attack or of asthma worsening.
- Regular exercise can improve lung capacity and strengthen your heart.

CONVENTIONAL TREATMENTS

Asthma is controlled and managed using a variety of different medicines that are tailored to individual needs. Two types of inhalers, which contain steroids and other medicines, are usually prescribed. A bronchodilator is used to treat the symptoms of asthma, and anti-inflammatory medicines help to prevent the symptoms. You may also be given a nebulizer—a device that helps you to use your inhaler effectively. For severe asthma attacks, a course of steroid medicines may be prescribed.

NATURAL REMEDIES

There are various natural remedies you can try for easing different aspects of asthma.

NUTRITIONAL MEDICINE Foods containing the naturally occurring substance sulfite, used as a food preservative, can trigger asthma in some people. Watch your diet and cut down on sulfite foods, such as beer, wine, processed foods, and shrimp. Sometimes food allergies can trigger asthma, so work with a nutritionist to try to identify and remove any potential allergens from your diet.

ALEXANDER TECHNIQUE Poor posture, especially hunching your shoulders and pushing the neck into the chest, can make the symptoms of asthma worse. Work with a qualified Alexander Technique practitioner to learn how to improve your posture and benefit your breathing.

YOGA Join a yoga class, because practicing yoga, especially stretching postures and breathing techniques, can be beneficial.

AROMATHERAPY Put a few drops of eucalyptus essential oil onto a tissue and gently inhale it to help your breathing (steam inhalation isn't recommended for asthmatics).

HELPFUL THERAPIES Buteyko breathing methods, which involves learning breathing exercises and techniques to reduce overbreathing, is beneficial. Find a qualified practitioner to teach you.

OSTEOPATHY An osteopath may be able to use soft tissue massage and manipulation techniques to relax the chest muscles and also to ease breathing problems.

Caution

- Don't abandon taking prescribed asthma medication.
- If you're having a severe asthma attack and are unable to breathe, dial 911 and request emergency medical treatment.

HERBAL REMEDIES

- If your asthma has been brought on by a cold or chest infection, then take one or two teaspoons of echinacea tincture with water two or three times a day for a week, or until the symptoms go.
- To ease the discomfort of a tight chest, take one teaspoon of cramp bark tincture with water three times a day for up to a week.

CALL YOUR DOCTOR

If you suspect that you may have asthma, call your doctor. Likewise, if you are asthmatic and your symptoms are getting worse or your medication is not working effectively, consult your doctor.

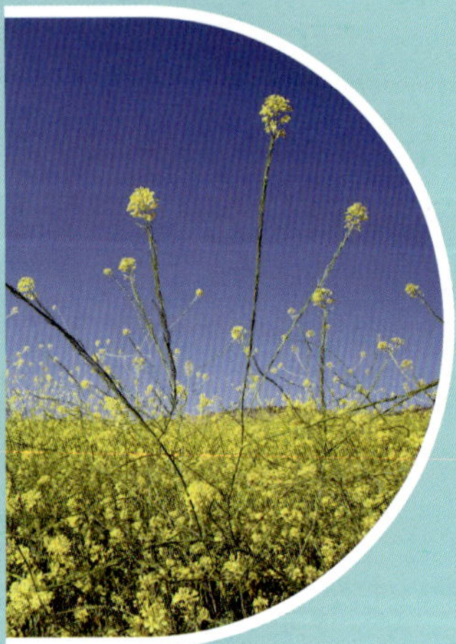

Hay Fever

Hay fever is an allergic reaction to pollen, which is produced by seasonal grasses, occurring usually in the spring and summer. Like asthma, it is on the increase, and the symptoms listed below are common to other allergic reactions, including house dust mites, exhaust fumes, and atmospheric pollution.

SYMPTOMS

- Sore, swollen, itchy, and stinging eyes
- Stuffed-up nose and sinuses
- Streaming nose
- Frequent bouts of violent sneezing
- Itching of the roof of the mouth
- Itching in the ears
- Mild form of asthma with tightness in the chest

Did You Know?

Cutting back on your daily intake of dairy products may reduce mucus production and relieve hay fever symptoms. However, if you consume less milk, yogurt, and cheese, you must find other sources of calcium and other missing nutrients.

PREVENTION

As always, prevention is better than cure and the only real way to prevent hay fever is to avoid inhaling allergenic material. Although this is not practical, you could try the following measures.

- Keep the windows shut and avoid going outside early in the morning, late in the evening, and just before and after thunderstorms, when pollen counts are higher and more likely to trigger attacks.
- Don't open your car windows when you are traveling; if it's a hot day, turn on the air-conditioning to stay cool. Make enquiries about getting a pollen filter fitted to your car.
- Some people with hay fever claim that wearing wraparound sunglasses to protect their eyes from pollen is also helpful.
- Smear some petroleum jelly around and just inside your nostrils to trap pollen and help prevent inhalation.
- You can take conventional antiallergy medication before an attack (see opposite), or you can use a natural antihistamine, such as ginkgo biloba or nettle (three times daily).

Quick Fix

You can quickly soothe sore, itchy eyes with a cool, damp washcloth.

CONVENTIONAL TREATMENTS

Antihistamines are commonly used to prevent allergic reactions. These are available as nose sprays, pills, and eye drops, or as syrups for young children. Although antihistamines are reasonably effective, they can cause drowsiness and other side effects. Check the packaging for details or ask the pharmacist or your doctor for advice.

Healing Foods

Find a source of locally produced organic honey and have four teaspoons a day to help relieve hay fever symptoms. It is important that it is made by bees collecting the pollen from flowering plants in your area.

Herbal Remedies

The usual remedies use cleansing and strengthening herbs for the respiratory tract.

- Take up to eight 200-milligram eyebright capsules to relieve symptoms.

Homeopathic Remedies

You can buy "over-the-counter" homeopathic hay-fever tablets or try:

Allium cepa 6C: Take one tablet twice daily to relieve watering eyes and running, sore nose

Euphrasia 6C: Take one tablet twice daily to relieve watery, sore eyes, and running nose with frequent sneezing

Sabadilla 6C: Take one tablet twice daily to relieve irritated eyes, blocked nose, and violent sneezing.

NATURAL REMEDIES

You can experiment with a whole range of natural remedies to discover what works best for you. Here are some of the options you might consider.

ACUPRESSURE Points 41 and 47 may increase mucus drainage; points 50 and 51 may help stop bouts of sneezing.

AROMATHERAPY Place a drop of either basil or melissa oil in a handkerchief for instant relief from blocked sinuses and a stuffed-up nose.

NUTRITIONAL MEDICINE Eat more citrus fruit, berries, and vegetables. They are good sources of vitamin C and help protect mucus membranes. Oily fish and flaxseed oil contain omega-3 fatty acids, which can counter inflammatory reactions triggered by pollen allergy.

CALL YOUR DOCTOR

If your symptoms do not diminish as a result of taking natural remedies or over-the-counter antihistamines, consult your doctor.

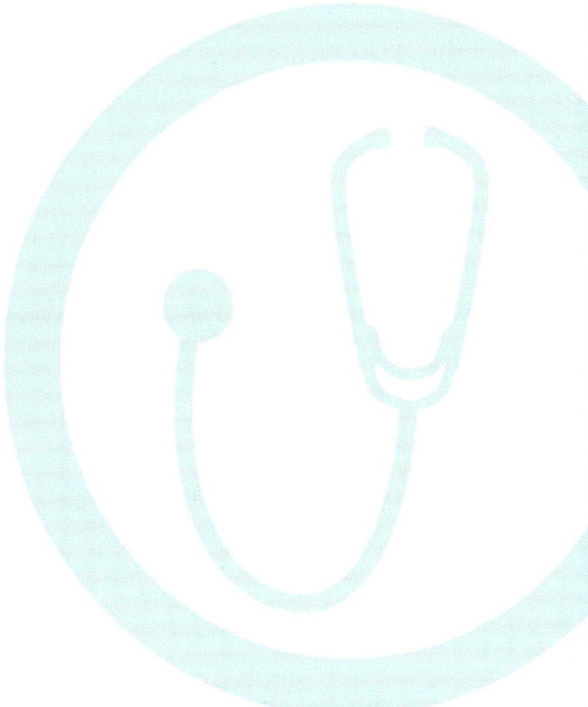

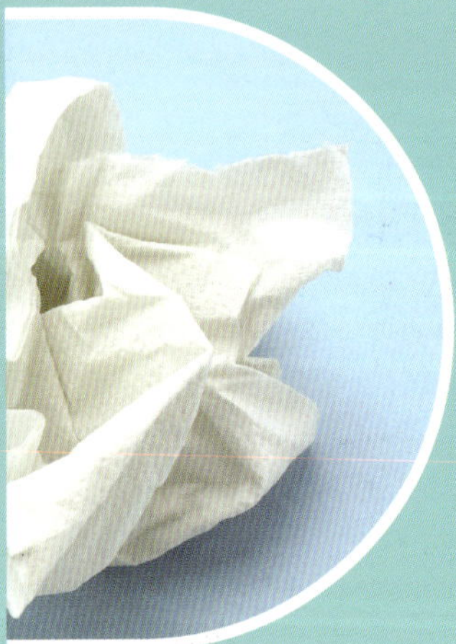

Common Cold

Colds are viral infections of the upper respiratory tract and affect us all at some time or another. Although they are so common and highly contagious, there is no known cure. Colds are annoying and debilitating but most disappear within five days, unless there are complications.

SYMPTOMS

- ▷ Blocked nose
- ▷ Runny nose and sneezing
- ▷ Possible sore throat
- ▷ Possible fever
- ▷ Tickly cough
- ▷ Headaches

Did You Know?

There are around 200 different cold viruses, which are transmitted by sneezing, coughing, or hand-to-hand contact.

PREVENTION

Colds may be a sign that you are run down and need to boost your immune system. The best ways to prevent them include the following:

- Eat a healthy diet that contains vitamin C (citrus fruits, leafy green vegetables, tomatoes, and bell peppers) and zinc (shellfish, meat, and pumpkin seeds)
- Take a vitamin C supplement every day
- If possible, avoid crowded, overheated places when cold viruses are circulating in winter
- Do not rub your eyes and nose after hand contact with people who have colds
- Get outside and get plenty of fresh air and exercise
- Stay relaxed and calm and try not to get stressed or overtired.

CONVENTIONAL TREATMENTS

There are many over-the-counter cold and cough remedies, but they can only relieve the symptoms at best, not cure your cold. These range from painkillers for headaches to decongestants. Antibiotics will not work unless there is a secondary bacterial infection.

NATURAL REMEDIES

Most people have their own tried and tested homemade remedies for relieving the unpleasant symptoms of colds. These include the following:

- Squeeze the juice of a lemon into a cup of hot water and stir in one teaspoon honey. If desired, add some grated fresh ginger
- Drink plenty of fluids to replace any lost through sneezing and sweating (if you have a fever)
- Gargle with saltwater
- Eat onions and garlic for their decongestant and antiseptic properties—make a French onion soup or just bake some whole in a little olive oil.

HERBAL REMEDIES Make a herb tea with some elderflower (for stuffed-up nose and catarrh), hyssop (for coughs), and peppermint (for reducing mucus). Taking echinacea and goldenseal drops every day in water helps to boost the immune system as well as relieving irritation of the mucous membranes.

AROMATHERAPY

- Add three drops each lavender, eucalyptus, and thyme oils to a bowl of boiling water and inhale the steam.
- Or sprinkle a couple of drops of eucalyptus, pine, or lavender oil onto a handkerchief.
- Before going to bed, have a soothing bath and add a few drops of tea tree, eucalyptus, pine, or lavender oil to the water.

HOMEOPATHIC REMEDIES

These can be helpful in relieving cold symptoms.

Aconite 6C: Take one tablet every four hours at the beginning of a cold to relieve a stuffed-up nose and frequent sneezing.

Natrum muriaticum 6C: Take one tablet every three to four hours for a cold that starts with sneezing with white or clear discharge.

CALL YOUR DOCTOR

Most colds do not necessitate a visit to the doctor and will clear up of their own accord in a few days. However, you should make an appointment if you experience any of the following symptoms:

- You have shortness of breath
- Your cough gets progressively worse and won't go away
- You have persistent fever for more than a week
- You have a compromised immune system (for example, due to HIV) or chronic respiratory and/or heart disease.

IMMEDIATE RELIEF

There is no quick fix for a cold, but you can clear a blocked nose and make breathing easier by steam inhalation. Add some eucalyptus drops to a heatproof bowl of boiling water, cover your head with a towel, bend over the steam, and inhale deeply.

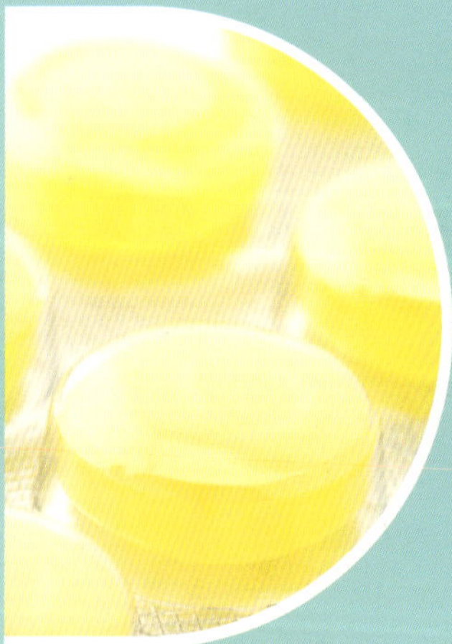

Coughs

Coughing is one of your body's natural defense mechanisms, a reflex action used by the respiratory system to clear the airways and remove or prevent infection. It may be caused by irritation of the throat or larynx, an increase in catarrh or saliva, or excess sputum, usually due to bacterial infection. Many coughs are just dry and irritating—a by-product of a cold—but they can be persistent and more serious.

SYMPTOMS

- ▷ Dry tickly throat
- ▷ Dry, barking cough
- ▷ Deep, painful cough
- ▷ Clear or colored mucus
- ▷ Possible sore throat

Did You Know?

Some people think that taking garlic capsules every day helps to prevent and relieve coughs. Garlic is decongestant and antibacterial.

PREVENTION

The best way to prevent unwanted coughs and respiratory problems is not to smoke and to avoid passive smoking situations. You can also:

- Exercise regularly to strengthen your lungs
- Try to avoid pollution, smog, and traffic fumes, or wear a face mask when you are cycling in heavy city traffic
- Wear a protective face mask when tackling any dusty housework and home improvements
- Do not sleep in air-conditioning
- Put a humidifier in centrally heated rooms.

CONVENTIONAL TREATMENTS

You can choose from a wide array of cough mixtures and lozenges, which claim to soothe and loosen coughs. However, there is little evidence for their efficacy. Deep, painful, and persistent coughing may be a symptom of a lower respiratory infection and might require antibiotics.

NATURAL REMEDIES

For centuries, people have treated coughs with homemade medicines, herbs, and nutritional remedies.

- Eat less dairy foods (milk, yogurt, cheese) to reduce mucus formation.
- Try to eat some garlic, leeks, and onions every day by adding them to soups, stews, casseroles, etc.
- Apply a mustard pack to your chest.
- Slice some onions thinly into rings and layer them up in a bowl with brown sugar sprinkled between the layers. The following day, drain off the liquid and drink a teaspoonful at a time.
- Add freshly squeezed lemon juice and honey to hot water.
- Swallow one teaspoon honey, letting it trickle down your throat.

HERBAL REMEDIES Many herbs are traditionally used to treat coughs. You can make a herbal tea for chesty coughs with white horehound, thyme, coltsfoot, cowslip, and peppermint, whereas marshmallow root can help ease dry coughs. You can also make herbal steam inhalations with eucalyptus and peppermint.

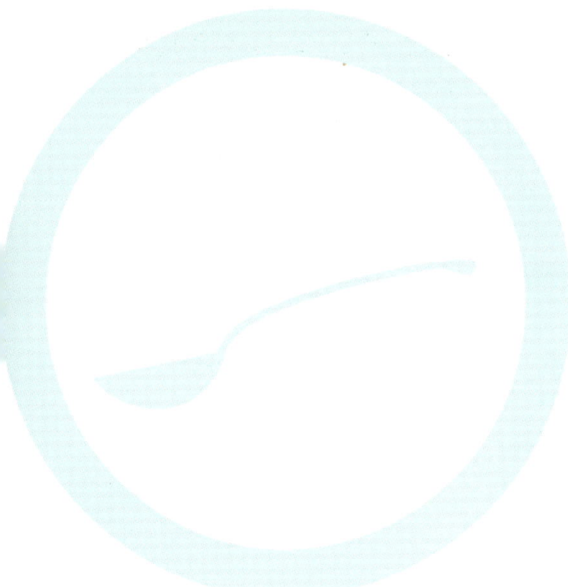

AROMATHERAPY

- Add three drops of eucalyptus, cypress, thyme, or sandalwood oil to steaming hot water and inhale deeply to soothe the airways.
- Mix eucalyptus, sandalwood, or frankincense oils with a carrier oil and rub gently into the chest and throat, or heat the oil in a special burner and breathe in the fragrance.
- You can also use tea tree oil as a gargle—just add two to three drops to a cup of warm water and gargle three times a day.

HOMEOPATHIC REMEDIES

The following remedies can be helpful in relieving cough symptoms. Choose the appropriate remedy for your symptoms.

Bryonia 6C: Take one tablet three times daily for dry, painful coughs.

Stannum 6C: Take one tablet three times daily for chesty coughs with greenish mucus.

CALL YOUR DOCTOR

If your cough does not clear up and becomes progressively worse or you cough up blood-stained mucus, you must see your doctor. Coughs may be a sign of a more serious, underlying condition and this needs checking. If accompanied by a bacterial lung infection, you may be prescribed antibiotics.

Quick Fix

Sucking herbal cough lozenges may be soothing and bring instant relief in a coughing fit, although they will not cure your cough.

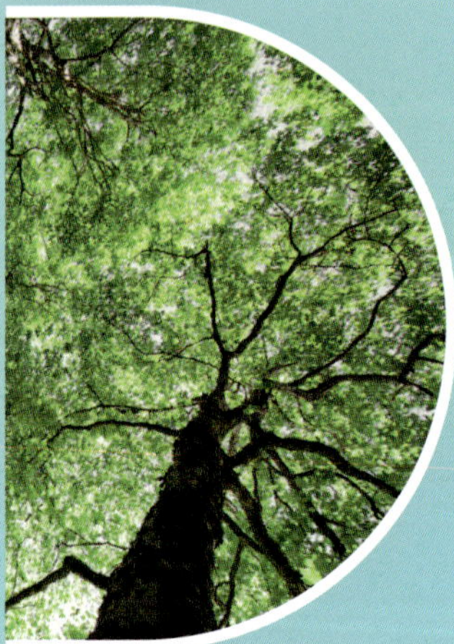

Bronchitis

Bronchitis affects the main airways of the lung (the bronchi). It causes inflammation and irritation, the production of more mucus than is normal, and a hacking cough. It is common during the winter months, particularly after a cold, influenza, or sore throat, but as well as infections, it can also be caused by environmental factors.

SYMPTOMS

- A bad, hacking cough
- Coughing up yellowy mucus
- Wheezing
- Breathlessness
- A sore throat
- Blocked nose and sinuses
- Headaches
- Chills or a fever
- General aches, pains, and feeling unwell

PREVENTION

Good hygiene is beneficial, because bronchitis is often caused by a virus spread via coughing or sneezing. Wash your hands frequently or use antibacterial gel on them if you're in contact with people who have colds or flu.

- If you work in an environment where you could be exposed to breathing in irritating substances, protect your lungs by wearing a mask on your face.
- Damp or cold environments can also lead to bronchitis, so try to avoid such circumstances.
- If you're a smoker, quit smoking; cigarette smoke can make you more susceptible to bronchitis.
- If you have a low immune system, try to eat a healthy balanced diet, so that your body gets a good dose of essential nutrients.

Did You Know?

A humidifier can help keep the air in a room moist and aid your breathing. If you don't have one, you can create the same effect by simply placing a pot of water on a radiator.

CONVENTIONAL TREATMENTS

Drinking plenty of fluids not only keeps you hydrated but also helps to thin the mucus and make it easier to cough up. Painkillers can ease any aches, pains, or headaches. Over-the-counter cough medicines may provide some relief. It also helps to get plenty of rest and, where possible, have fresh air in a room. If your doctor thinks that you could have an increased risk of developing pneumonia, antibiotics may be prescribed.

NATURAL REMEDIES

There are various natural remedies that may help ease the symptoms of bronchitis.

HERBAL REMEDIES Use expectorant herbs, such as elecampane and thyme, to encourage coughing and rid yourself of mucus. A herbalist can make up a tincture for you. Take echinacea, along with garlic, for their infection-fighting abilities, and try ginseng supplements to help reduce bronchial inflammation.

AROMATHERAPY Steam installation can provide much-needed relief for the congestion of bronchitis. Lean your head over a bowl of hot water to inhale. Add a drop of eucalyptus oil to clear your nasal passages, or lavender to relax your muscles and help your breathing. If you have no oils, then simply breathe in the steam. Inhale several times a day as required.

OSTEOPATHY An osteopath may be able to provide help for chronic bronchitis by working on the shoulder muscles, neck, and back to ease any congestion and clear the air passages.

NUTRITIONAL MEDICINE

- Include plenty of garlic in your diet, because it's good for your immune system.
- Avoid eating processed foods and dairy products while you have bronchitis, because they can encourage more mucus to form.
- Eat plenty of vitamin C—or take vitamin C supplements—because it can help thin the mucus.

CALL YOUR DOCTOR

The symptoms of bronchitis are similar to those of pneumonia, which can be more serious. Don't try to self-diagnose—call your doctor, especially if your symptoms change. This is especially important if you have any other lung or heart conditions.

Helpful Supplements

- Colloidal silver has natural antibiotic properties and can work with viruses and bacteria.
- Where bronchitis is triggered by an allergic reaction, such an environmental factor, taking the antioxidant supplement quercetin can be beneficial.

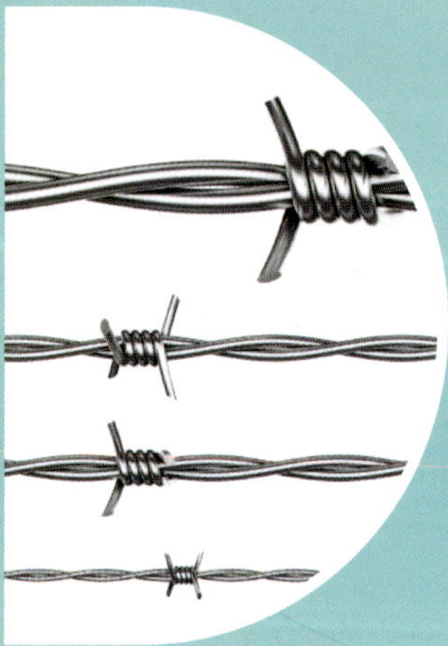

Sore Throat

Most sore throats are due to minor bacterial or viral infections and clear up after a few days. They are more common in winter, often accompanying the common cold or influenza, and are spread by airborne droplets, through coughing and sneezing, or by hand-to-hand contact. However, they can also be caused by allergies, such as hay fever, or irritation from smoking.

SYMPTOMS

- Throat feels sore with pain at back
- Difficulty swallowing
- Throat looks red
- Tonsils may be swollen and coated
- Possible swollen lymph nodes in neck
- May be fever, headache, pain in ears

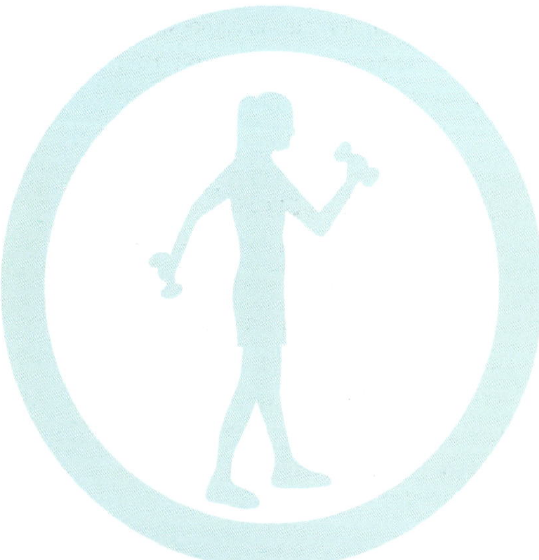

PREVENTION

Most sore throats are caused by viruses, so there are few preventive measures that you can take. However, you can reduce your chances of getting one and decrease the incidence and severity by:

- Eating a healthy diet
- Giving up smoking and avoiding smoky environments
- Drinking plenty of fluids, especially water
- Wrapping up warmly in winter and wearing a scarf to protect your throat from cold
- Staying healthy, relaxed, and stress-free to prevent becoming rundown and more susceptible to infections
- Not sharing towels or drinking or eating utensils with anyone who already has a sore throat.

Did You Know?

Most home remedies, especially honey, lemon, and cider vinegar taken three times daily, are more effective in relieving sore throats than conventional over-the-counter preparations.

CONVENTIONAL TREATMENTS

You can easily treat a sore throat yourself with over-the-counter painkillers, such as acetaminophen, or by using a saltwater mouthwash and consuming plenty of fluids and soft foods. However, if the cause is bacterial instead of viral, your doctor may prescribe a course of antibiotics.

NATURAL REMEDIES

The most common homemade remedy for a sore throat is to add the juice of a lemon and two teaspoons honey to a cup of hot water. Stir well to dissolve the honey and sip. Other remedies you can try include the following ones.

- Boost your immune system with raw fruit and fruit juice—drink plenty of citrus and pineapple juice.
- Take vitamin C and garlic capsules every day.
- Gargle with lemon juice and hot water or some cider vinegar and hot water.
- Swallow one teaspoon honey, letting it trickle down your throat.

AROMATHERAPY Add a few drops of tea tree or myrrh oil to a massage carrier oil or cream and gently massage them into your throat before wrapping a scarf around it to keep it warm.

Quick Fix

Suck antiseptic pastilles or natural herbal lozenges to ease a sore throat, or even some ice cubes, which are very soothing.

HERBAL REMEDIES

- You can gargle with echinacea, sage, thyme, rosemary, or make them into a tea and sweeten with honey, if desired.
- Marshmallow root or slippery elm tea will ease and soothe a sore throat.
- Make a sage infusion (see page 142) and, after straining, add one teaspoon each cider vinegar and honey. Use as a soothing gargle four times daily.
- In addition, try taking one 200-milligram capsule echinacea four times a day.

HOMEOPATHIC REMEDIES

The following can be helpful in relieving a sore throat.

Belladonna 30C: Take one tablet four times daily for three days for sudden onset with red, dry painful throat and difficult swallowing.

Phytolacca 30C: Take one tablet four times daily for three days for intense dryness, burning in throat, pain in ears on swallowing, and dark red tonsils.

SEE YOUR DOCTOR

You should see the doctor if you experience the following symptoms:

- You have a temperature above 100.4°F
- You have difficulty swallowing
- You have had a sore throat for more than two weeks
- You have a rash and/or vomiting.

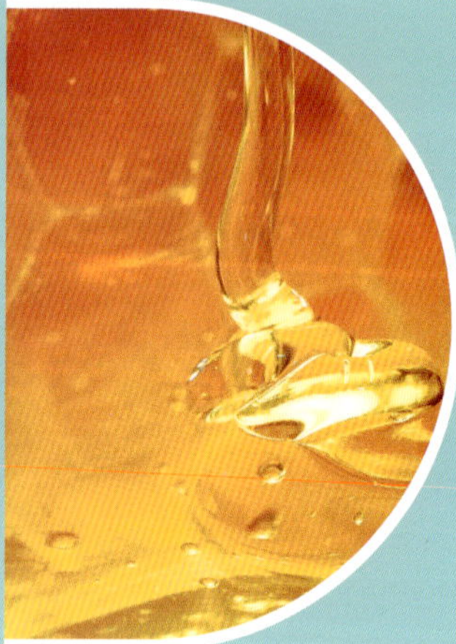

Tonsillitis

This is an inflammation of the tonsils, which is due to acute infection. The tonsils are lymph nodes on either side of the back of the mouth, and their function is to protect against upper respiratory tract infections. If they become infected, they get inflamed and swollen with fluids and white blood cells, making swallowing painful and eating difficult.

SYMPTOMS

- Sore throat
- Swollen, possibly coated, tonsils
- Difficulty swallowing
- Swollen lymph nodes in the neck
- Possible fever
- Headache and earache
- Breath smells unpleasant

Did You Know?

If you have recurrent bouts of tonsillitis on a regular basis your doctor may recommend an operation to remove your tonsils (a tonsillectomy).

PREVENTION

Eating a healthy, varied diet, staying warm in cold weather, and supporting the immune system with echinacea capsules (up to 600 milligrams four times a day) will help keep you healthy and ward off respiratory and throat infections. In addition, you can:

- Avoid sharing utensils or towels with anyone who has a sore throat
- Wear a scarf in winter
- Boost your immune system with zinc and selenium—eat five Brazil nuts and a handful of pumpkin seeds every day
- Give up smoking.

CONVENTIONAL TREATMENTS

The usual treatment for tonsillitis is to drink plenty of fluids, take over-the-counter painkillers, such as acetaminophen, and eat soft food. Gargling with saltwater or dissolved painkilling tablets may bring some relief, as will sucking ice cubes or sore throat lozenges. If the cause is viral, you will have to rest and wait for the illness to run its course. However, if it caused by a bacterial infection, your doctor may prescribe antibiotics.

NATURAL REMEDIES

Many of us practice natural medicine to treat tonsillitis and throat infections without even realizing it. The traditional remedy is a soothing drink of hot water mixed with honey and freshly squeezed lemon juice.

NUTRITIONAL MEDICINE Because swallowing is painful, eat blended vegetable soups made with onions, leeks, and garlic (antiseptic qualities), cabbage, bell peppers, broccoli, and tomatoes (good sources of vitamin C), and carrots and sweet potatoes (for beta-carotene content).

AROMATHERAPY Add a few drops of tea tree, thyme, and lavender essential oils to a heatproof bowl of hot water. Cover your head with a towel and bend over the bowl, inhaling the steam.

HERBAL REMEDIES

- Make a gargle by blending four tablespoons of honey, six tablespoons of lemon juice, four tablespoons of apple cider vinegar, one crushed garlic clove, and one teaspoon of grated ginger.
- Alternatively, gargle with raspberry leaf tea or add a teaspoonful of chopped fresh sage leaves to a cup of boiling water, then cover and steep for 10 minutes, strain, and use as a gargle when cool.

HEALING FOODS

- To soothe a painful, inflamed throat and tonsils, you can freeze pineapple juice in small containers and insert a wooden or plastic stick. Unmold and suck the ice pops.
- Honey has natural antiseptic qualities, so swallow one teaspoonful four times a day.

HOMEOPATHIC REMEDIES

The medicine selected depends on the symptoms presented. However, if there is no response within 24 to 36 hours, you should consult your doctor.

Lachesis 30C: Take one tablet four times a day for three days to relieve swollen dark red or purple tonsils, which start on the left side and with pain shooting to the ear when swallowing

Phytolacca 30C: Take one tablet four times a day for three days to relieve dark red or purple tonsils with white pus, burning in the throat with pain worse on the right side.

CALL YOUR DOCTOR

Consult your doctor if you experience any of the following symptoms:

- Your sore throat persists for more than two weeks
- You have difficulty swallowing and cannot eat
- You have a fever above 100.4°F
- You have a rash and/or vomiting
- You have an illness that lowers your immunity (such as HIV) or you are undergoing immuno-suppressive treatments, such as chemotherapy or steroids.

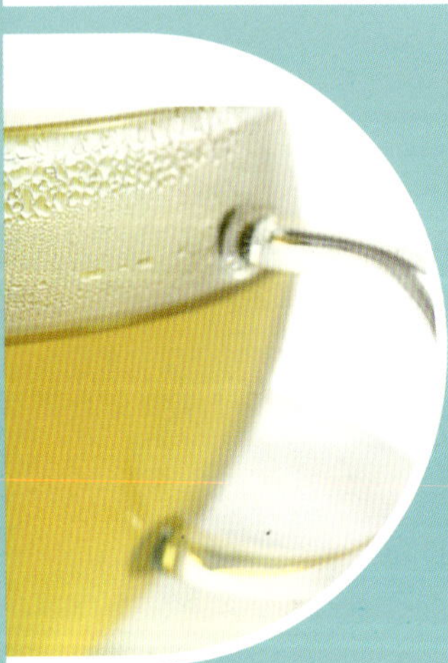

Sinusitis and Congestion

When you can't breathe properly, you realize how much you take clear nasal passages for granted. Sinusitis occurs if the sinuses become infected or inflamed, causing large amounts of mucus to block them. Nasal congestion may also be due to allergies, or the after effects of colds or flu.

SYMPTOMS

SINUSITIS

- ▷ Pain above eyebrows, in upper jaw, around eyes and nose
- ▷ Earache or even neck pain
- ▷ A feeling of pressure in your face
- ▷ A blocked nose
- ▷ A headache
- ▷ Green or yellow mucus
- ▷ Mucus that drains from the back of your nose into your throat
- ▷ May cause a sore throat or cough
- ▷ Reduced sense of smell
- ▷ Fever

CONGESTION

- ▷ Being unable to breathe through your nose
- ▷ Headache
- ▷ Stuffy head
- ▷ Nasal discomfort
- ▷ Disturbed sleep

PREVENTION

- Chronic sinusitis is often linked to allergies, so identifying the potential allergens and doing your best to avoid them could prevent future bouts. Common allergens include dust, pollen, spicy foods, and alcohol.
- Irritants, such as household chemical sprays or cleaning products, can trigger sinusitis, so avoiding these may help.
- Eating healthily and taking remedies, such as echinacea, to boost your immune system during the winter, when colds and flu are rife, may reduce your risk of sinusitis and congestion. Both are common after catching a cold.

Did You Know?

Viral or bacterial infections are a common cause, but sinusitis can also be triggered by allergies, irritants, or nasal polyps.

CONVENTIONAL TREATMENTS

Painkillers can be used to help relieve the pain and bring down a fever, if you have one. Nasal decongestants may relieve the symptoms of a blocked nose. Some are available over the counter, but your doctor may also prescribe steroid nasal sprays. If your sinusitis could be caused by a bacterial infection, antibiotics may be prescribed. For cases of chronic sinusitis that keep occurring and do not respond to treatment, surgery may be needed as a last resort. If nasal polyps are found to be blocking the nose and are causing recurring sinusitis, these may need to be surgically removed.

NATURAL REMEDIES

The old-fashioned home remedies for dealing with sinus problems were to eat plenty of onions, leeks, and garlic every day. If you don't like the flavor and smell of garlic, you can take it in capsule form.

NUTRITIONAL MEDICINE Dairy products are associated with the production of mucus, so it may be beneficial to cut down on the amount of dairy products you consume.

AROMATHERAPY Put a drop of lavender, tea tree, or eucalyptus essential oil into a base carrier oil, such as sweet almond oil, and gently massage it into your face. This can help ease the discomfort felt from sinusitis.

ACUPRESSURE Pressing the acupoints on the large intestine meridian, which are located around the bottom of the nose, can help relieve the symptoms of sinusitis. Acupuncture can also help.

HERBAL REMEDIES

- For chronic sinusitis, which may be due to an infection, take a daily echinacea capsule to boost your immune system and help fight the infection.
- Take pippali supplements, or a tincture, to ease sinus headaches.

HOMEOPATHIC REMEDIES

There are various homeopathic remedies that could help ease symptoms.

Kali Bich 6C, if you are experiencing a feeling of pressure around the bridge of your nose and have thick nasal mucus.

Sticta Pulmonaria 6C, for cases of chronic sinusitis and times when you don't have any mucus discharge.

CALL YOUR DOCTOR

You can treat mild sinusitis yourself, but if the condition is debilitating and very painful or persistent, call your doctor.

Quick Fix

Put a few drops of eucalyptus essential oil in a bowl of steaming water. Lean over, covering your head with a towel, and inhale deeply for 5 to 10 minutes. This should provide some relief from congestion. Repeat several times a day. Alternatively, add the oil to a warm bath.

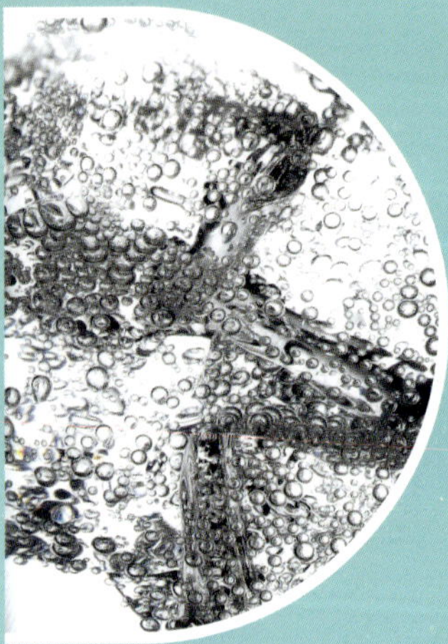

Hiccups

Hiccups are a reflex reaction, which occurs when your diaphragm suddenly contracts. As it contracts, the top of the windpipe closes immediately, causing the characteristic "hic" noise. Short bouts of hiccups are relatively common and harmless and often have no apparent cause. Although cases of persistent hiccups lasting longer than 48 hours are rare, they can sometimes be caused by acid reflux, medication, or an underlying disease.

SYMPTOMS

- An involuntary "hic" noise
- Persistent hiccups can cause tiredness, exhaustion, disturbed sleep, embarrassment

PREVENTION

Sometimes hiccups just occur—there doesn't seem to be any major reason why—but many other cases can be prevented.

- Overeating, eating a meal too quickly, or suddenly having a particularly cold or extremely hot drink are all associated with bouts of hiccups, so avoiding these may reduce the risk.
- If you're prone to frequent hiccups, it may be worth avoiding carbonated drinks, because these are linked to hiccups.
- Stress and overexcitement can bring on hiccups. If you're experiencing stress, find ways to relax.
- Smoking a lot or drinking alcohol are also known causes of hiccups, so give up smoking and drink less.

Did You Know?

The record for the longest running case of hiccups is held by Charles Osborne, an American who had hiccups for 68 years—from 1922 to 1990.

CONVENTIONAL TREATMENTS

While hiccups rarely need medical treatment, there are various self-help methods you can use to relieve the symptoms. Not everything works for everyone, but you could try the following.

- Hold your breath for a short period of time to stop hiccups—you may have to keep repeating this a number of times for it to work.
- Pull your knees up to your chest.
- Sip on some ice cold water, suck an ice cube, bite on a lemon, or drink a small amount of vinegar. All these can sometimes work—most probably due to the sudden shock to your system of tasting something cold, sour, or strange.
- Lean forward, with the aim of compressing your chest.
- If you're feeling athletic, do a headstand, because it could help get the diaphragm out of the spasm.

NATURAL REMEDIES

Try the following natural approaches to dealing with hiccups to find out what works for you.

HERBAL REMEDIES Slowly drinking spearmint or fennel tea, or sucking on a small piece of ginger, can help to stop hiccups.

NUTRITIONAL MEDICINE Some research suggests that a lack of magnesium may be linked to recurrent hiccups, so you could try taking magnesium supplements if you're susceptible to hiccups, or eat foods that are rich in magnesium, such as spinach or broccoli.

HYPNOTHERAPY If you are regularly prone to hiccups, or experience persistent hiccupping, then being hypnotized by a professional hypnotherapist could help ease your symptoms.

HELPFUL THERAPIES

The biochemic tissue salt, Mag Phos, has antispasmodic properties and can help relieve hiccup spasms. Take four 6C tablets when hiccups occur, or dissolve in hot water and sip every 5 to 15 minutes for the duration of the hiccup attack.

CALL YOUR DOCTOR

In cases where you experience persistent hiccups, for 48 hours or longer, your doctor may prescribe medication to bring the hiccups under control. The length of time you will need to take the medication will vary from weeks to months, depending on the severity of the hiccups.

IMMEDIATE RELIEF

The holistic therapy of yoga, which uses postural exercises, relaxation, and breathing, can help relieve the spasm of hiccups. For instant relief, try lying on the floor with your arms at your side. Breathe in slowly and deeply, holding your breath for 10 seconds, before exhaling. Repeat 20 times.

Using Herbs at Home

Using herbs in infusions (teas), decoctions, compresses, and tinctures is simple when you know how. You can turn your kitchen into a pharmacy and make them yourself at home. It's easy, not expensive, and does not take long to do—just follow the step-by-step instructions below.

HERBAL INFUSIONS

You can make an infusion (tea) from the dried or fresh leaves and flowers of plants. Drink them hot or cool, sweetened with a little honey to taste, if desired. Alternatively, they can be used as a gargle or mouthwash, or even added to the bathwater.

1. Use one teaspoon of dried herbs or two teaspoons fresh herbs per cup of water.
2. Warm a ceramic, glass, or stainless steel teapot (not an aluminum one) with hot water and then pour the water away.
3. Add the herbs and cover with water that is nearly boiling. Cover the pot and let steep for 10 to 15 minutes.
4. Strain the liquid, discarding the herbs, and drink or use as required.

HERBAL DECOCTIONS

These are similar to infusions but you can use the woody parts of the plant (stems, bark, and roots) as well as the leaves and flowers. Instead of brewing, the herbs are simmered gently in the water until the liquid reduces.

1. Coarsely chop or crush the herbs and place them in an enamel, stainless steel, or glass saucepan—do not use an aluminum, copper, or nonstick pan.
2. Cover the herbs with water—use one-and-a-quarter cups for every teaspoon of herbs.
3. Bring to a boil, then reduce the heat and simmer gently for 10 to 15 minutes, until the liquid has reduced by one-third.
4. Strain immediately and drink or use while the decoction is still warm.

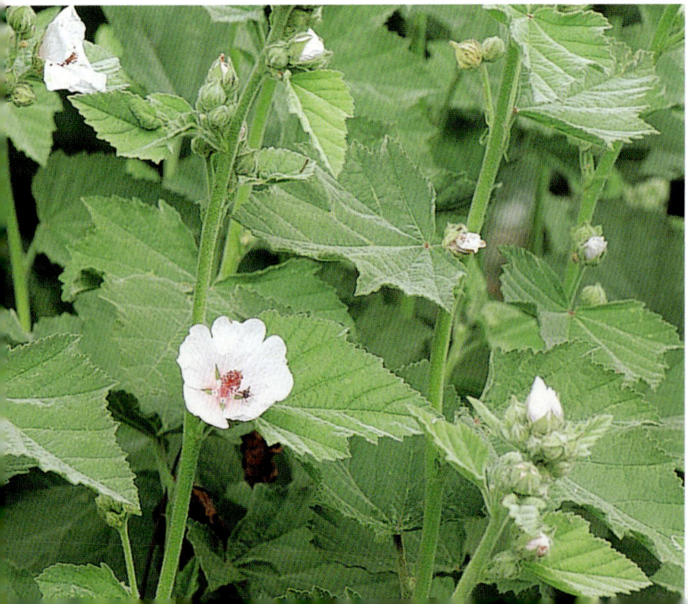

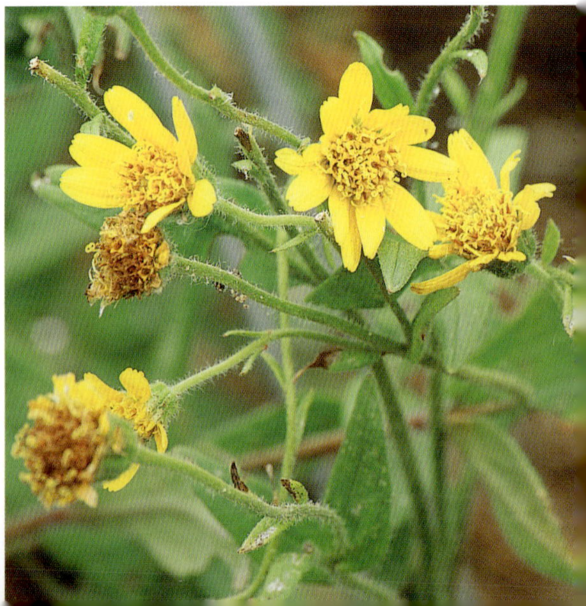

HERBAL COMPRESSES

These are useful in reducing inflammation and speeding up healing. Herbal compresses are usually used hot for treating sprained muscles and aching joints, but you can also use cool ones for relieving feverish headaches.

1 Make a hot herbal infusion or decoction (see opposite).
2 Take a clean pad of cotton gauze or cloth and dip it into the hot liquid to soak it up.
3 Gently squeeze out any excess liquid and then apply the compress to the affected area.
4 When it starts to cool down, apply a fresh one.

HERBAL TINCTURES

These are similar to cold infusions but alcohol is used instead of water, preserving the herbs and making them more concentrated. You can use vodka, brandy, or other alcohol, or apple cider vinegar.

1 Chop the herbs or use dried ones. Place eight ounces fresh herbs or four ounces dried herbs in a large glass jar or container with a screw-top lid.
2 Add two-and-a-half cups alcohol and cover the jar tightly.
3 Place the jar in a dark cupboard away from direct light and shake occasionally—at least three times a day—for two weeks.
4 Strain the liquid into dark-colored jars and seal securely. Store the jars in a cool, dark place until required.

HERBAL POULTICES

These are commonly used to treat inflammation, skin irritations and itching, arthritis, and aching joints, strained muscles, and ligaments. They may also be used in first aid for treating wounds and drawing out pus.

1 Take some fresh herbs and chop finely—or use dried herbs. Mix to a pulp or paste with a little hot water.
2 Put the herbal paste on some clean cotton gauze or thin cloth and fold it over to enclose the herbs.
3 Apply the hot poultice to the affected area and cover with some plastic wrap and a towel to retain the heat and moisture.
4 Replace the poultice as and when required.

HERBAL INHALATIONS

You can use a herbal infusion (tea) for these (see opposite). Use them for treating respiratory and chest infections, stuffed-up nose, catarrh, and sinusitis.

1 Make some hot tea with the appropriate herbs.
2 Pour the hot, steaming tea into a bowl and place on a table.
3 Put a large towel over your head and lean forward over the bowl, so your face is enclosed within the towel.
4 Breathe deeply and slowly, inhaling the steam, for a few minutes to clear your head and nasal passages.

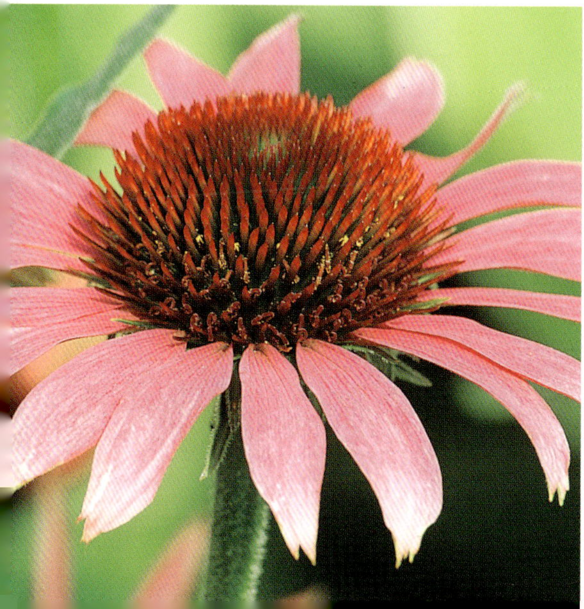

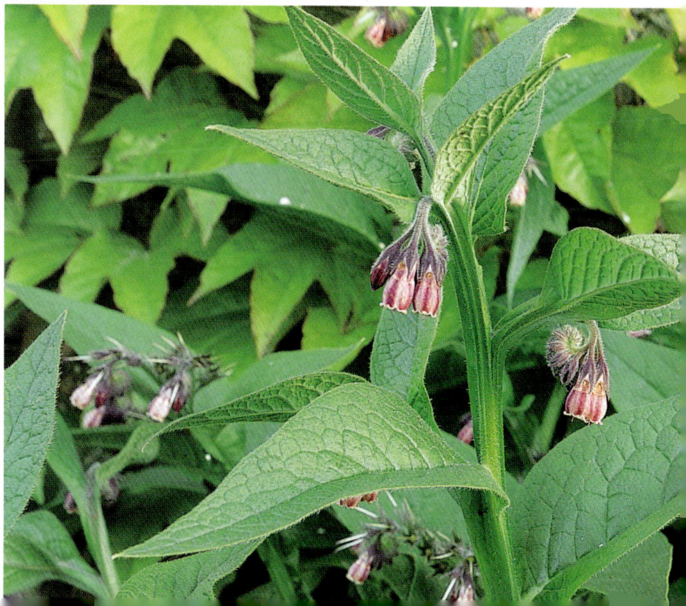

Immune System Problems

The immune system is one of the defense mechanisms your body uses to protect it against microorganisms that cause diseases. The key components of the system are the skin, mucus membranes, saliva, lymph nodes and vessels, spleen, adenoids, tonsils, thymus gland, and white blood cells. These are all designed to either repel or prevent germs from entering the body via the skin, mouth, nose, and other openings, and to destroy any invasive viruses, bacteria, parasites, and fungi that do cross these barriers.

To maintain optimum health and avoid infection or disease, you need to boost your natural immunity to germs and keep all these specialized defense mechanisms in efficient working order. In order to achieve this, your innate immunity and adaptive immunity must work together.

Your innate immune system consists of the key components (listed above) that you were born with. It attempts to repel invading disease-causing microbes and to fight any that breach its natural protective barriers. Your adaptive immunity is the one that you acquire from exposure throughout your life to different germs and diseases.

Signs of whether your immune system is functioning effectively include inflammation and swelling (blood flow to the infected area increases to fight the infection) and a raised temperature or swollen lymph nodes.

Eating a healthy diet that contains all the essential nutrients, getting regular exercise, getting enough sleep, managing stress, having good, supportive relationships with your family and friends, and avoiding exposure to toxic chemicals (in processed foods, cigarettes, alcohol, recreational drugs, and environmental pollutants) can all help you to stay healthy, fight off infections, and build a strong immune system.

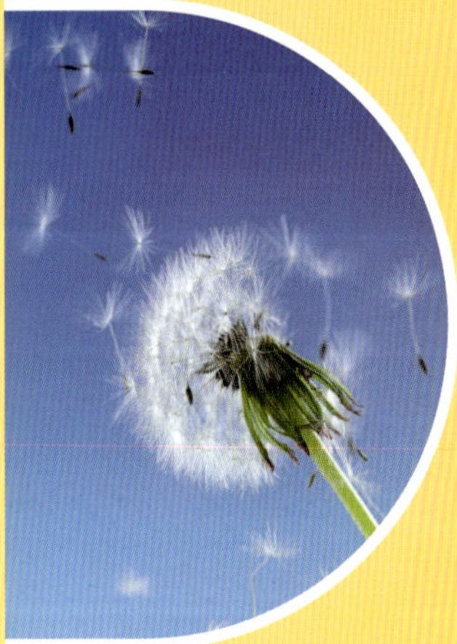

Allergies

An allergy is an adverse immune reaction to a substance or substances that are normally harmless. These substances are known as "allergens"; they cause the immune system to overreact and produce a special type of antibody (IgE) to attack the invading material, while histamines are released that cause the symptoms of an allergic reaction. Common allergens include foods, medicines, pollens, spores, household chemicals, insects, animals, and dust mites.

SYMPTOMS

Symptoms vary between people, but some of the most common include the following:

- Sneezing and rhinitis (runny nose)
- Wheezing
- Excess catarrh
- Urticaria (hives)
- Coughing
- Swelling
- Itchy eyes, ears, lips, throat, and palate (roof of mouth)
- Shortness of breath
- Vomiting and diarrhea

PREVENTION

There is little that can be done to prevent allergies, apart from avoiding the allergens in question. The cause of allergies is unclear; however, they have been linked to overuse of antibiotics and other medicines, low intake of fruit and vegetables, and an imbalance in the bacteria in the digestive tract, so taking steps to address these issues may help. There is also some evidence to suggest that breast-feeding can reduce allergies in susceptible children.

CONVENTIONAL TREATMENTS

Allergies may be treated with antihistamines, nasal or topical steroids, and cromolyn sodium (which prevents the release of inflammatory chemicals). These can be used alone or in combination. Emergency treatment requires epinephrine in the form of an injectible pen.

Did You Know?

About 20 percent of the U.S. population will develop an allergy at some point in their lives. Allergies tend to run in families, so if both parents have allergies, there's a 60 percent chance their children will have allergies. If neither parent has an allergy, there's still a 15 percent chance of a child having an allergy.

NATURAL REMEDIES

The traditional remedy is to take a little local honey in a cup of warm water with two tablespoons of apple cider vinegar to reduce the reaction to allergens. This is particularly useful during the hay fever season.

HERBAL REMEDIES Teas made from chamomile, elderflower, red clover, and yarrow can reduce allergic reactions. Garlic has been traditionally used to boost immunity, either added to cooking or taken as capsules.

AROMATHERAPY Place a few drops of Roman chamomile in a vaporizer to treat an allergic reaction. Lavender oil in some light carrier oil can be used in a gentle massage of the chest or the affected area to reduce spasm.

HEALING FOODS Foods that support your immune system include those that are high in vitamin C (fresh fruit and vegetables, in particular), zinc (eggs, nuts, and seeds), vitamin A (fish and brightly colored vegetables), and the B vitamins (seafood, beans, whole grains, and nuts). You can take a vitamin C supplement to boost your body's defenses.

HOMEOPATHIC REMEDIES

Treatment will be undertaken on a constitutional basis (see page 202); however, the following remedies can address specific symptoms.

Urtica 30C will help with hives.

Pulsatilla 30C will help with thick catarrh and itching eyes.

Arsenicum 30C is for sneezing and itching eyes.

CALL YOUR DOCTOR

Many allergies respond well to self-help and natural remedies, but it is wise to call your doctor to get an accurate diagnosis. If you have a severe allergic reaction to any substance (anaphylactic shock), you must seek urgent medical advice. Symptoms can include swelling of the throat and mouth, difficulty swallowing or speaking, severe breathing difficulties, a drop in blood pressure, and loss of consciousness.

Flower Remedies

- During a sudden allergic reaction, offer Rescue Remedy or Emergency Essence.
- Beech is a basic essence for treating all allergies and conditions related to intolerance.
- Holly helps in cases of strong immune reactions, such as severe fits of sneezing or irritation.

Caution

Anaphylaxis (anaphylactic shock) is an extreme and severe allergic reaction. The whole body is affected, often within minutes of exposure to the allergen. This type of reaction is a medical emergency, and an ambulance must be called immediately.

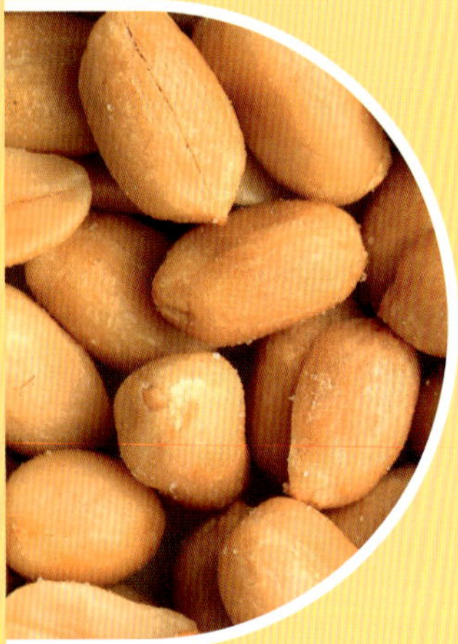

Food Allergies

Food allergies occur when your immune system becomes confused, and instead of ignoring harmless food proteins that make their way into the bloodstream, it triggers a reaction that causes histamine to be released. This is the chemical that is responsible for such symptoms as hives, skin rashes, and swelling. Anaphylaxis, or "shock," is a severe, life-threatening reaction.

SYMPTOMS

- A rash (particularly around the mouth)
- Tingling of the mouth and tongue
- Urticaria (hives)
- Swelling of lips or face
- Vomiting and diarrhea
- Running nose
- Wheezing
- Eczema
- Stomach pain
- Headaches
- Breathing problems, pallor, or loss of consciousness are anaphylactic reactions

PREVENTION

The incidence of food allergies is increasing. The most common allergens (known as the "big eight") are peanuts (and tree nuts), sesame seeds, wheat, soybeans, dairy produce, fish, shellfish, and eggs. Exclusive breast-feeding for the first six months of a baby's life can reduce the incidence of food allergies. Otherwise, avoiding the problem foods entirely is the best way to prevent attacks. There is some evidence that encouraging bowel health by eating a fiber-rich diet can help to prevent allergies.

CONVENTIONAL TREATMENTS

Antihistamines are offered to deal with symptoms if an attack occurs or, in an emergency, epinephrine pens (EpiPens) can be used. Supplements may be prescribed to make up for shortfalls in your diet.

Did You Know?

Most serious food allergies begin in infancy or the preschool years, but they are often outgrown. If you have a family history of food allergies or other allergic conditions, you are between 15 and 60 percent more likely to develop one yourself.

NATURAL REMEDIES

There are many natural treatments that you can try, depending on your symptoms.

HERBAL REMEDIES

- Horsetail tincture contains good levels of calcium, which is believed to be deficient in people who develop food allergies.
- Stinging nettle (infusion or juice) can help reduce the allergic reaction and supplement calcium.
- Agrimony tincture can ease bowel irritation and the recovery of damaged mucous membranes.
- To soothe gastric sensitivity and to heal mucous membranes, take goldenseal tincture three times a day in a little liquid.

NUTRITIONAL MEDICINE

- Probiotics may be important in the control of food allergies because they improve digestion, helping the intestinal tract to control the absorption of food allergens; they also change the immune system response to food in the digestive tract.
- A multivitamin and mineral pill will help you get any nutrients that may be deficient; vitamins A, C, and E are important for immune response.
- The nutrient quercitin (found in apples and onions) is rich in bioflavonoids and can reduce allergic reactions by reducing histamine release.
- Zinc is important for a healthy immune response.
- Essential fatty acids (EFAs) have been shown to reduce inflammation and support the immune system. They are also responsible for general repair in the body, including the digestive tract. Flaxseed oil, cold-water fish oils, and borage oil can be taken in capsule form.

HOMEOPATHIC REMEDIES

Constitutional treatment will be required to get to the root of the allergies, and also to encourage healing of the digestive tract and a healthy immune response. Many people with allergies will be offered bowel nosodes to encourage bowel health.

Apis 30C can be used to treat hives.

Lycopodium 30C, for digestive complaints that follow eating suspect foods.

Aconite 30C can be taken at the first sign of an attack.

Arsenicum 30C is ideal for people who are highly sensitive to many foods and respond by becoming ill, restless, and exhausted, with breathing problems and digestive disorders.

CALL YOUR DOCTOR

Breathing problems, pallor and loss of consciousness are anaphylactic reactions, and a medical emergency (see page 147). If you experience any of these, seek urgent medical help as they could be life-threatening.

Caution

Anaphylactic shock is a medical emergency and should be treated immediately. Do not delay. Call an ambulance.

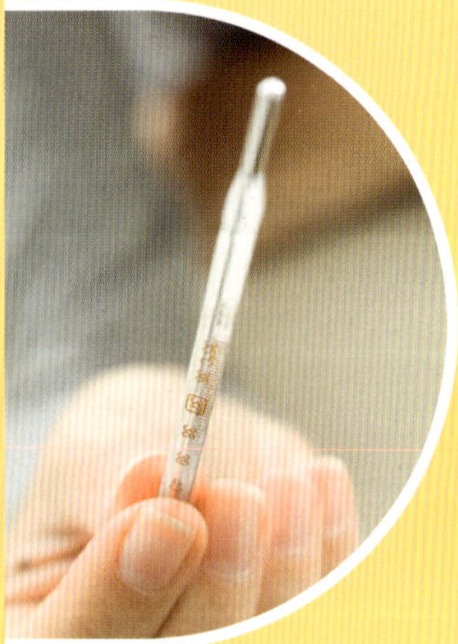

Fever

A fever is the body's reaction to an acute viral or bacterial infection. Raising the temperature helps to create an inhospitable environment for viral or bacterial invaders, and it also stimulates the production of disease-fighting white blood cells. Technically speaking, a fever is a body temperature above the normal of 98.6°F. In most cases, fevers are nothing to worry about unless they are accompanied by other symptoms.

SYMPTOMS

- Chills
- Aching muscles
- Listlessness and fatigue
- Elevated body temperature
- Red cheeks
- Feeling hot and/or cold
- Shivering and shaking

PREVENTION

A fever is actually a positive symptom, in that it provides evidence that your body is hard at work fighting off infection. There is nothing that can be done to prevent a fever, but you can keep yourself cool when it sets in to prevent overheating.

CONVENTIONAL TREATMENTS

Acetaminophen and aspirin are the two most common medications that are used to bring down a fever, with ibuprofen a close third. Note that children should not take aspirin because it can cause a rare but serious condition known as Reye's syndrome.

NATURAL REMEDIES

If you have a fever, you can try one of the following natural remedies.

FLOWER REMEDIES Rescue Remedy can be taken to ease any distress and calm you down. Chicory, Hornbeam, and Cherry Plum are useful for all illnesses that may cause fever and, in particular, childhood illnesses.

HERBAL REMEDIES

- Yarrow and lime flowers are calming and cooling, and encourage sweating when you feel hot.
- Cinnamon, ginger, and angelica can be used to produce heat when you are shivering.
- Hyssop, along with licorice root and thyme, have traditionally been used to lower a high temperature.

AROMATHERAPY

- Tea tree encourages the body to sweat, while also helping to encourage the immune system to fight off invaders, such as bacteria and viruses.
- Lavender and peppermint are cooling oils and help to soothe and bring down your temperature.
- Try sage, pine, rosemary, and eucalyptus in a vaporizer in your room to support your immune system and open the airways.

Self-Help

- Always drink plenty of fluids to avoid becoming dehydrated. Babies, in particular, can dehydrate quite quickly.
- Avoid eating heavy meals, which will divert the energy required for healing to your digestive system; instead, eat little and often. Fresh fruit and vegetable juices or vegetable soups contain immune-boosting vitamin C.
- Don't take fever-reducing medication for fevers under 102°F, unless suggested by your doctor. It's usually best to let your fever run its course, so your body can do the job of fighting infection.

HOMEOPATHIC REMEDIES

There are a number of homeopathic remedies that will be useful, according to the symptoms.

Belladonna 30C, for fever with a red, hot face and staring eyes.

Phytolacca 30C helps when there are painful ears and swollen glands, better on taking cool drinks.

Aconite 30C is ideal for a fever that comes on suddenly.

Ferrum phos 30C, for fever with a slow onset.

Gelsemium 30C can help when you feel drowsy and chilly, with aching limbs.

Merc sol 30C is suggested where there is yellow discharge with a fever.

CALL YOUR DOCTOR

If the fever lasts longer than a few days or your temperature is over 104°F, you should call your doctor to ascertain and treat the cause. Feverish babies under three months should always be seen by a doctor immediately; over three months, wait for 24 hours to see if it resolves.

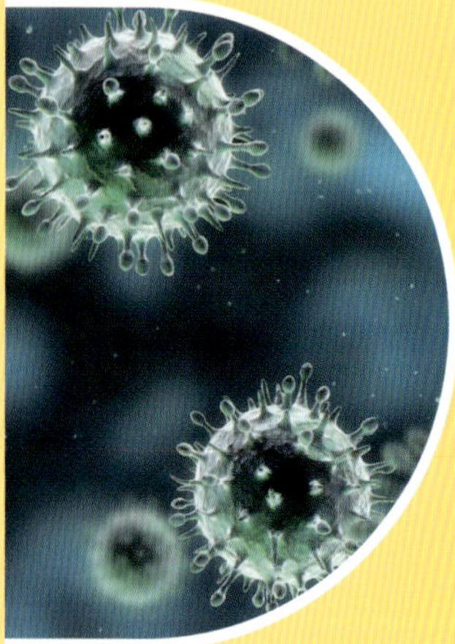

Influenza

Influenza is a viral disease of the upper respiratory tract, which is spread by the contaminated droplets infected people emit when they cough or sneeze. There are a number of different types of flu, some of which confer immunity once you overcome them, and others that mutate constantly, so your body cannot build up resistance.

SYMPTOMS

- A high fever, possibly accompanied by shivering
- A sore throat
- Possibly a cough
- A running nose and sneezing
- Breathlessness
- Weakness
- Headache
- Stiff or aching joints and muscular pains
- Nausea and loss of appetite

PREVENTION

- Always wash your hands after touching surfaces that others have touched, such as handrails on public transport.
- Antiflu vaccines may work in the short-term for virulent, current strains, but, because the viruses constantly change, so too will the vaccines used against them.
- Boost your immune system by adopting a healthy diet and lifestyle.

CONVENTIONAL TREATMENTS

Conventional treatments for influenza consist of symptom-reducing medicines, such as acetaminophen, cough suppressants, decongestants, pain relievers, and occasionally antihistamines. Antibiotics should never be offered for flu, because they have no effect on viruses. In severe cases, antiviral medication may be offered.

NATURAL REMEDIES

Barley water is the traditional natural remedy for relieving high fever—particularly when the cause of the fever is infection and inflammation. It also works to increase levels of the immune-boosting B vitamins and to keep you hydrated.

SELF-HELP Get plenty of rest, and aim to stay in bed for at least 48 hours. Don't push yourself; give your body time to fight off the infection and recover. Drink plenty of fluids, including vitamin C-rich fresh fruit and vegetable juices.

HERBAL REMEDIES

- Fenugreek seeds crushed in a lemon and honey hot drink will help to bring down fever and soothe aching limbs.
- Echinacea is an immune stimulant that appears to activate your infection-fighting capacity when taken at the onset of a cold or flu; you can take it in tincture form.
- Ginger contains almost a dozen antiviral compounds; it helps to reduce pain and fever, suppresses coughing, and it has a mildly sedative effect to encourage rest. Grate some fresh ginger root into a hot honey and lemon drink, or look for tincture or pill forms.

Flower Remedies

- Crab Apple promotes purification of your blood, and helps you get strong enough to fight off infection.
- Olive is for overwhelming fatigue.
- Walnut can help to strengthen your immune system against invaders.
- Rescue Remedy or Emergency Essence can both help to soothe and calm you, promoting restful, restorative sleep.

AROMATHERAPY

- Use a eucalyptus or peppermint essential oil inhalation to unblock sinuses and your chest.
- Add one to two drops of tea tree and geranium oils to a few tablespoons of a light carrier oil, and massage into your chest and head to reduce symptoms and fight infection.
- Oils that act to bring down fever include chamomile, melissa, and tea tree.

HOMEOPATHIC REMEDIES

Choose remedies according to your symptoms.

Gelsemium 30C, when muscular weakness, aching, and heaviness are the most predominant symptoms.

Rhus tox 30C, when there is aching in the joints instead of the muscles, and if you are restless and can't find a comfortable position.

Bryonia 30C, for a bad headache and dry cough; if you feel intensely irritable and just want to lie still.

Eupatorium perfoliatum 30C, for very intense aching in the back and limbs with shivering chills.

Belladonna 30C, for a high fever, with red cheeks and staring eyes.

CALL YOUR DOCTOR

Most cases of flu get better of their own accord without medical intervention. However, if you have asthma, chronic bronchitis, or heart disease, or have difficulty breathing or a cough that gets persistently worse, you should see your doctor. Secondary chest infections and pneumonia can be complications.

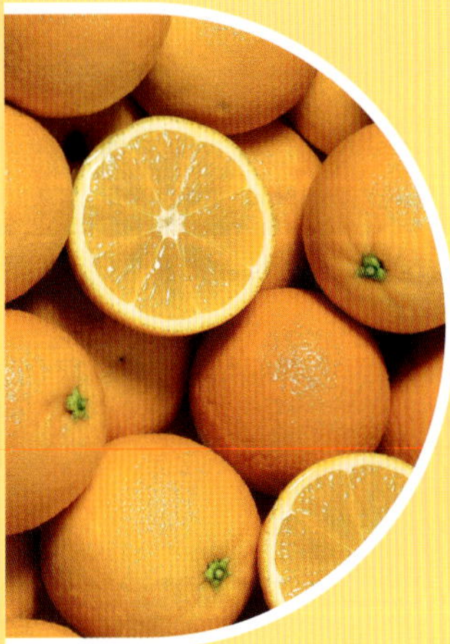

Mononucleosis

Often shortened to "mono," mononucleosis is caused by the Epstein-Barr virus (a herpes virus), which multiplies in the white blood cells, harming the immune system's efficiency. The virus is often transmitted via saliva, hence its nickname of the "kissing disease." Symptoms may last for only six weeks, but recovery is slow, and fatigue and low energy levels may linger for months. Most people are exposed to mono by the age of 18 years and become immune.

SYMPTOMS

- Fever
- Fatigue
- Enlarged lymph nodes in the neck
- Inflamed throat and tonsils
- Little energy
- Sometimes a mild rash of small, slightly raised red spots

PREVENTION

Taking steps to boost your immune system will make it more probable that you will resist the infection and develop antibodies instead. However, there is nothing that can be done to prevent mononucleosis apart from avoiding close contact with infected people.

CONVENTIONAL TREATMENTS

Almost all cases resolve within about four to six weeks without any medical treatment. Bed rest and plenty of fluid are normally suggested. In rare cases, corticosteroid medicines are needed to reduce severe inflammation, particularly if your tonsils are swollen.

NATURAL REMEDIES

There are numerous natural remedies that may help to alleviate the symptoms and aid recovery.

FLOWER REMEDIES Olive will be helpful if you feel exhausted on all levels. Mustard is ideal for any depression, and Gorse will help with feelings of hopelessness.

HERBAL REMEDIES

- Herbs to promote healing include cleavers, echinacea, and nettles, all of which stimulate immune activity as well as fighting infection.
- Infusions of yarrow and elderflower will help to control fever, and induce sweating.
- Licorice supports the adrenal glands, which are under pressure in this illness, and also has some antibacterial and antiviral properties, which can help to prevent secondary infections.
- Tonic herbs, such as ginseng, may help your recovery.

AROMATHERAPY

- Eucalyptus, lavender, rosemary, and tea tree oils encourage the immune activity and fight the virus.
- Black pepper oil stimulates the spleen, which is involved in the production of new blood cells.
- Thyme oil is a powerful stimulant and is widely used to combat fatigue and lethargy. It can also stimulate a sluggish appetite.

HOMEOPATHIC REMEDIES

Constitutional homeopathic treatment is recommended, but the following remedies may be useful, taken up to six times daily, for two days.

Belladonna 30C, for sudden high fever, with red face and agitation.

Mercurius 30C, for tender glands and smelly sweat.

Calcarea iodata 30C, for chilliness, sweating, a sour taste, and fatigue.

Cistus 30C, for chilly feeling, with painful neck and glands, exacerbated by cold air and mental exertion.

Baryta carb 30C, for swollen glands.

NUTRITIONAL MEDICINE

EVENING PRIMROSE OIL has a beneficial effect on the immune system and encourages healing.

ROYAL JELLY will help fight feelings of fatigue and depression, and stimulate the immune system.

MAGNESIUM deficiency is common in many cases of mononucleosis, and can be the result of a stressful lifestyle that caused you to become rundown. Take a daily supplement.

VITAMIN C stimulates the production of the white blood cells that produce antibodies against mononucleosis. It is also an anti-inflammatory that helps to relieve a sore throat and aching muscles. Take a daily supplement, or eat citrus fruit and plenty of green vegetables.

ZINC stops the Epstein Barr virus from replicating and entering your cells, and is also a powerful anti-inflammatory. Take a daily supplement.

CALL YOUR DOCTOR

If you suspect that you may have mononucleosis, call your doctor. A blood test will confirm whether you have the disease.

Caution

Mononucleosis makes a relatively profound attack on the immune system, and you will need to work on building it back up again, probably for several months.

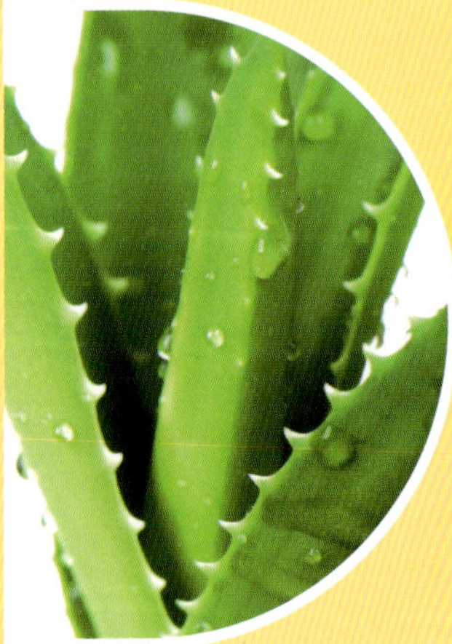

Chicken Pox

Chicken pox is a particularly contagious viral infection, caused by the herpes-zoster virus, that appears most often in childhood. It is characterized by pimples that fill with fluid to become blisters. Eventually, the blisters dry up and form scabs, which may cause scars. The blisters are itchy, but scratching should be discouraged to prevent infection. The incubation period is from 10 to 14 days, and infected people are contagious from just before the pimples appear.

SYMPTOMS

- Headache
- Fever
- General malaise
- Pimples, usually starting on the torso and spreading to most parts of the body, including the mouth, anus, vagina, and ears

Did You Know?

One bout of chicken pox normally gives lifetime immunity against the illness, but the virus that causes chicken pox (varicella zoster) can lie dormant for years, then resurface as shingles (see page 158) in adults.

CONVENTIONAL TREATMENTS

Your doctor may suggest calamine lotion to ease the itching, and acetaminophen or ibuprofen to relieve symptoms and reduce the body temperature. In most cases, children will recover within about 10 days. In severe cases, antiviral medication may be offered. There is a vaccine against chicken pox offered to children after they reach one year old.

NATURAL REMEDIES

There are many traditional remedies for chicken pox. For example, a witch hazel compress can be applied directly to the pimples, or a little added to your bath, to ease discomfort. You can also add baking soda to a bath to ease itching. Tie a handful of oatmeal in a cheesecloth or an old stocking, and hang it under the running water when you fill the bathtub. Not only will this soothe the itching, but it will also encourage healing of the skin. Try dabbing some vitamin E oil on the pimples when they begin to dry up to help prevent scarring.

HERBAL REMEDIES

- Infusions of nettle are ideal for treating chicken pox because nettle is a strengthening herb that will help to heal the skin.
- Aloe vera gel, dabbed on the pimples, can cool and help to promote healing.
- Calendula cream can be applied to the pimples to soothe and encourage healing, as well as to prevent scarring. A handful of calendula flowers can also be added to a bath.
- Echinacea can help to support the immune system and reduce the duration of the illness.

AROMATHERAPY

- A few drops of Roman chamomile can be used in the bath to soothe.
- Essential oil of lavender can be dabbed directly on pimples to ease the itching and to encourage healing. Lavender also has an antibacterial action, which will help prevent a secondary infection.

HOMEOPATHIC REMEDIES

Homeopathic remedies can be effective. Try the following, depending on the symptoms presented.

Variolinum 30C can be taken once in cases where there is an epidemic of chicken pox, before your child acquires the illness, and symptoms should be less severe.

Rhus tox 30C can be taken for a few days after contact with an infected child, and then again as soon as the first spots appear.

Aconite 30C is useful in the early stages of the illness.

Belladonna 30C is useful for fever.

CALL YOUR DOCTOR

When fever lasts for more than a couple of days, or there is an obvious chest infection accompanying the rash, call your doctor. Very rarely, chicken pox pneumonia can occur as a secondary infection.

Flower remedies

- Chicory, Hornbeam, and Cherry Plum can help relieve some of the discomfort.
- Impatiens can ease irritability.
- Crab Apple may be diluted and applied directly to the pimples to encourage healing.
- Olive is useful for convalescence.

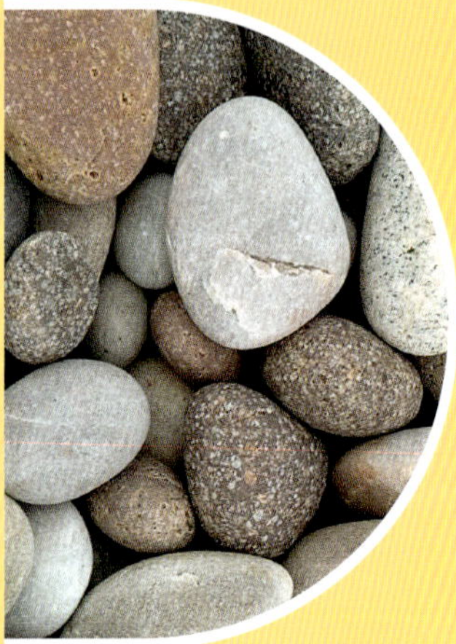

Shingles

Shingles is an extremely painful disease caused by the herpes zoster virus (also the chicken pox virus). Following an attack of chicken pox, the virus remains dormant in the body. Many years later, a drop in the efficiency of the immune system may cause reactivation of the virus—this time in the form of shingles—causing acute inflammation in the ganglia (a mass of nerve cells) near the spinal cord.

SYMPTOMS

- ▷ The first sign of shingles is sensitivity in the affected area, then pain
- ▷ Pain can be itching, tingling, throbbing, aching, or stabbing
- ▷ There may be fever and nausea
- ▷ A rash of small blisters develops on the fourth or fifth day, usually on one side of the body and in a linear pattern
- ▷ These turn yellow within a few days, form scabs, then drop off, sometimes leaving scars.
- ▷ In some cases, there may be persistent pain for months or years (postherpetic pain)

Did You Know?

Shingles can be passed on by direct contact with fluid from the blisters, until they eventually dry up and crust over. This can also cause chicken pox in people who haven't had it before, but shingles isn't triggered by contact with someone who has chicken pox.

PREVENTION

Shingles tends to strike when you are run-down, so be sure that you get plenty of rest, eat well, get some exercise, and reduce your stress levels.

- Avoid direct contact with anyone else who has shingles.
- Boost your immune system by increasing your intake of vitamins and minerals (in particular, vitamins A, B, and C, and the mineral zinc).
- Take probiotics, the healthy digestive bacteria that can help to ward off infection.

CONVENTIONAL TREATMENTS

Antiviral medicines, such as acyclovir, are offered to reduce the severity of the active stage. Analgesic medicines, including capsaicin creams, may be offered if the pain is severe. If you develop, or are at an increased risk of, postherpetic neuralgia, you may be prescribed medication, such as amitriptyline, which is usually used as an antidepressant but also acts on your nerves and can help to control pain.

NATURAL REMEDIES

You can try some of the following natural remedies for treating shingles.

HERBAL REMEDIES Oats, St. John's wort, and vervain have a direct impact on the health of your nerves. Make an infusion of any of these and sip throughout the day. Ginseng encourages overall health and restores nervous stability, as well as combats the effects of stress.

AROMATHERAPY Chamomile, eucalyptus, melissa, lavender, and tea tree are all useful antiviral oils, which can be used in the bath, in a massage, or applied as a compress. Lavender, applied undiluted to painful areas, can soothe and encourage healing.

HOMEOPATHIC REMEDIES

The following remedies can be taken once every two hours for up to 10 doses.

Arsenicum 30C, for burning pains worse between midnight and 2 a.m., with skin eruptions and a restless, chilly, and anxious state.

Lachesis 30C, when the left-hand side of the body is affected with swelling.

Rhus tox 30C, for red, blistered, and itching skin—better for movement and warmth.

NUTRITIONAL MEDICINE

- Eat plenty of vitamin B-rich foods, such as whole-grain cereals, nuts, seeds, and yeast extract, which aid the nervous system.
- High-dose vitamin C supplementation has been shown to reduce pain as well as help to dry up and heal the blisters. Take the highest dose you can without triggering diarrhea.
- Supplementation with vitamin E is now known to reduce the long-term symptoms associated with shingles. Take a supplement, broken into three doses, with food. Vitamin E oil, applied directly to the sores, will encourage healing.

CALL YOUR DOCTOR

Shingles is extremely painful and can cause serious complications and permanent damage if it affects your eyes. Always call your doctor for an accurate diagnosis, medical advice, and treatment.

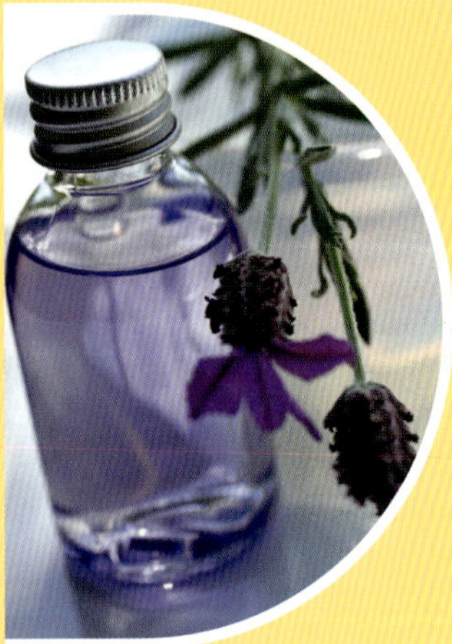

German Measles

German measles (rubella) is a viral infection characterized by a mild rash and swollen lymph glands (usually in the back of the neck or behind the ears), and is most common in children. The incubation period is 14 to 21 days, and the disease can be spread from seven days before the rash appears, although it is most contagious once the rash is present. The condition only lasts three to five days.

SYMPTOMS

- Mild fever
- Swollen, tender lymph nodes
- An itchy rash that appears first on the face and spreads downward—usually beginning with pinprick pink or pale red dots that join together to form evenly colored patches
- Headaches
- Loss of appetite
- Mild conjunctivitis
- A runny nose
- A sore throat

PREVENTION

The main line of defense is the rubella vaccine, which is normally given to children at 12 to 15 months as part of the MMR vaccine. A second dose is provided between the ages of four and six years of age. Apart from this, it's difficult not to acquire this contagious disease once you have been in contact with an infected person; however, cases are less common since immunization against the disease began.

CONVENTIONAL TREATMENTS

Your doctor may suggest acetaminophen to bring down any fever and reduce discomfort. Don't give aspirin to children, because it can cause a rare but serious condition called Reye's syndrome. Creams and ointments can be prescribed if the rash is very itchy; these include calamine lotion and mild steroid preparations.

NATURAL REMEDIES

The following natural treatments may help to ease the symptoms of German measles.

AROMATHERAPY A few drops of lavender oil on the bedclothes, or on a handkerchief near the bed, eases symptoms and is calming. For a buildup of phlegm, a few drops of tea tree or eucalyptus oil in a vaporizer will encourage easier breathing.

FLOWER REMEDIES Rescue Remedy will ease distress, and help to calm. Chicory, Hornbeam, and Cherry Plum are indicated for childhood illnesses.

NUTRITIONAL MEDICINE Eat plenty of raw fruits and vegetables to cleanse the system. Increase your intake of foods containing vitamin C and zinc to aid the action of the immune system. Acidophilus taken during and after any illness encourages the growth of healthy bacteria in the digestive tract.

HERBAL REMEDIES

- Hot yarrow tea, cooled and drunk several times daily, will relieve symptoms.
- An infusion of elderflower combined with peppermint will help to cool a fever and calm you—and your child.
- A high fever can be treated with an infusion of catmint, taken as required.

Self-Help

Frequent, tepid baths will relieve any itchiness and bring down a fever. Add some Epsom salts or baking soda to the water.

HOMEOPATHIC REMEDIES

Homeopathic remedies are useful in all cases of rubella. Choose the appropriate one for you.

Pulsatilla 30C, when there is thick yellow discharge from the nose and hot, red eyes.

Belladonna 30C, for fever, a bright red rash, and hot face.

Phytolacca 30C, for painful ears and swollen glands, better on taking cool drinks.

Aconite 30C if there is a high fever and not too much mucus.

Merc sol 30C where there is yellow discharge from the nose and a fever.

CALL YOUR DOCTOR

Contact your doctor immediately if you suspect you or your child is infected. The symptoms in small children may be mild, but if a pregnant woman comes into contact with the condition, there is a serious risk of miscarriage and birth defects.

Caution

If you are pregnant and are unsure of your immune status, ask your doctor.

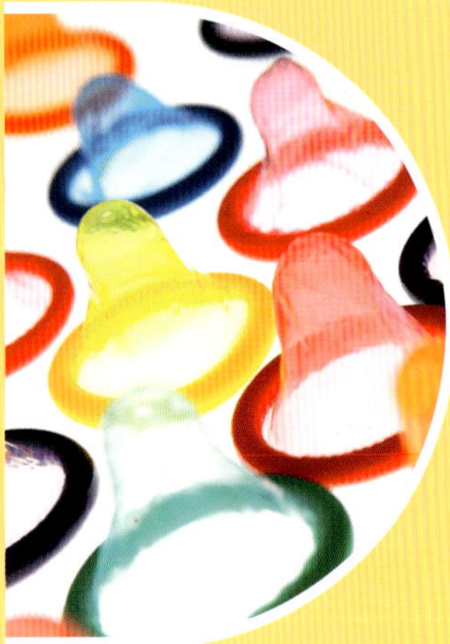

Herpes Simplex

Herpes simplex (HSV) is a virus of which there are two main strains. Oral herpes (HSV-1) causes cold sores around the lips or nose; genital herpes (HSV-2) affects the genitals, buttocks, or anal area. HSV-2 is usually, but not always, sexually transmitted. HSV-1 is transmitted by contact with infected saliva, and it is possible to carry the virus without experiencing any symptoms whatsoever.

SYMPTOMS

- ▷ Blisters or ulcers, usually on the mouth, lips, gums, or genitals
- ▷ Enlarged lymph nodes in the neck or groin area (although usually only at the time of the initial infection)
- ▷ Fever (during the first episode)
- ▷ Fever blisters
- ▷ Genital lesions, which burn or tingle
- ▷ Mouth ulcers

Did You Know?

Most people with genital herpes have five to eight outbreaks per year, but not everyone has recurrent symptoms; over time, the number of outbreaks usually decreases. Oral herpes can recur monthly or only once or twice a year. You may be able to anticipate an outbreak if you notice a tingling sensation (a prodrome).

PREVENTION

Once you have the herpes simplex virus, you will carry it for life, but you can prevent attacks by:

- Eating a healthy diet, with plenty of fresh fruit (especially citrus fruit which are rich in vitamin C and bioflavonoids) and vegetables, whole-grain cereals, and good-quality proteins to boost your immune system
- Not kissing anyone who has a cold sore or sharing towels and facecloths with them
- Applying sunblock to lips to protect them from sunshine and cold winds
- Using a condom to reduce the risk of catching or spreading herpes.

CONVENTIONAL TREATMENTS

Some cases are mild and may not need treatment. If cold sores are particularly troublesome, your doctor may prescribe idoxuridine paint or the antiviral medicine acyclovir (in pill or cream form), or another antiviral agent. Genital herpes can be treated with antiviral medication, such as acyclovir or valacyclovir. Topical antibiotic ointments also may be applied to prevent secondary bacterial infections.

NATURAL REMEDIES

At the first sign of cold sores appearing around the mouth, rub the area with a cut slice of lemon. To relieve blisters and other symptoms, try the following.

AROMATHERAPY Bergamot, eucalyptus, and tea tree oils will help to treat the blisters and should be applied at the first sign of a sore. Lavender oil will help to heal blisters as they begin to erupt and can be used until they heal.

HOMEOPATHIC REMEDIES

Homeopathy can help avoid recurring cold sores, but constitutional treatment will be required. The following remedies may help, depending on the symptoms.

HSV-1

Natrum mur 30C, for deep cracks in the lower lip, dry mouth, and puffy burning sores.

Rhus tox 30C, for mouth and chin sores, and ulcers at the corner of the mouth.

Sempervivum 30C, for ulcers in the mouth and bleeding gums; worse at night.

Capsicum 30C, for cracks at the corners of the mouth, pale lips, rash on chin, blisters on tongue, and bad breath.

HSV-2

Apis mel 30C, may prevent the blisters from appearing (stop if blisters do appear).

Rhus tox 30C, when you feel a stinging sensation.

Arsenicum 30C, for small blisters that burn.

HERBAL REMEDIES

- St. John's wort tincture applied at the first sign of tingling should help stop a cold sore from appearing.
- Apply calendula tincture or ointment to blisters to ease pain.
- Echinacea or goldenseal can help to combat the infection and boost your immune system.
- Lemon balm tea can be effective, because it has considerable antiviral activity against herpes simplex.

CALL YOUR DOCTOR

If you experience recurrent attacks of cold sores around your mouth or nose, you should call your doctor. If you experience any of the other symptoms that are listed opposite, especially in the genital area, make an urgent appointment. You may need antiviral medicines.

Caution

The virus can be dangerous in newborn babies, or in people with a weakened immune system. HSV is believed to be more contagious when blisters are present, but it can be transmitted without active lesions.

Eat Your Way to Health

The saying "you are what you eat" is very true—eating too much of the wrong foods can play a significant role in a variety of health conditions. If you are interested in eating more healthily, here are the main food groups that make up a healthy, well-balanced diet, and those that you should avoid.

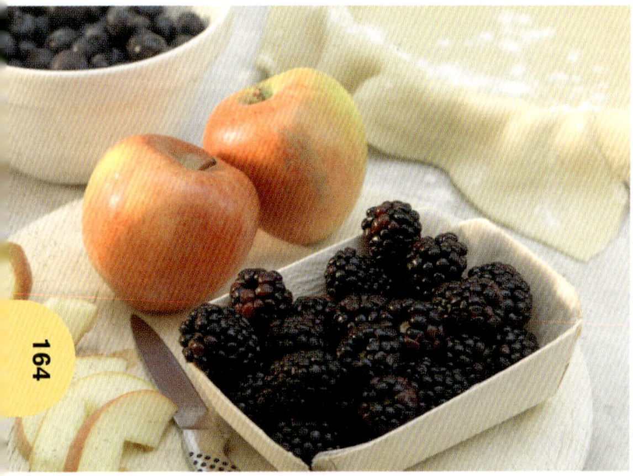

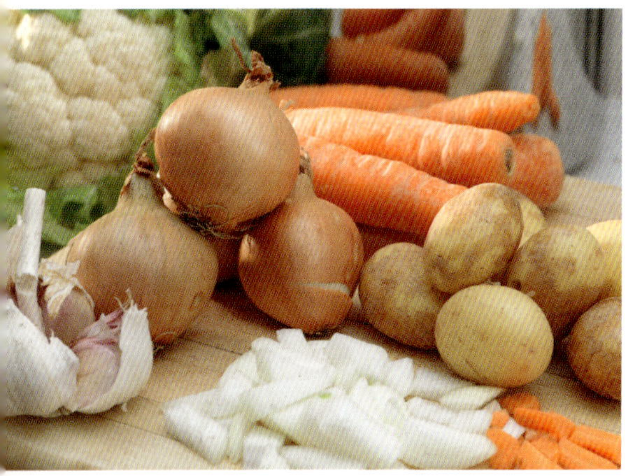

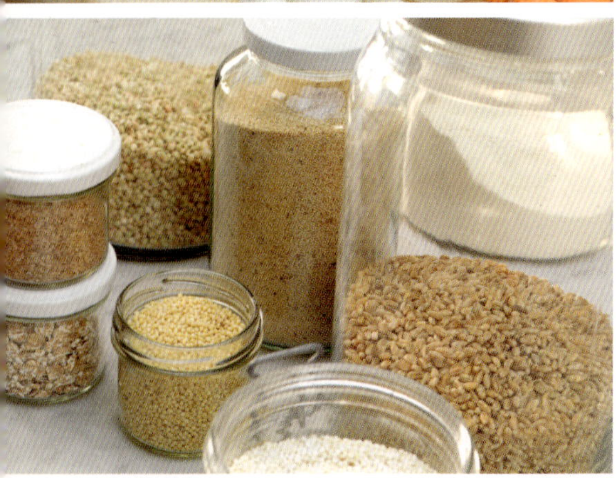

FRUITS AND VEGETABLES

Fruits and vegetables are an important source of many essential vitamins and minerals. Ideally, you should aim to eat at least five portions of fruits and vegetables each day.

These five portions are easily achieved, especially if you spread them out throughout the day. One portion is equivalent to one apple, one banana, three heaping tablespoons of vegetables, or a slice of melon. As well as fresh fruit and vegetables, you can include dried, canned, or frozen options, plus one glass of fruit or vegetable juice.

STARCHY FOODS

About one-third of your daily diet should be made up of starchy foods (carbohydrates), such as bread, potatoes, pasta, and cereals. They are a good source of essential nutrients, plus they provide you with energy and fuel for your body.

Whole-wheat bread and whole-grain cereals, such as brown ice or whole-wheat pasta, contain more fiber than their white counterparts, so, ideally, you should eat them regularly.

MEAT, EGGS, FISH, AND BEANS

The third important food group to include in your healthy diet is protein, which comes in the form of meat, fish, eggs, and beans. Meat is packed full of vitamins and minerals, including iron and zinc, and it's a good source of vitamin B12. Fish has plenty of vitamins and minerals, too, and oily fish, such as fresh salmon, tuna, sardines, herring, or mackerel, is particularly good for your health.

Aim to eat three to five servings of protein daily. For ultimate health, avoid fatty cuts of meat and opt for lean types instead, or trim the fat off before you cook it (and remove the skin from chicken). Ideally, include two portions of fish in your diet each week, one of which should be an oily fish. For vegetarians and other nonmeat eaters, good sources of protein include eggs, tofu, beans, nuts, and seeds. Even if you do eat meat, aim to include some vegetarian source of protein in your diet, because diets high in red meat have been linked to health problems.

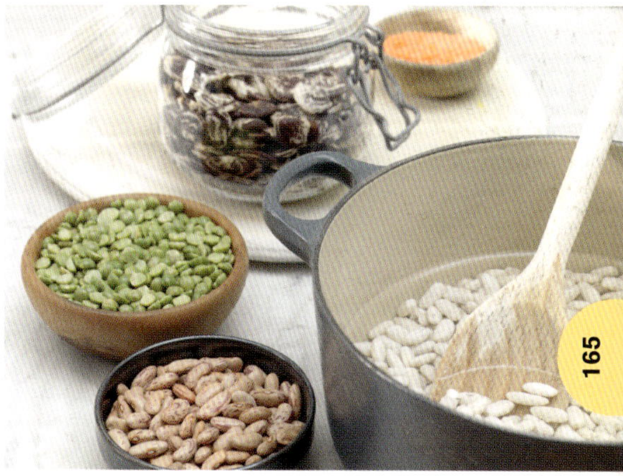

DAIRY PRODUCTS

Dairy products, such as milk, yogurt, and cheese, are important nutritional elements and are good sources of protein and calcium, which is good for your bones. Aim to have about two-and-a-half cups of skim or low-fat milk each day. Eating a small container of yogurt or a matchbox-size piece of cheese provides you with the same amount of calcium as a cup of milk.

Note Many cheeses and yogurts are high in fat, so opt for lower-fat, healthier versions instead.

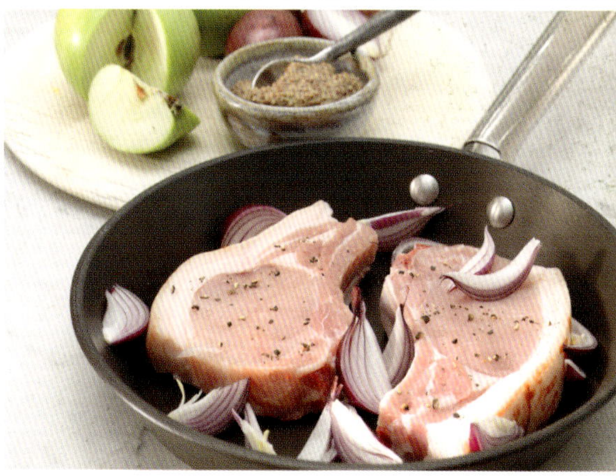

SUGAR AND FAT

Although your body needs some fat, foods containing sugar and fat should be eaten in limited quantities. Where possible, opt for low-fat or reduced-sugar foods, and choose fats that are rich in monounsaturated fatty acids, such as olive oil, instead of saturated ones, such as butter.

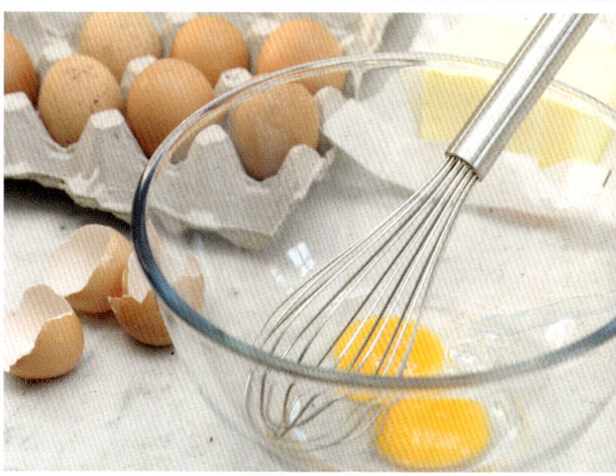

Digestive Problems

In the digestive tract, which extends from the mouth to the anus, food is digested and processed, and waste products are eliminated. The nutrients in the food you eat (protein, fats, carbohydrates, vitamins, and minerals) are absorbed into the bloodstream and carried around the body to the cells.

Digestion begins when you start chewing the food in your mouth. It passes down the esophagus into your stomach, where it is churned and partly digested with gastric juices to a semiliquid consistency. It passes into the small intestine, where the nutrients are broken down into molecules and pass into the blood vessels and lymphatic system. The undigested residues enter the large intestine, where water and minerals are absorbed back into the body and the liquid digestive products are turned into semisolid waste. The waste (feces) passes into the rectum for storage and is subsequently expelled through the anus.

It is a complicated process and a variety of digestive problems can occur, ranging from relatively harmless ones, such as indigestion and constipation, to far more serious conditions, such as inflammatory bowel disease. The system has its own built-in defense mechanisms, however, and can react rapidly against irritants, such as contaminated food (food poisoning or gastroenteritis) or alcohol, through vomiting or diarrhea.

To stay fit and healthy, you need to look after your digestive system, which means eating plenty of fiber-rich, whole-grain cereals, fruits, and vegetables to provide the bulk to carry away body waste and keep stools soft. Good personal hygiene, eating regular meals, and a variety of nutritious foods will all help to prevent many common digestive problems.

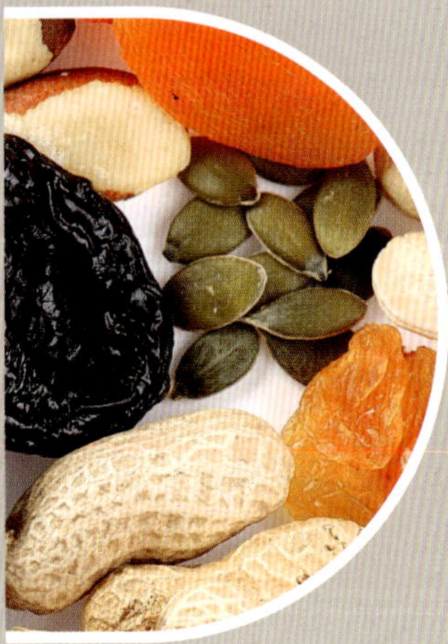

Constipation

Most doctors define constipation as having a bowel movement less than twice a week, although some say that a movement every four or five days is adequate. However, constipation is not so much about regularity as stools. Do you have to strain to pass stools more than one-quarter of the time? Do you feel a sense of incomplete emptying after a bowel movement? And, most importantly, are your stools hard? If so, you probably are experiencing constipation.

SYMPTOMS

- Straining on the toilet
- Flatulence
- Bloating
- Stomach/abdominal pain and cramps
- Lethargy
- Headaches

PREVENTION

- The single most effective way to prevent constipation is to be sure that your diet is rich in fiber; this means eating plenty of fresh fruits and vegetables, whole-grain cereals, and fewer refined convenience foods.
- Also important is water to bulk up the fiber and encourage healthy evacuation–drink at least eight glasses a day.
- Some foods, particularly milk and milk products, tend to delay things in the large intestine, causing constipation. Try abstaining from dairy produce for two weeks to see if it makes any difference.
- Regular exercise will help to stimulate bowel movements.

CONVENTIONAL TREATMENTS

You can buy over-the-counter laxatives in your local pharmacy. Apart from adopting a high-fiber, high-fluid regime, laxatives and suppositories are the usual conventional treatments for constipation. Natural or vegetable laxatives are available.

NATURAL REMEDIES

Treatment is generally based on the cause of your constipation, but the follow natural remedies should be useful for treating symptoms.

HERBAL REMEDIES Laxative herbs can be drunk as herbal infusions up to three times daily; these include licorice, marshmallow root, and senna. Aloe vera is also a powerful laxative. Take just one teaspoon of gel a day, or drink a small glass of aloe vera juice three times daily.

AROMATHERAPY

- Massage a drop of marjoram or fennel oil, which has been diluted in grapeseed oil, into the abdomen, to relieve constipation.
- Rosemary and mandarin (as well as any other citrus oils) stimulate peristalsis, which is the rhythmic movement along the digestive tract. Use in a warm abdominal massage, or add five drops of each to your evening bath.

NUTRITIONAL MEDICINE

- Acidophilus supplements will encourage the health of the intestines, and make bowel movements more normal.
- Eat dried apricots and figs as snacks, and add seeds and bulking agents, such as bran and psyllium husks, to your breakfast cereal.
- Prunes, or dried plums, are a classic laxative remedy; soak them overnight and eat them for breakfast with a little yogurt with live cultures.

HOMEOPATHIC REMEDIES

In homeopathy, constipation is regarded as a constitutional problem, but the following remedies can help with occasional symptoms.

Lycopodium 30C, when there is flatulence but no need to open bowels for long periods of time. Hard stools, passed with pain.

Nux vomica 30C, for constipation that alternates with diarrhea.

Silicea 30C, when there is a burning sensation after a bowel movement.

Causticum 30C, for a stitchlike pain accompanying a bowel movement.

Bryonia 30C, for large, hard, dry stools, with congestion in the abdomen causing distension, and a burning feeling in the rectum.

Alumina 30C, for no desire to open the bowels until the rectum is full; stool may be covered in mucus.

CALL YOUR DOCTOR

If laxatives are not having any effect, or you are suffering from abdominal pain, weight loss, blood in your stools, or pencil-thin bowel movements, you should see your doctor to ensure that there is not an obstruction or another problem. There are many possible causes of constipation, some of which are minor and others that are more serious. Always consult your doctor immediately if a child under three is constipated.

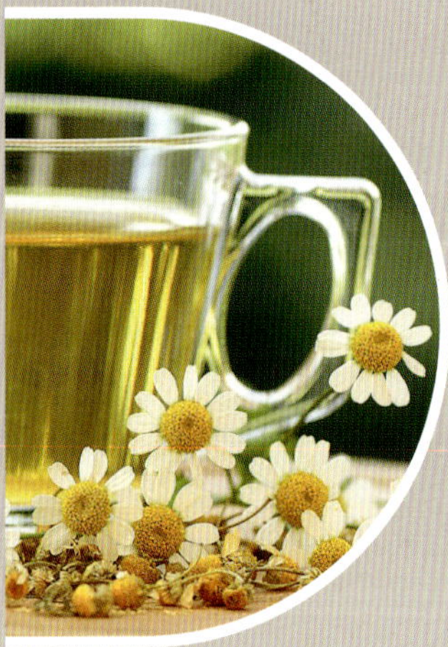

Diarrhea

Diarrhea, defined as the profuse evacuation of watery stools at least three times a day, may be accompanied by vomiting and abdominal pain and is usually due to a viral or bacterial infection, parasites, or toxins in the bowel, when it is known as gastroenteritis. It can also be caused by a long-term condition, such as irritable bowel syndrome or Crohn's disease (see pages 178–181), and may be an indication of a food allergy (see pages 148–149).

SYMPTOMS

- Urgent need to have a bowel movement
- Liquid stool, at least three times per day
- Sometimes cramping or abdominal pain
- Sometimes nausea or vomiting
- May be loss of appetite

PREVENTION

Basic personal hygiene can help to prevent diarrhea.

- Pay close attention to washing your hands, especially after going to the bathroom, touching pets, and gardening.
- Always make sure that you wash your hands with soap and water before and after touching food, especially raw meat or poultry.
- Good food hygiene and refrigeration of food can also help to prevent diarrhea.

CONVENTIONAL TREATMENTS

Medical advice is usually to eat more carbohydrates and to take plenty of fluids for 24 to 48 hours. Antidiarrheal medicines, such as loperamide, can relieve symptoms by slowing down the movement of bowel contents, and sometimes by increasing water absorption from the digestive tract. An electrolyte mixture (rehydration fluid) may be suggested if there is any dehydration.

NATURAL REMEDIES

Natural treatments will address the symptoms and encourage normal, healthy bowel movements.

AROMATHERAPY Massage your abdomen with a few drops of antiseptic and relaxing oils, such as chamomile, lavender, and neroli, to ease diarrhea; this is particularly helpful if diarrhea is linked to anxiety. If an infection is suspected, use eucalyptus or tea tree oil instead. Add fennel and ginger oils (one drop of each) to a warmed carrier oil, such as grapeseed, to deal with any abdominal pain or cramping.

HERBAL REMEDIES

- Peppermint and blackberry leaf tea act as astringents in the digestive tract and can help to ease the condition.
- An infusion of meadowsweet provides a gentle treatment for diarrhea because it tones the lining of the small intestine.
- Chamomile, drunk as an infusion, may reduce intestinal cramping and ease the irritation and inflammation associated with diarrhea.
- Calendula ointment can be applied to sore buttocks to soothe and heal.

Good Kitchen Hygiene

To minimize the risk of diarrhea and food poisoning, always:

- Use separate cutting boards for raw meat, poultry, fish, and vegetables
- Cover raw meat and poultry and keep them separate from other foods in the refrigerator
- Wash knives and kitchen utensils carefully
- Always wash your hands with soap and warm water after handling food, especially raw meat and poultry.

NUTRITIONAL MEDICINE

- Taking a probiotic, such as acidophilus, during and after an attack can help to build up healthy bacteria in your digestive tract.
- Increasing your fiber intake during an attack of noninfectious diarrhea is now known to alleviate diarrhea by making stools more solid. Try taking psyllium seed, or eating whole-grain cereals.
- Avoid dairy products for the duration of the attack, because they promote mucus in the digestive tract, which can help pathogens proliferate.
- Eat plenty of apples; they contain the soluble fiber pectin, which helps to bulk out stools and also heal the digestive tract.

HOMEOPATHIC REMEDIES

Chronic diarrhea should be treated constitutionally, but acute attacks may be treated with one of the following remedies.

Aconite 30C, for diarrhea that comes on suddenly, with a distended abdomen.

Pulsatilla 30C, for diarrhea that is worse at night, and made worse by rich foods.

Colocynth 30C, for diarrhea accompanied by griping pains, with yellowish, thin, and copious stools.

Argentum nit 30C, for diarrhea caused by anxiety, characterized by belching and cravings for sweet and salty food.

CALL YOUR DOCTOR

Call your doctor urgently if a baby or child with diarrhea shows symptoms of dehydration, including a sunken fontanelle (the soft spot on top of the head), unresponsiveness, drowsiness, prolonged crying, glazed eyes, or a dry mouth. For adults, if diarrhea contains blood, lasts longer than five days, or occurs after foreign travel, call your doctor.

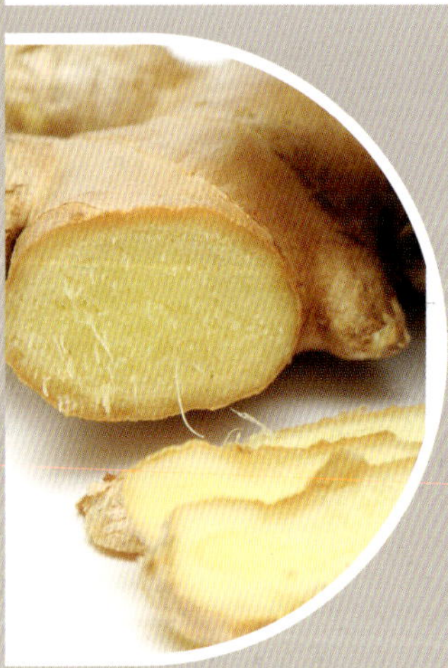

Nausea and Vomiting

Nausea and vomiting can be symptoms of gastroenteritis, inner ear infection, pregnancy, motion sickness, food poisoning, migraine, overeating (especially the wrong kinds of foods), heat exhaustion, and medication, as well as many other health problems. A constant feeling of nausea with no vomiting but with a headache and abdominal pain may also be related to stress or anxiety.

SYMPTOMS

Nausea and vomiting are symptoms rather than ailments in their own right, but they are characterized by the following:

- Feelings of sickness
- Sometimes dizziness
- Emptying of stomach contents
- Retching

PREVENTION

Careful hygiene (hand washing after dealing with pets, going to the bathroom, or preparing food) is important, and avoiding sharing towels can also help to prevent infections from being passed on. In reality, however, the cause of the nausea and vomiting must be addressed to prevent them from occurring.

CONVENTIONAL TREATMENTS

A fluid-only diet is usually recommended for 24 hours, with fluid replacement solutions offered in the event of dehydration. A variety of antinausea medications (antiemetics) can be prescribed, although many of these are not appropriate for children and pregnant women or while breast-feeding.

Did You Know?

In children, vomiting can be the result of coughs or colds (due to excess mucus) or a raised temperature.

NATURAL REMEDIES

Treatment should be offered according to the cause of the nausea and vomiting, but the following natural remedies may be useful.

AROMATHERAPY The essential oils of peppermint or lavender can be used in a vaporizer and inhaled to alleviate nausea and vomiting. Similarly, thyme or tea tree can be used for their antiseptic properties. Massage the stomach and chest with a few drops of lavender or chamomile in a light carrier oil to calm and reduce any spasm.

FLOWER REMEDIES Rescue Remedy or Emergency Essence will be useful for prolonged or distressing vomiting; it will help to reduce panic and calm the mind and body. Holly or Beech may help if the vomiting is linked to fearfulness, stress, and emotional problems.

HERBAL REMEDIES

- Make a cup of very weak black currant or chamomile tea and drink lukewarm, in small sips. This will help to soothe the digestive tract.
- Chewing a little fresh or candied ginger will help to settle the stomach and is particularly useful for motion sickness or pregnancy-related nausea.
- Echinacea, peppermint, and thyme can be drunk as infusions or added to a footbath when there is infection at the root of the illness.

HOMEOPATHIC REMEDIES

These can be effective. If the condition is chronic, constitutional treatment is indicated. There are remedies that will help for acute attacks.

Arsenicum 30C is the best one to try first, when nausea and vomiting are accompanied by diarrhea, and symptoms seem to be worse between midnight and 2 a.m.

Nux vomica 30C, when nausea is made better by vomiting, and may be caused by overindulgence (after a party, for example).

Tabacum 30C, for nausea and vomiting relieved by uncovering the abdomen. This is a good one for motion sickness.

Phosphorus 30C, for cravings for cold water, which is then vomited, and burning pains in the stomach.

Pulsatilla 30C, for vomiting after rich fatty food, with tearfulness.

Arnica 30C, when vomiting follows a head injury.

Aconite 30C, when vomiting and severe pain last for more than an hour, and are not relieved by vomiting.

CALL YOUR DOCTOR

Any case of vomiting that continues for longer than 24 hours, or occurs in a child who is under the age of three months, should be seen by a doctor. Children dehydrate quickly, and if there is floppiness, a sunken fontanelle (the soft spot on top of the head) in a baby, or fewer wet diapers, make sure that you see your doctor urgently. Blood in the vomit should also always be investigated.

Quick Fix

For immediate relief for nausea, try wearing an acupressure wristband. They are sold in pharmacies for treating motion sickness.

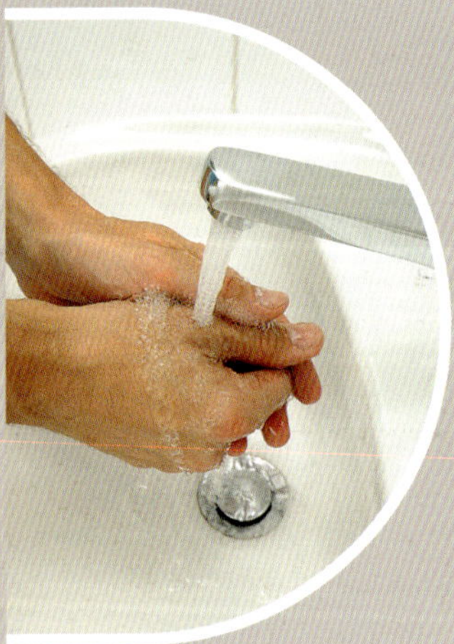

Gastroenteritis and Food Poisoning

Gastroenteritis is an infection of the digestive tract, caused either by a virus, such as the norovirus, or by bacteria, as in food poisoning. It is highly infectious, but most people only experience mild symptoms, lasting a few days.

SYMPTOMS

- ▷ Nausea and vomiting
- ▷ Diarrhea
- ▷ Abdominal pain
- ▷ Headaches
- ▷ High temperature
- ▷ Possible dehydration

PREVENTION

- Wash your hands after going to the bathroom and after touching any surfaces in public places.
- Avoid direct contact with the body fluids of a person with gastroenteritis: use separate towels, don't share cups or plates, and make sure the toilet is cleaned thoroughly after each bout of vomiting or diarrhea they have experienced.
- To avoid food poisoning, practice good food hygiene rules.
- Prepare and store raw and cooked foods separately.
- Make sure food is thoroughly cooked through, especially poultry, pork, and eggs.
- Don't eat foods that are past their expiration date.
- Wash your hands before preparing food and after contact with raw meat and poultry.

Did You Know?

You can ease back into eating again when you start to get your appetite back with the BRAT diet. Eat the following foods.

- **B**ananas—ripe ones
- **R**ice—must be plain, boiled
- **A**pples—raw ones
- **T**oast—preferably dry whole wheat without butter.

CONVENTIONAL TREATMENTS

People with mild to moderate cases of gastroenteritis should stay at home and make sure they get plenty of fluids. Rehydrating salts, available over the counter, are recommended for vulnerable groups, such as the elderly, or after prolonged bouts of gastroenteritis. For severe cases, your doctor might prescribe loperamide to reduce diarrhea. Antibiotics may sometimes be prescribed to prevent secondary infections in the most vulnerable groups.

NATURAL REMEDIES

There are many treatments to soothe the digestive tract and restore normal function. Natural remedies focus on helping your digestive system to recover normal function after an attack of gastroenteritis or food poisoning.

NUTRITIONAL MEDICINE Eat small, easily digested meals, including plain, nonfatty foods, such as clear soups, dry toast, boiled rice, and bananas. Avoid smoking, alcohol, caffeine-containing drinks, and spicy or fatty foods.

AROMATHERAPY Massage a few drops of chamomile and geranium essential oils, blended with a light carrier oil, into the abdomen to bring relief from discomfort. Use a blend of basil, oregano, and lavender in the bath.

HERBAL REMEDIES

- Take probiotics after any kind of stomach upset to restore the balance of healthy bacteria in the digestive tract.
- Garlic tablets and manuka honey have an antibacterial effect, which could help in cases of bacterial infection.
- Powdered ginger added to a hot drink can help to ease nausea and has an anti-inflammatory effect on the digestive tract.
- Slippery elm powder mixed with hot water will help to soothe the digestive lining after an infection.

HOMEOPATHIC REMEDIES

Homeopathic remedies can be taken hourly, as required. As always, choose the appropriate remedy for the symptoms presented.

Arsenicum 30C, for burning pains in the abdomen and great thirst.

Pulsatilla 30C, for symptoms worse at night, and tearfulness.

Baptisia 30C, if a salmonella infection is suspected, with stools that are dark, bloody, and smelly, nearly liquid.

Phosphorus 30C, for a burning sensation when stools are passed, with vomiting and cravings for cold water, which is then vomited.

Sulfur 30C, for burning diarrhea that is worse around 5 a.m., with a red and itchy anus.

CALL YOUR DOCTOR

If your symptoms last longer than three days, contact your doctor. If there is blood in your stools or vomit, seek medical advice immediately. You should also get help if you have any symptoms of dehydration, such as an inability to pass urine, dry mouth, and eyes that appear sunken. Gastroenteritis can be dangerous in the elderly, the very young, or those who have other health problems that weaken the immune system, so a close eye should be kept on them.

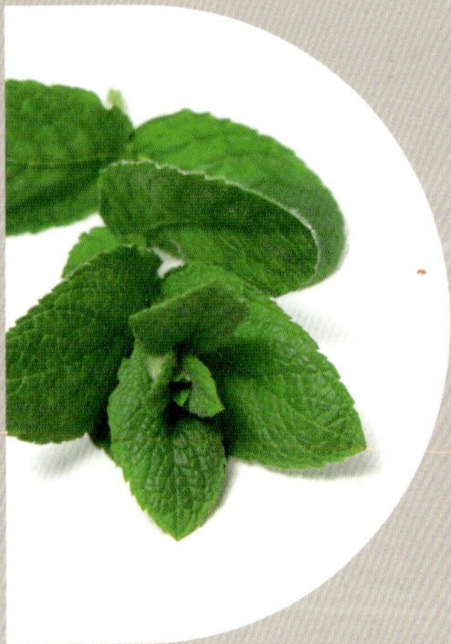

Indigestion and Heartburn

Indigestion, or dyspepsia, is a burning pain in the upper abdomen caused by a reflux of stomach acid irritating the lining of the esophagus. Heartburn has the same cause but tends to be felt just behind the breastbone.

SYMPTOMS

- A burning pain in the throat, chest, or stomach that is worse when you are lying down
- Sour acidic taste in the mouth
- A sore throat

Did You Know?

Acid reflux is a common problem that affects many people and it is seldom serious, but in the long term it may lead to the lining of the digestive tract becoming damaged.

PREVENTION

- Don't smoke, because the chemicals in cigarette smoke irritate the digestive lining.
- Keep your weight down.
- Avoid foods that bring on indigestion, such as rich, spicy, fatty dishes, chocolate, pastry, acidic fruit juices, alcohol, and caffeine-containing drinks.
- Eat small meals and don't stuff yourself full.
- Wear loose clothing, without tight waistbands.
- Don't eat too late at night; always make sure that at least three hours elapse after a meal before you go to bed.
- Raising the head of the bed with wooden blocks can help prevent acid reflux.

CONVENTIONAL TREATMENTS

Antacids, which are available over the counter in pharmacies, neutralize stomach acids and ease symptoms, but you shouldn't take them long term or exceed the stated dosage. For severe, recurrent indigestion, your doctor might prescribe proton pump inhibitors (PPIs) or H2 antagonists (such as nizatidine) that inhibit the production of stomach acid. Promotility agents, such as metoclopramide, are for particularly severe symptoms; they work by speeding up the rate at which the stomach empties.

NATURAL REMEDIES

There are plenty of ways to lessen the effects of acid reflux. The traditional remedy to ease heartburn and indigestion is two or three teaspoons of apple cider vinegar in a glass of water before meals. The vinegar lowers the acidity of stomach acids but lets them digest food efficiently.

HELPFUL THERAPIES Both acupressure and reflexology may be helpful in relieving indigestion.

NUTRITIONAL MEDICINE Baking soda is a natural antacid and you can mix a little with water in a glass for instant relief.

HERBAL REMEDIES

- Licorice powder containing a substance called glycyrrhizin is effective at soothing indigestion. Don't take it if you have any other health problems, however, because there can be interactions.
- Aloe vera juice has anti-inflammatory, pain-killing properties.
- Peppermint tea can relieve mild indigestion when sipped after a meal.
- Marshmallow root tea can coat and soothe the lining of the esophagus.

AROMATHERAPY

- Neroli, peppermint, and chamomile oils have a healing and soothing effect on the digestive system; use in the bath or mixed with a carrier oil for a light massage of the abdominal area.
- Chamomile and lavender oils can be used in the same way for relief of cramping and wind. Inhaling peppermint oil from a vaporizer can help with flatulence.
- Heartburn can be relieved by massaging your abdomen with a few drops of neroli or chamomile in a warm carrier oil, such as grapeseed.

FLOWER REMEDIES

- Impatiens is ideal if you tend to do everything too quickly and pay the consequences later.
- Olive will help with fatigue caused by overindulgence.
- Oak is good for persistent indigestion caused by an inability to change poor lifestyle habits.

HOMEOPATHIC REMEDIES

For relief of symptoms, try one of the following.

Nux vomica 30C, for heartburn, discomfort, and flatulence, especially after a heavy meal or overindulgence.

Carbo veg 30C can help if you have a full, heavy feeling, and feel sleepy after eating.

Lycopodium 30C relieves tiredness and bloating after eating, and helps when you have a burning in your throat.

CALL YOUR DOCTOR

If you are suffering recurrent bouts of indigestion, if it is particularly painful, or if it suddenly feels worse than it has felt before, see your doctor.

Caution

Taking aspirin or NSAIDs, such as ibuprofen, to relieve the pain of indigestion will only make it worse.

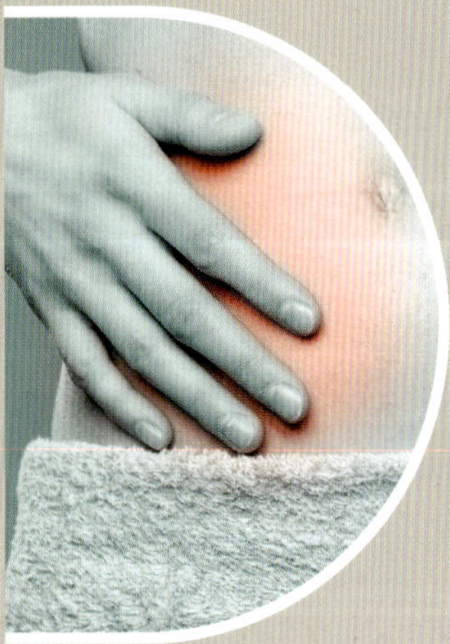

Inflammatory Bowel Diseases

Crohn's disease and ulcerative colitis are both chronic, remittent conditions in which inflammation of the lining of the bowel causes uncomfortable and potentially dangerous symptoms.

SYMPTOMS

- ▷ Diarrhea, with blood and/or mucus in the stools
- ▷ Abdominal cramps, especially after eating
- ▷ Relapsing and remitting episodes
- ▷ Fever and joint pain
- ▷ Weight loss
- ▷ Vitamin and mineral deficiencies
- ▷ Fatigue

Did You Know?

No one is entirely sure about the causes of Crohn's disease and ulcerative colitis, but it seems that there may be a genetic element as well as some environmental triggers.

PREVENTION

- Keep a food diary and note down which foods make your symptoms worse, so you can avoid them. One study found that the commonly implicated foods were wheat, milk, yeast, corn, egg, potato, rye, tea, coffee, apples, mushrooms, oats, and chocolate.
- Eating six small meals instead of three large ones a day can help. Focus on high-vitamin, low-sugar foods.
- If you are a smoker, quitting can ease the symptoms of Crohn's disease.

CONVENTIONAL TREATMENTS

Mild to moderate cases of Crohn's disease and ulcerative colitis may be treated with aminosalicylates, which reduce inflammation. If the symptoms are more severe, however, steroids, such as budesonide and prednisolone, may be given during active episodes, but there are potential dangers if they are used for a long term. Immune system suppressants, such as azathioprine, may be prescribed during a nonactive phase to try to prevent relapses.

NATURAL REMEDIES

Before taking any natural treatments alongside the conventional ones, discuss them with your practitioner to avoid interactions.

NUTRITIONAL MEDICINE Several studies have indicated that fish oils ease symptoms and prevent relapses, so it's worth taking daily fish oil capsules. Zinc, selenium, vitamin B12, and folic acid deficiencies are common, so take a good multivitamin and mineral supplement to replace all these.

FLOWER REMEDIES Try Rescue Remedy or Emergency Essence when you experience any pain or discomfort. Blend the Bach flower remedies Impatiens, Willow, Agrimony, and Wild Oat with a little water, and sip throughout the day to encourage healing and deal with symptoms.

HERBAL REMEDIES

- Probiotic supplements with healthy digestive bacteria are useful.
- Some people swear by drinking a small glass, about half a cup, of aloe vera juice three times a day.
- Licorice root powder containing glycyrrhizin can have a soothing effect on the bowel.
- Garlic powder tablets can help to deal with any fungal growth in the digestive system.
- Slippery elm powder can be mixed with a little warm water to soothe and heal inflammation of the digestive tract.

Reduce Stress

Take steps to reduce the stress levels in your life. Identify the main stressors and try to deal with them by changing your daily routines, or take up some form of relaxation therapy, such as yoga or meditation.

AROMATHERAPY

- Massage a blend of lavender and peppermint into the abdomen, or add it to the bath to relieve conditions associated with stress, and also to relax any spasms.
- A few drops of juniper or cedarwood oil added to the bath have an antispasmodic, sedative, and tonic effect.
- Essential oil of basil can help to reduce symptoms, used in the bath or simply inhaled from a vaporizer when you feel discomfort.

HOMEOPATHIC REMEDIES

Treatment should be constitutional, but the following remedies may be useful.

Argentum nitricum 30C, if you are anxious and experience flatulence and diarrhea.

Ignatia 30C, if your bowels are particularly sensitive during periods of emotional distress.

Podophyllum 30C, for abdominal pain that is better for heat and when lying down; often explosive diarrhea.

CALL YOUR DOCTOR

Always consult your doctor if there is blood in your stools, if you have recurrent diarrhea or abdominal pain, or if you lose weight for no obvious reason.

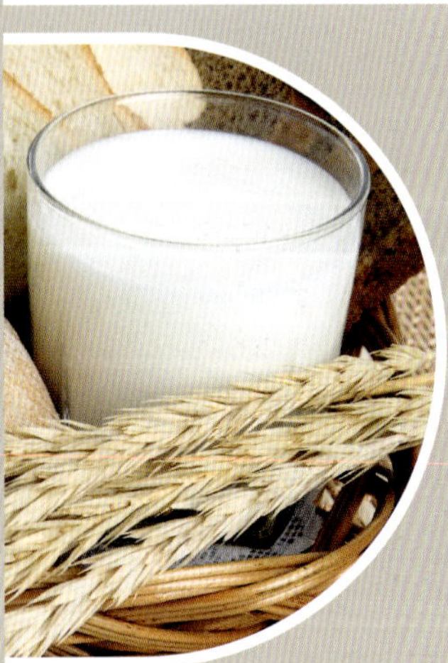

Irritable Bowel Syndrome

About one-third of the population are affected by irritable bowel syndrome (IBS) at some point in their lives, but only half of them will consider it severe enough to consult their doctor. It's a chronic condition, but, fortunately, plenty can be done to relieve it and to prevent recurrence.

SYMPTOMS

The following should last for at least six months before a diagnosis of IBS is confirmed:

- ▷ Abdominal pain that is relieved by defecation
- ▷ Bloating
- ▷ Constipation or diarrhea

You may also have at least two of the following:

- ▷ Needing to strain to pass stools
- ▷ Feeling the bowel movement is incomplete
- ▷ Having to rush to the bathroom for a bowel movement
- ▷ Fewer than three bowel movements a week
- ▷ More than three bowel movements a day
- ▷ Excess flatulence

PREVENTION

- Keep a food diary and find out which foods improve symptoms and which make them worse.
- Eat small, regular meals and chew your food properly.
- Drink eight large glasses of water a day, and cut down on tea, coffee, alcohol, and carbonated beverages.
- Get 30 minutes of exercise five days a week to stimulate the normal functioning of your digestive system.
- Stress make the symptoms of IBS worse, so try to relax and reduce the amount of stress in your life.

CONVENTIONAL TREATMENTS

Your doctor will probably recommend making lifestyle changes before prescribing medication, but antispasmodic medicines can help. Bulk-forming laxatives might be prescribed for constipation, and loperamide may be offered for IBS-related diarrhea.

NATURAL REMEDIES

There are different types of IBS so visit a practitioner for an individual diagnosis, but the following natural remedies could help.

FLOWER REMEDIES Impatiens will help with attacks that come on as a result of stress or overindulgence.

NUTRITIONAL MEDICINE

- Some IBS symptoms are caused by the action of intestinal bacteria on fiber, so it's worth trying a very low-fiber diet for a while, then gradually reintroducing foods that contain fiber until you find a level you can tolerate.
- A gluten-free diet can be helpful.
- Other possible irritants can include dairy products, eggs, yeast, onions, potatoes, and chocolate. Exclude them all, then reintroduce one at a time to see which, if any, cause symptoms.
- Many people with IBS report that symptoms are eased by taking probiotics.

HERBAL REMEDIES

- Cynara artichoke supplements seem to be effective at reducing pain and bloating, and results can be seen within 10 days.
- Agrimony and hops can be blended into an infusion and drunk before meals to regulate digestion and ease discomfort.
- Wild yam and cramp bark can be taken in either capsule or tincture form to ease painful spasms and cramps.

HOMEOPATHIC REMEDIES

Constitutional treatment will be necessary, but the following remedies should help in the short term.

Argentum nitricum 30C, for digestive upsets accompanied by nervousness, bloating, nausea, and greenish diarrhea.

Asafoetida 30C, for a feeling of constriction in the digestive tract and a bloated abdomen, but inability to pass wind.

Colcynthis 30C, for cutting pains and cramping that are worse before diarrhea.

Lycopodium 30C, for chronic digestive discomfort and bowel problems, with bloating and a feeling of fullness that comes on early in a meal.

Podophyllum 30C, for abdominal pain and cramping followed by watery, offensive diarrhea.

CALL YOUR DOCTOR

If any change in your bowel habits lasts longer than six weeks, or if there is blood in your stools, consult your doctor. You should also seek medical advice if you have a family history of bowel cancer, or if you are over 60 years old.

Pilates

This is an exercise system that works to strengthen the abdominal and pelvic muscles. If you are prone to constipation, Pilates can help you to push more effectively.

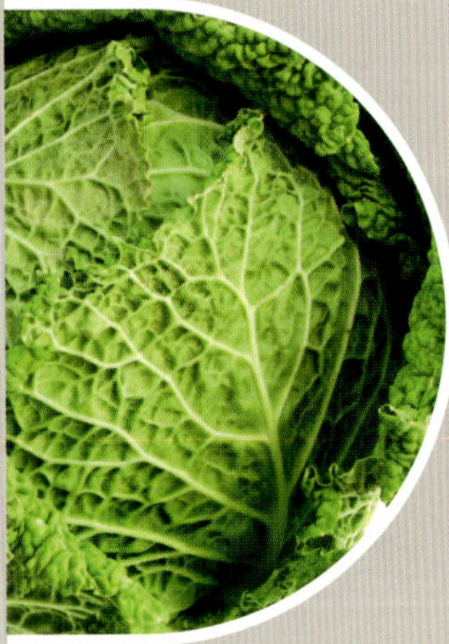

Peptic Ulcers

A peptic ulcer is an area of damage to the lining of either the stomach or the wall of the small bowel, caused when the layer of mucus that normally protects them from stomach acids is compromised. The most common cause is a bacteria called *Helicobacter pylori,* but NSAIDs (nonsteroidal anti-inflammatory drugs), such as aspirin, naproxen, and ibuprofen, taken over long periods of time, can also be a factor. They also tend to run in families.

SYMPTOMS

- ▷ Acute abdominal pain, usually just below the breastbone
- ▷ Burning pain extending into the back
- ▷ Pain that is worse immediately after eating
- ▷ Heartburn
- ▷ A bitter taste in your mouth
- ▷ Nausea or vomiting
- ▷ Regurgitating food

Did You Know?

Stress seems to play an important role and, if you have peptic ulcers, you should reassess your life to introduce more relaxation and try to eliminate any stressful situations and relationships. Consider signing up for a stress management course.

PREVENTION

- Avoid food and drink that exacerbate symptoms, including spicy foods and alcohol.
- Smoking is a known cause of ulcers, so giving up can help to prevent them.
- Alcohol can cause peptic ulcers, so only drink in moderation.
- Avoid NSAIDs—ask your pharmacist for advice on the other options.
- Drink a large glass of water before each meal to dilute stomach acids.
- Stress caused by injury or trauma is another cause of peptic ulcers. You may not be able to prevent these happening but you can take steps to manage the stress effectively.

CONVENTIONAL TREATMENTS

The two types of medication offered for the treatment of ulcers include proton pump inhibitors (PPIs) and H2 blockers, both of which are designed to reduce the production of acid in your stomach. If bacteria is responsible, you will also be offered antibiotics.

NATURAL REMEDIES

Most natural treatments are designed to heal the digestive tract and ease symptoms.

AROMATHERAPY Althea soothes mucous membranes and relieves gastritis and peptic ulcers. Use a few drops of this oil in an abdominal massage or in the bath.

HERBAL REMEDIES

- Antibacterial herbs, such as echinacea, red clover, and thyme, can be drunk daily as an infusion to combat any bacteria present.
- Manuka honey heals and strengthens the stomach lining and kills harmful bacteria.
- Slippery elm encourages the health of the mucous membranes, and can be taken in capsule, tincture, or infusion form. Meadowsweet has a similar effect.
- An infusion of chamomile can help to relieve the pain, particularly if it is sipped just after meals.
- Powdered licorice containing glycyrrhizin can help to heal peptic ulcers by increasing the production of the mucus that lines the stomach.

NUTRITIONAL MEDICINE

- Increase your intake of EFAs (essential fatty acids), which are natural anti-inflammatories, and protect the lining of the entire gastrointestinal tract. Fish oil or flaxseed supplements may be useful.
- Fresh cabbage juice and raw cabbage can strengthen the lining of the stomach.
- A diet rich in dietary fiber (psyllium or flaxseeds) can help to protect the digestive tract.
- Zinc is crucial to the health of your stomach lining, so eat plenty of whole grains, shellfish, and pumpkin seeds or take supplements.
- Vitamin C will promote healing of ulcers—take a supplement, or better, increase your intake of vitamin C-rich foods.

HOMEOPATHIC REMEDIES

Argentum nitricum 30C is ideal for ulcers with gnawing pain and belching.

Arsenicum 30C is indicated for ulcers with a burning feeling that is worse for food and drink.

Hydrastis 30C may be appropriate if the symptoms include gastritis and abdominal pain.

Nux vomica 30C may help if symptoms are worse after heavy meals, alcohol, and stimulants, such as coffee or tobacco.

CALL YOUR DOCTOR

Call your doctor if you have difficulty swallowing food, have lost weight, notice blood in your vomit or feces, or experience sudden, extreme abdominal pain.

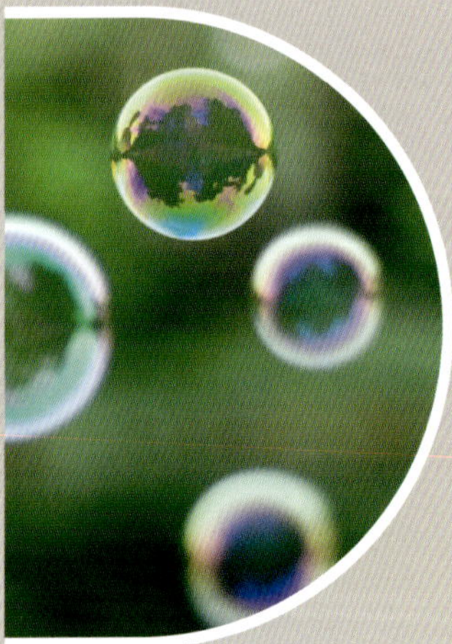

Flatulence

Every human being passes gas, but some people do so in excessive quantities. Bowel gases come from the air that we swallow while eating, from carbonated drinks, and from the digestion of foods in the intestine. If the digestive system is not working efficiently and foods decompose in the digestive tract, gas can have a sulfurous smell and there may be abdominal bloating as well.

SYMPTOMS

- ▷ Frequent passing of gas
- ▷ Foul-smelling gas
- ▷ Embarrassing intestinal noises
- ▷ Bloating

PREVENTION

- Avoid gas-producing foods, such as beans, lentils, cauliflower, cabbage, broccoli, and cucumber, as well as carbonated drinks.
- Reduced-calorie products that contain sugar substitutes, such as sorbitol and fructose, can also cause flatulence, as can fruit juices.
- Eat small meals of easily digestible foods, such as potatoes, rice, yogurt, and bananas.
- Eat slowly and chew each mouthful thoroughly.
- Keep a food diary to see which foods exacerbate symptoms.
- Get plenty of exercise, which will help your digestive system to work more efficiently.
- Avoid chewing gum and smoking, both of which cause you to swallow air.

CONVENTIONAL TREATMENTS

A supplement called alpha-D-galascitosidase can improve the way in which you digest carbohydrates. To help alleviate the symptoms of gas, try over-the-counter tablets or capsules containing simethicone.

NATURAL REMEDIES

Excess gas can be a symptom of irritable bowel syndrome (see pages 180–181), so the remedies listed there may help, or you can try the following.

TRADITIONAL REMEDIES Try drinking the juice of a lemon in a glass of water with a half teaspoon of baking soda to quieten a noisy digestive system.

NUTRITIONAL MEDICINE Some people are lactose intolerant and don't have the correct enzymes to break down milk products. Try avoiding them for a few weeks to see if your symptoms improve. You could also try excluding wheat- and gluten-containing products to see if this makes a difference.

HERBAL REMEDIES

- Drink peppermint tea after a meal or take peppermint oil capsules to aid digestion.
- Probiotics should help.
- There are plenty of herbs you can use in your cooking that have an antiflatulent effect. Basil, dill, turmeric, rosemary, coriander, cloves, cardamom, fennel seeds, caraway seeds, and anise seeds are all good.
- Chamomile tea can relieve spasms and discomfort associated with gas.

AROMATHERAPY

- Marjoram, ginger, and fennel will help your body to disperse gas and calm any associated pain. Add a few drops of each to a light carrier oil and massage into your abdomen.
- Massaging your abdomen with a drop of fennel oil in a light carrier oil can help to release trapped gas and encourage healthy digestion.

HOMEOPATHIC REMEDIES

Choose the appropriate remedy for the symptoms.

Carbo veg 30C, for feelings of heaviness, sleepiness, and belching after meals, with offensive-smelling flatulence.

Lycopodium 30C, for a bloated, rumbling abdomen, and when passing gas eases abdominal discomfort.

Colocynthis 30C, for cutting, cramping pain in the stomach that is relieved by bending double.

Chamomilla 30C, for searing pains caused by gas; you'll feel worse for warmth.

Ipecac 30C, for pains that feel like a hand clutching your intestines, with pains moving from left to right.

CALL YOUR DOCTOR

If you have abdominal pain and bloating that won't clear up after a few weeks; if you have blood in your stools; or if you keep getting persistent diarrhea or constipation, consult your doctor.

IMMEDIATE RELIEF

To relieve trapped gas, kneel on the floor, then lean forward, so that your forehead touches the floor, with your arms straight forward, palms face down.

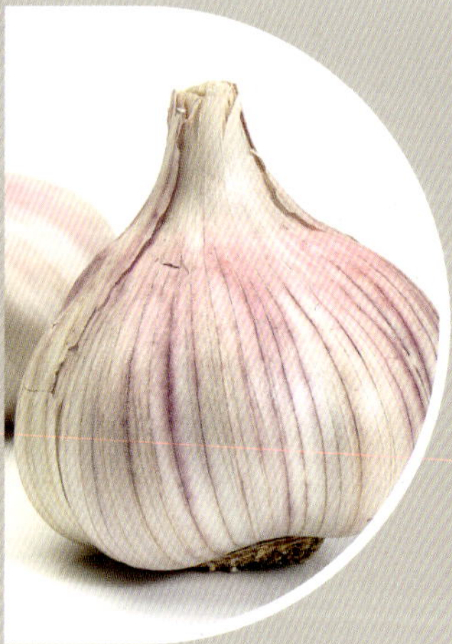

Intestinal Worms

Infestations of worms in the digestive system are common throughout the world, particularly in young children, who usually contract them at school. Worms can sometimes be seen around the anus or in the feces, and they inflame the area of the bowel or rectum where they attach themselves. The most common worms in humans in the United States are pinworms. Other types of worms occur, too, such as hookworms in tropical countries.

SYMPTOMS

- Diarrhea
- Bad breath
- Dark circles under the eyes
- Restlessness at night
- Anemia
- Itching around the anus

PREVENTION

- Encourage children to wash their hands regularly, particularly after going to the bathroom, dealing with pets, or handling food.
- Avoid scratching the anus area.
- Worms thrive on sugar, so keep it to a minimum in your diet.
- Changing the bedclothes regularly and washing them at a high temperature can prevent the spread of worms.

CONVENTIONAL TREATMENTS

Over-the-counter preparations are available to stun or kill worms, which are then excreted in the feces. These are chosen according to the type of worm present. Only one or two doses are normally required. Laxatives may sometimes be offered to aid the expulsion of worms living in the intestines.

Did You Know?

Tapeworms are segmented, flat worms that humans can get from eating undercooked, infected meat or sometimes from food prepared by an infected person. Tapeworms may cause nausea, weakness, diarrhea, abdominal pain, and other symptoms, or no symptoms at all but are visible in feces. Call your doctor if you think you have tapeworms.

NATURAL REMEDIES

Some natural treatments depend on the type of worm present but the following remedies will all help to rid you of an infestation.

FLOWER REMEDIES Rescue Remedy is good for discomfort or distress. Rub into the pulse points, and around the anus to relieve itching. Crab Apple is excellent if you feel unclean or polluted.

AROMATHERAPY Rub a drop each of eucalyptus, lavender, and tea tree oil into a bland ointment, such as petroleum jelly or chickweed. Rub around the anus to prevent itching and to prevent eggs from being laid. This is particularly helpful at night.

HERBAL REMEDIES

- A teaspoon each of cayenne pepper and senna can be combined in a cup of yogurt with live cultures and taken by the teaspoon before meals. The former stuns the worms and the latter encourages their expulsion.
- Wormwood tea will stun the worms, but should only be taken under the supervision of a registered herbalist.
- Garlic is toxic to worms. Crush and add it to a tablespoon of honey and take before meals, followed by a tincture of laxative herbs, such as licorice and dandelion root to aid expulsion.

NUTRITIONAL MEDICINE

- Acidophilus tablets can be taken for several weeks to improve the health of the bowel.
- Carrots, turnips, and apples are traditional remedies used to clear worms. Grate them together and take three times daily.
- Ripe pumpkin seeds are useful in the treatment of intestinal worms, especially tapeworms. One tablespoon of the seeds should be peeled and crushed, and then infused in a cup of boiling water and drunk. This will kill the parasites and help to expel the worms.

HOMEOPATHIC REMEDIES

Select the appropriate remedy for your symptoms.

Cina 30C may alter the balance of the body, so that you expel pinworms naturally.

Teucrium 30C, for itchy buttocks and nose, worse in the evening and with restless sleep.

CALL YOUR DOCTOR

Conventional treatment is always necessary for any tapeworm infestations. Call your doctor if treatment is not effective after two courses, or if you begin to lose weight.

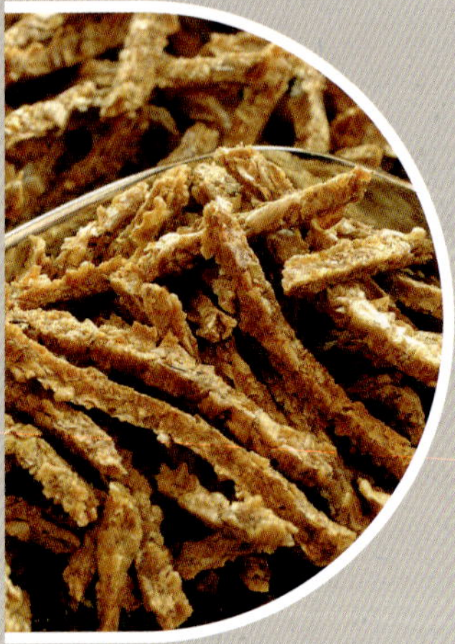

Hemorrhoids

Hemorrhoids, which are also commonly known as piles, are enlarged and swollen blood vessels in or around the lower rectum and anus. They are caused by increased pressure on the blood vessels in the area, as a result of being overweight, lifting heavy objects, pregnancy, constipation, or prolonged diarrhea, or simply aging.

SYMPTOMS

- Bleeding when passing stools
- An itchy feeling around the anus
- Intense pain, particularly when passing a stool
- Bright red bleeding after passing a stool
- Discharge of mucus when passing a stool
- Straining and feeling as though bowels are still full after a movement

PREVENTION

- Include plenty of fiber in your diet to make sure that bowel movements are efficient and you don't strain.
- Avoid lifting heavy articles, and try to maintain a healthy weight.
- Drink plenty of water to keep stools soft.

CONVENTIONAL TREATMENTS

You can choose from a number of over-the-counter preparations that act as anti-inflammatories and help to reduce pain and itching. Creams containing corticosteroids can be prescribed to reduce the inflammation. If pain is intense, analgesic ointments can be prescribed. Long-term hemorrhoids may be addressed by banding, in which a tight elastic band is placed around the bottom of the hemorrhoid. There are a number of other options available, including surgery.

NATURAL REMEDIES

There are plenty of remedies that can help with symptoms and encourage healing.

TRADITIONAL REMEDIES Witch hazel or lemon juice can be applied neat to hemorrhoids to reduce swelling and bleeding.

AROMATHERAPY A warm bath with 10 drops of bergamot (or a compress, with a few drops of this oil) will help to reduce pain and act as an antiseptic. Myrrh oil is cooling and anti-inflammatory; use in the same way.

HERBAL REMEDIES

- Calendula cream or ointment will encourage healing and relieve itching.
- Horse chestnut relieves swelling and inflammation, and helps to strengthen vein walls. Take in tea or capsule form, or apply externally as a compress.
- Butcher's broom contains anti-inflammatory and vein-constricting properties, and has traditionally been used for the treatment of hemorrhoids and varicose veins. Take in tea or capsule form.
- A strong, warm infusion of yarrow can be applied to the affected area to soothe and heal.
- Aloe vera gel is soothing for burning and pain.

NUTRITIONAL MEDICINE

- Increasing your fiber intake is the most important step you can take. Try psyllium, ground flaxseeds, or ispaghula husks.
- Bioflavonoids stabilize and strengthen blood vessel walls and decrease inflammation. They have been found to reduce anal discomfort, pain, and discharge during an acute attack of hemorrhoids. Boost your intake of bioflavonoids by eating more citrus fruit, grapes, berries, and whole grains, or take a daily supplement.

HOMEOPATHIC REMEDIES

Treatment should be constitutional, but the following remedies will help.

Hamamelis 30C can be taken two or three times daily to treat the cause of hamorrhoids.

Aloe 30C, for hemorrhoids that are swollen and protrude like a bunch of grapes and are soothed by cold compresses.

Calc fluor 30C, for hemorrhoids with bleeding and itching, or sore internal piles.

Nux vomica 30C, for itching, painful hemorrhoids, with a constricted feeling in the rectum and chronic constipation.

Pulsatilla 30C, for itching, uncomfortable hemorrhoids that will probably protrude.

CALL YOUR DOCTOR

Always call your doctor if you experience profuse bleeding, or if the hemorrhoids become hard and dark in color (which means that a clot may have formed within them).

IMMEDIATE RELIEF

Apply some ice, never directly to the skin but wrapped in a clean towel, for a local anaesthetic effect. This helps to relieve the irritation as well as the pain.

TOP 20 Superhealing Foods

The everyday foods you eat can help to keep you healthy and prevent or treat some common medical problems.

1 HONEY

Nutrients The B vitamins, minerals (depending on plant sources), antioxidants

Good for Sore throats, coughs, and colds; healing wounds; hay fever

Caution Don't give honey to children under 12 months because it can cause infant botulism

2 GINGER

Nutrients Vitamins A and B2 (riboflavin), iron, phosphorus, potassium

Good for Nausea, food poisoning, motion sickness; vertigo; respiratory ailments; menstrual pain; lowering blood cholesterol

3 GARLIC

Nutrients The B vitamins, vitamins A and C, calcium, potassium, iron, selenium

Good for Fighting infection; relieving colds, bronchitis, congestion; fungal infections; protecting against food poisoning; lowering cholesterol and high blood pressure; asthma; diarrhea, and indigestion

4 ONIONS

Nutrients Vitamin C, potassium

Good for Chest infections; lowering blood pressure; diabetes; preventing cancer

5 CARROTS

Nutrients The B vitamins, vitamin A (beta-carotene) and C, iron, fiber

Good for Eye health, healthy skin; gum disease; asthma and respiratory problems; protecting against cancer

6 BROCCOLI

Nutrients Vitamins C and K, calcium, potassium, fiber

Good for Protecting against cancer and infections; improving cognitive function

7 WATERCRESS

Nutrients Vitamins A and C, folic acid, calcium, iron, potassium, lutein

Good for Protecting against cancer; urinary infections; good eye health and reducing risk of cataracts and age-related macular degeneration

8 AVOCADOS

Nutrients Vitamins B2 (riboflavin) and E, fiber

Good for Healthy skin and treating skin problems; fighting stress; good digestion; boosting immune system; lowering cholesterol levels

9 TOMATOES

Nutrients Vitamins A and C, iron, antioxidant lycopene, folic acid

Good for Preventing cancer (especially prostate); chronic fatigue syndrome; aiding memory and fighting dementia

10 APPLES

Nutrients The B vitamins, vitamins C and E, fiber, potassium, antioxidants

Good for Fiber helps digestion; food poisoning; lowering blood pressure and cholesterol

11 BANANA

Nutrients Vitamin B6, potassium, zinc, fiber

Good for Digestive ailments, constipation, diarrhea; convalescing after illness; relieving muscular cramping

12 CITRUS FRUITS (LEMONS, LIMES, ORANGES, PINK GRAPEFRUIT)

Nutrients Vitamin C and bioflavonoids, folic acid (oranges)

Good for Boosting body's natural immunity; treating coughs, colds, flu, sore throats; arthritis; lowering cholesterol; protecting against heart disease and cancer; gum disease

13 BERRIES

Nutrients Vitamin C, antioxidants

Good for Fighting infection; preventing heart disease and cancer; urinary tract infections (cranberries and blueberries); respiratory tract infections; improving short-term memory loss (blueberries)

14 SEEDS (PUMPKIN, SUNFLOWER, FLAXSEEDS)

Nutrients Vitamin E, zinc

Good for Healthy nervous system; good digestion; reducing risk of dementia and enhancing memory and thinking skills

15 NUTS

Nutrients Protein, the B vitamins, vitamin E, zinc, selenium, magnesium, iron, healthy oils, folic acid

Good for Healthy nervous system, fatigue and stress; lowering cholesterol; preventing memory loss

16 WHOLE GRAINS

Nutrients protein, the B vitamins, vitamin E, folic acid, fiber, zinc

Good for Constipation; protecting against bowel disease, heart disease, cancer, diabetes; high blood pressure

17 OATS

Nutrients Protein, vitamins B6 and E, magnesium, fiber

Good for Treating constipation; lowering cholesterol and blood pressure; protecting against colon cancer

18 BEANS AND LEGUMES (LENTILS, DRIED PEAS)

Nutrients Protein, the B vitamins, fiber, calcium, iron, magnesium, zinc

Good for Constipation; protecting against cancer, bowel and heart disease

19 YOGURT WITH LIVE CULTURES

Nutrients Protein, vitamins A and D, calcium

Good for Stomach ailments, food poisoning, constipation; fighting fungal infections; boosting the immune system

20 OILY FISH

Nutrients Protein, vitamins A, B12, and D, omega-3 fatty acids, iodine

Good for A healthy heart and preventing heart disease; healthy nervous system; protecting against memory loss and Alzheimer's disease

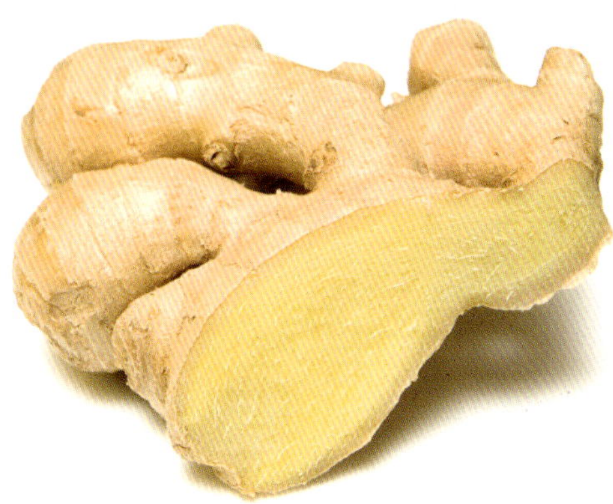

Urinary Problems

The urinary system performs some important functions in the body: filtering the blood, expelling waste products and excess water, and maintaining the correct balance of blood flow and pressure, and fluids and minerals. It is composed of the bladder, kidneys, two ureters, and the urethra (the tube through which urine passes leaving the body).

The kidneys purify the blood by filtering out waste products and toxins. While the cleaned blood returns to the heart, the filtered liquid is turned into urine to be channeled through the ureters into the bladder, where it is stored before being expelled by the body through the urethra.

Most of the time, your waterworks will function efficiently and well, but the urinary tract is susceptible to infection, especially in women, because of its location near the anus and vagina. If bacteria enter the urethra, other parts of the system, such as the bladder and kidneys, can become infected, too, if the problem is left untreated. Difficulty in passing urine, pain when you urinate, or an increase in the volume of urine can be symptoms of more serious disorders and will warrant medical investigation.

Drinking plenty of fluids, especially cranberry juice, eating a high-fiber diet, good personal hygiene, and going to the bathroom promptly when you feel the need to urinate (at least once every three hours during the day) can all help to prevent urinary tract infections and keep your system flushed out and healthy.

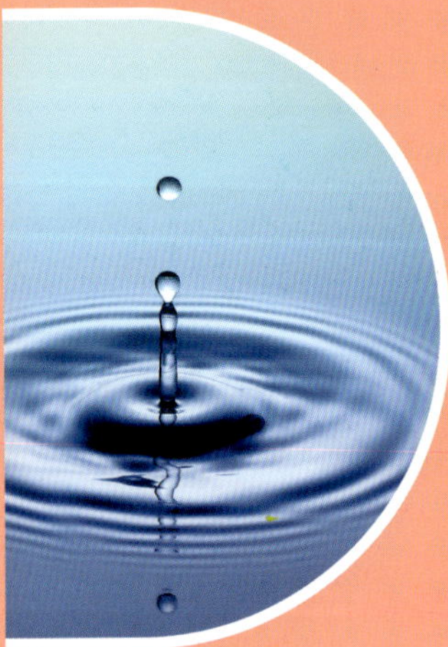

Incontinence

Incontinence is an involuntary loss of bladder control, leading to the unplanned leakage of urine. It can be embarrassing and awkward, especially with stress incontinence, because it can occur when coughing, sneezing, or making sudden movements. Stress incontinence becomes more common as people get older, especially in women, with about one in five over-40s experiencing it.

SYMPTOMS

- ▷ A sudden release of urine—from a few drops to your whole bladder
- ▷ A sudden urge to urinate (known as urge incontinence and caused by an overactive bladder)

Did You Know?

This is not solely a women's problem; men can develop incontinence, too, especially when prostate problems are an issue.

PREVENTION

One of the common causes of stress incontinence is weakened pelvic floor muscles—the muscles that hold the pelvic organs in place. These muscles get weaker after having children and after menopause. Regularly practicing Kegel exercises, especially after childbirth and as you get older, can help to reduce the chance of incontinence and accidental leakages. Gadgets are available to do Kegel exercises, but you can simply learn to do the exercises yourself.

NOTE If you're not sure which are your pelvic floor muscles, try stopping a stream of urine when you are urinating. The muscles you use are the same ones you want to strengthen.

kegel EXERCISE

1 Sit or stand with your knees apart and tighten your pelvic floor muscles. Hold while counting to five, then relax. Repeat five times.

2 Tighten your muscles again, but this time for only a few seconds before releasing. Repeat this faster muscle action for up to five minutes. Aim to do the exercises for five minutes every day, gradually increasing the amount of time you hold your muscles.

CONVENTIONAL TREATMENTS

Various types of incontinence pads are available to save some of the embarrassment of an unexpected leakage. Strengthening the pelvic floor muscles is commonly recommended for anyone experiencing stress incontinence, as is losing weight if you're overweight. In some cases, anticholinergic or antimuscarinic medication, in addition to exercises, may be prescribed. For anyone who is severely affected, surgery may be required.

Electrical stimulation, involving the use of a specially designed electrical device, is sometimes used to help the pelvic floor muscles become stronger. If a urine or kidney infection is suspected to be the cause of urge incontinence, then antibiotics may be prescribed.

NATURAL REMEDIES

The following natural remedies may be helpful in treating and relieving incontinence.

AROMATHERAPY The essential oil cypress has astringent and relaxing properties. Mix a few drops with a base carrier oil, such as sweet almond oil, and gently massage into your lower abdomen.

HOMEOPATHIC REMEDIES Take Causticum 6C to help symptoms of involuntary incontinence as a result of sneezing, coughing, or laughing. Pulsatilla 6C or Ferrum Phos 6C may help incontinence that occurs when lying down in bed.

NUTRITIONAL MEDICINE Simple dietary amendments may help to reduce the symptoms of incontinence. Cut back on caffeine, because it has diuretic properties, avoid drinking carbonated drinks, and eat less tomato-base foods, because they could irritate the bladder.

HELPFUL THERAPIES Biofeedback, a method that encourages people to learn to improve their health by gaining control over bodily functions, may offer some help with incontinence. Find a local practitioner and see if it works for you.

HERBAL REMEDIES

Some herbs may help people with incontinence. You can try the following remedies.

- Ginkgo supplements or tincture can help a weak bladder and incontinence.
- Try taking varuna to help improve muscle tone and bladder control.
- Take healing horsetail tincture to help the urinary system.
- For men with incontinence linked to prostrate problems, take the herb saw palmetto. Supplements are available and should be taken as directed on the packaging.

CALL YOUR DOCTOR

Many people are too embarrassed to seek medical help, but if your symptoms are severe or interfering with your daily life, call your doctor.

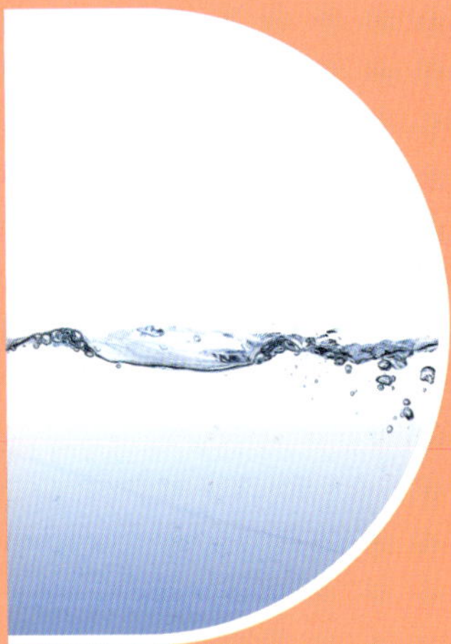

Water Retention

Water or fluid retention can affect anyone, but it's particularly common in women around the time of a menstrual period or during pregnancy, and it can get worse as you get older. Even though it may be caused by underlying heart or kidney diseases, water retention is seldom linked to other health problems and, although a nuisance when it happens, it is not a serious concern.

SYMPTOMS

- Swelling of the feet and ankles
- Swelling around the abdomen
- Swelling in the hands
- Swelling in the face
- You may weigh more in the evening than in the morning
- The need to loosen clothing or shoes

PREVENTION

- If you are prone to water retention, especially around your ankles and legs, it can be useful to wear support stockings to try to prevent fluid buildup from occurring. This is especially pertinent if you tend to sit down for long periods or spend a lot of time traveling in cars or planes.
- Putting your legs up in a raised position—for example, propped up on a footstool or on a couple of cushions—can help to prevent the swelling from recurring.
- Leading a healthy lifestyle, including eating a varied, well-balanced diet and getting regular exercise, can help to prevent water retention.
- Maintain a healthy weight for your height and build. People who are overweight are more at risk of fluid retention.
- Avoid standing still for long periods of time, because this can trigger water retention.

Did You Know?

Water retention can sometimes be caused by not drinking enough, so make sure you drink eight glasses of water a day to keep your body completely hydrated.

CONVENTIONAL TREATMENTS

Diuretics or water tablets are often prescribed to relieve water retention. They work by increasing the amount of urine the kidneys produce, making you need to go to the bathroom more often. Sometimes the tablets can cause side effects, such as feeling dizzy when you stand up. If water retention occurs during pregnancy, do not take diuretics—consult your doctor for advice. If you are overweight, your doctor may suggest losing weight, because this can help reduce water retention, too. Support or compression stockings may be advised, especially if your job involves a lot of standing around or traveling.

NATURAL REMEDIES

The following natural therapies and remedies may help to relieve the condition.

NUTRITIONAL MEDICINE If you eat a lot of salt, or regularly add salt to your meals, then cutting down on salt consumption can have a positive effect on reducing fluid retention. Include more naturally potassium-rich foods in your diet. They can help reduce the salt levels in your body and relieve areas of swelling. Bananas are a good option, as are tomatoes.

AROMATHERAPY Add a few drops of soothing lavender or rosemary essential oil to a carrier oil, such as sweet almond, and gently massage the area affected by water retention. Repeat daily as necessary.

HERBAL REMEDIES

- Dandelion is one of nature's best diuretics, so try drinking dandelion tea or using a tincture.
- Another diuretic herb available in tincture format is corn silk. A one-milliliter tincture should be diluted in a teaspoon of water three times a day. A professional herbalist will be able to mix you up a special blend for the ultimate diuretic remedy.

CALL YOUR DOCTOR

If you have persistent swelling around the abdomen or in your feet and ankles, possibly accompanied by breathlessness or fatigue, call your doctor. Fluid retention can sometimes be linked to underlying kidney or heart conditions, and some tests and investigations may be required.

IMMEDIATE RELIEF

You can ease the discomfort of swollen feet or ankles by making up a warm, soothing footbath and then soaking your feet in the water with a few drops of rosemary essential oil added.

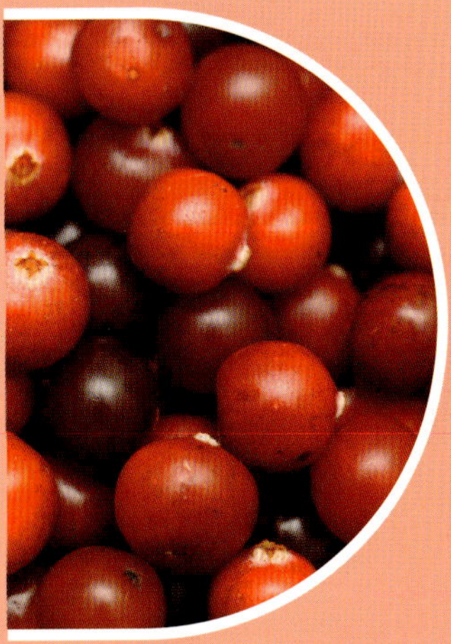

Cystitis

This bladder condition occurs due to infections or irritations of the bladder, or lower urinary tract. It is more common in women than men—up to 40 percent of women will get cystitis at some point in their life—and it can trigger a range of uncomfortable symptoms. One of the main causes is bacteria, such as *E. coli*, which gets in the urethra from other areas of your skin and travels up into your bladder.

SYMPTOMS

- ▷ Frequent urination
- ▷ Pain or burning when urinating
- ▷ Feeling like you need to keep urinating, but not being able to
- ▷ Blood in urine
- ▷ Cloudy or dark urine
- ▷ Feeling unwell as a whole
- ▷ Pain or discomfort in your lower back or lower abdomen

PREVENTION

There are various ways in which cystitis can be prevented, particularly if you are prone to it.

- Wear cotton underwear and loose clothing.
- Try to empty your bladder before and after having sex.
- Drink more fluid, particularly water, every day.
- Empty your bladder frequently, or at least once every three hours, instead of hanging on.
- Avoid using scented products in the bath, such as bubble bath, because it may cause irritation.
- Avoid spermicidal products—speak to your doctor about alternatives.
- Reduce any stress in your life and eat a healthy diet that is rich in vitamin C—a poor diet and stress can both lower your immunity to infections.

CONVENTIONAL TREATMENTS

Over-the-counter painkillers can be used to help relieve the pain of cystitis. If you have an infection, your doctor may prescribe antibiotics for three to six days. If cystitis occurs repeatedly, additional investigations may be required.

NATURAL REMEDIES

Various natural remedies can help ease the symptoms and discomfort of cystitis. Here are some options.

HERBAL REMEDIES The herb bachu has natural antiseptic and diuretic properties and can help soothe the pain and burning feeling that cystitis produces. Corn silk is another diuretic and yarrow is a urinary antiseptic. Take individually, or choose a tincture that combines all three (a herbalist can make this up for you). The usual dosage is one milliliter tincture diluted in a teaspoon of water three times a day.

NUTRITIONAL MEDICINE Boost your immune system by taking vitamin C or echinacea.

HOMEOPATHIC REMEDIES

Cantharis 6C or Sarsapilla 6C can be taken for burning pain when urinating.

Merc cor 6C, for when urination is painful and you have blood in your urine.

CALL YOUR DOCTOR

Always call a doctor if you have any of the following:

- Your symptoms persist and don't improve within two to three days
- You have blood in your urine
- You have a high temperature, feel nauseous, and are vomiting
- You have severe abdominal or lower back pain
- You're diabetic, pregnant, or over 65 years of age
- You have, or have had, any other kidney related problems, such as kidney stones.

IMMEDIATE RELIEF

You can take regular, warm baths to help ease the pain and discomfort of cystitis, avoiding the use of any scented bath products.

Healing Drinks

- Drink two cups of pure unsweetened cranberry juice daily during an attack of cystitis. The juice contains an acid that helps acidify the urine and prevent bacteria from sticking to the bladder lining. If you don't like the taste, then opt for tablets containing cranberry extract instead.
- Marshmallow root also produces a similar effect by increasing levels of acid in urine and reducing the growth of bacteria. Brew a pot of marshmallow root tea and drink two to three cups daily.

Quick Fix

Add half a teaspoon of baking soda to a glass of water and drink it. This can help make your urine less acidic.

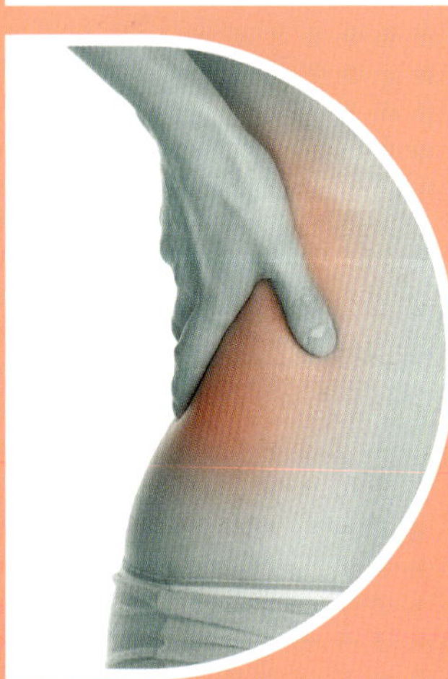

Kidney Stones

Kidney stones are solid masses that form in the kidney from substances found in the urine, such as calcium and acid. They can remain in the kidney, or travel through the urinary tract—small stones may pass out without causing much discomfort and you may not even know you have them. However, if a stone becomes large, moves into the ureter, and gets stuck, it can cause severe pain, infection, and, in some instances, damage to the kidneys.

SYMPTOMS

- Pain or aching on one or both sides of your back
- Spasms of severe pain
- Blood in the urine
- Cloudy urine
- Burning feeling when you urinate
- Fever or chills
- Vomiting

PREVENTION

About 50 percent of people who have had kidney stones develop more within the next 10 years. Once you have had one or more stones and know what type you are susceptible to, there are practical steps you can take to reduce your risk of additional kidney stones.

- If you've had a uric acid stone, then cutting down on the amount of meat you eat can help, because when meat breaks down it makes uric acid.
- If you've had a calcium oxalate kidney stone, it helps to cut down on foods that are high in oxalate, such as spinach, rhubarb, coffee, and chocolate.
- Drinking plenty of water—between 8 and 12 cups daily—can help reduce the levels of the substances that form kidney stones and flush them through your system.
- Keep active, get regular exercise, and aim to eat a healthy, balanced diet.

CONVENTIONAL TREATMENTS

Drinking a lot of water and just being active can sometimes be enough to flush a small stone through the body. Painkillers can be taken to help with the pain. If there's a kidney infection alongside the stones, antibiotics may be required. For large stones that are not passed through naturally, a treatment called extracorporeal shock wave lithotripsy is used under local anaesthetic to break down the kidney stones. If stones get stuck in the ureter or are very large, surgery may be required to remove them.

NATURAL REMEDIES

There are some helpful self-help home remedies for you to try. Try drinking dandelion or nettle tea. They both act as natural diuretics, helping your kidneys to function well. Use two tablespoons dried leaves, or you can buy them as tea bags. Ideally, drink two to three cups of dandelion or nettle tea daily.

HERBAL REMEDIES Use herbs with diuretic properties to increase and dilute your urine, such as herbal tinctures of stone root or parsley piert. To ease an inflamed urinary system, you can take a tincture of marshmallow and couch grass. Just dilute one milliliter tincture in a teaspoon of water three times a day.

NUTRITIONAL MEDICINE Take vitamin B6, vitamin K, and magnesium supplements, because they may help reduce the crystallization process that causes kidney stones to form. You can take vitamin A and the amino acid lysine to lower levels of calcium excretion.

HEALING FOODS

- Eat plenty of cranberries, or drink cranberry juice, to help any associated infection.
- Include bran in your diet, because it can reduce the absorption of calcium and lower levels of calcium in the urine.

CALL YOUR DOCTOR

If you are experiencing severe pain in the kidney region and any other symptoms of kidney stones, don't self-diagnose or try and treat it yourself—always see a doctor for a professional diagnosis and treatment.

Caution

Natural remedies can be helpful for future kidney stone prevention and for helping ease any further symptoms, but they should not be used as a first port of call.

TOP 20
Homeopathic Remedies

Homeopathy is a holistic treatment, which is based on the principle that "like cures like." Diluted natural substances are used to stimulate the body's natural defenses. The remedy used will depend on the ailment and symptoms, but treatment should always be on a constitutional basis, taking into account the patient's personality, emotional attributes, personal likes and dislikes, and physical features. It is better to consult a qualified homeopathic practitioner instead of making a diagnosis yourself.

1 ARGENTUM NITRICUM

Constitutional features Cheerful and outgoing when well; anxious when unwell

Used for Nervous disorders, anxiety, chronic fatigue syndrome, depression; and digestive problems, including indigestion and irritable bowel syndrome

2 ARSENICUM ALBUM

Constitutional features Restless and anxious with desire for order and tidiness

Used for Digestive problems, food poisoning, diarrhea, vomiting, peptic ulcers; and skin ailments, such as eczema and psoriasis; conjunctivitis; sore throat; and dandruff

3 BELLADONNA

Constitutional features Lively and sensitive but prone to sudden-onset illness

Used for Fever, headaches, neuralgia; arthritis; tonsillitis, earache; German measles; abdominal pain with nausea and vomiting

4 BRYONIA ALBA

Constitutional features For people in business working hard, who may feel angry or disappointed

Used for Acute illnesses; rheumatism, arthritis, sciatica and backache; headache; diarrhea, indigestion, and gastritis

5 CHAMOMILLA

Constitutional features Constitutional medicine, for hypersensitive people

Used for Toothache, teething, and earache; arthritis; painful periods; withdrawal symptoms after giving up caffeine, alcohol, or smoking

6 HEPAR SULPHURIS

Constitutional features Mentally and physically sensitive

Used for Skin conditions, acne, boils, abscesses; sore throat, coughs, bronchitis; neuralgia

7 IGNATIA

Constitutional features For idealists, romantics, grief, and disappointment

Used for Digestive problems, diarrhea, stomach cramps; headaches; coughs

8 IPECAC

Constitutional features Constitutional medicine

Used for Asthma; coughs; morning sickness, nausea, and vomiting

9 LACHESIS

Constitutional features Intense, competitive, talkative, prone to jealousy

Used for Depression; menopause; asthma; back pain, sciatica; neuralgia

10 MERCURIUS SOLUBILIS

Constitutional features Calm, reserved, susceptible to temperature changes

Used for Arthritis; colds, sore throat, tonsillitis, ear infections; canker sores; colitis

11 NATRUM MURIATICUM

Constitutional features Constitutional medicine, for sensitive people with suppressed emotions

Used for Back pain; colds; headache, premenstrual tension; canker sores, cold sores; eczema, psoriasis; irritable bowel syndrome; asthma

12 NUX VOMICA

Constitutional features Ambitious workaholics, impatient, competitive

Used for Stress, fatigue; sleep problems, insomnia; headache; asthma, hay fever; irritable bowel syndrome, peptic ulcers, colic

13 PHOSPHORUS

Constitutional features Enthusiasm for life, empathy for other people, fear of being alone

Used for Respiratory problems, bronchitis, coughs; digestive disorders, peptic ulcers, gastroenteritis; angina; nose bleeds

14 PULSATILLA

Constitutional features Emotional, timid, or symptoms due to hormonal changes and pregnancy

Used for Asthma, hay fever; arthritis, diarrhea, constipation, irritable bowel syndrome; morning sickness; period problems, postnatal depression; conjunctivitis; ear infections

15 RHUS TOXICODENDRON

Constitutional features Cheerful and lively when well; depressed and agitated when ill

Used for Rheumatism, arthritis, sprains, neck pain and stiffness; influenza; shingles, chicken pox; eczema

16 SABINA

Constitutional features Do not feel cold but intolerant of heat

Used for Heavy periods, nosebleeds; arthritis, gout; back pain

17 SANGUINARIA CANADENSIS

Constitutional features Regularly recurring conditions, such as migraine

Used for Allergies, asthma, hay fever; migraine, menopausal hot flashes; shoulder pain

18 SEPIA

Constitutional features Exhausted, feeling drained and dull

Used for Headaches; backache; constipation; fatigue, depression, premenstrual syndrome; cystitis, nausea in pregnancy

19 SILICA

Constitutional features Delicate, lacking stamina, sensitive, poor self-esteem

Used for Abscesses, skin infections; headaches

20 SULFUR

Constitutional features Intellectual, self-confident, self-absorbed

Used for Arthritis; acne, eczema, abscesses; conjunctivitis; diarrhea; tonsillitis; migraine; dandruff

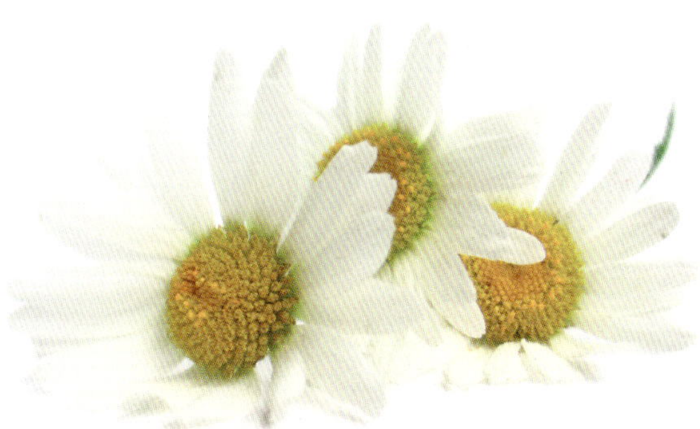

Emotional and Nervous Disorders

With so many people leading busy, stressful lives, it's no wonder that emotional disorders and psychological illnesses are common and can profoundly affect quality of life. Emotional health is shaped by personal experiences, relationships, and body image. People who feel valued and comfortable about themselves, who can manage stress, can forge strong, close relationships with family and friends, can adapt to changes in their lives, and can recover rapidly from setbacks also tend to be psychologically healthy and less likely to have emotional and nervous disorders.

Some health problems, such as headaches and migraines, are not indicative of your emotional health, but fatigue, anxiety, and insomnia may be a temporary reaction to a difficult stressful situation or symptomatic of deeper psychological disorders. Some health conditions, such as chronic fatigue syndrome (CFS), are still controversial and experts are divided on whether they are physical or entirely psychological illnesses.

You cannot eliminate stress, difficult situations, and trauma from your life, but you can take positive action to enable you to cope with them, to manage your condition, and to adapt accordingly. As with other aspects of your health, good nutrition and regular exercise have an important role to play. Natural remedies and therapies, including yoga, meditation, relaxation, massage, aromatherapy, herbal medicine, and homeopathy, are also helpful. In addition, depending on the problem and its severity, there are many conventional treatments, such as medication, counseling, cognitive behavioral therapy, and self-help groups.

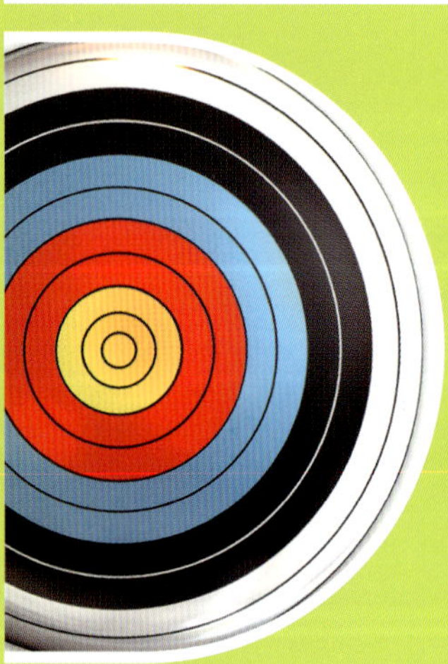

Headache

Most people experience the head and neck pain associated with a headache at some point. Headaches can be brought on by a variety of factors, including tiredness, hunger, stress, bad posture, sunlight, vision problems, or certain foods and drinks. They can vary according to the severity of the symptoms and the frequency with which they occur.

SYMPTOMS

- Mild to moderate pain on both sides of your head
- Pressure around your head
- Tightened neck muscles
- Pressure behind your eyes

PREVENTION

In order to prevent headaches, it helps to understand what is causing them, so that you can make the appropriate lifestyle changes.

- Note how often you get headaches, how severe they are, and how long they last. This will help you identify what triggers them. For example, you may find you get headaches when you are hungry, anxious, driving, or after working at a computer screen for long periods.
- Try to manage your stress levels. Stress is a frequent cause of tension headaches.
- Get regular exercise. Aim for 30 minutes of moderate physical activity five days a week. This helps to reduce stress and the likelihood of getting a stress-related headache.
- Are you using painkillers frequently? You may get withdrawal headaches when you are not taking them. Either stop taking the painkillers altogether, or try to wean yourself off them gradually.

Did You Know?

There are three main categories of headache, including tension headaches, cluster and migraine headaches, and sinus-related headaches. Tension headaches, caused by muscle contractions, are the most common. The frequency of headaches tends to drop as people get older.

CONVENTIONAL TREATMENTS

Try to identify the cause of your headaches and eliminate it. Over-the-counter painkillers can be taken for most headaches, such as acetaminophen, aspirin, or ibuprofen. Antidepressant medicines, such as amitriptyline, may be prescribed for preventing migraine headaches. Cognitive behavioral therapy (a talking treatment) can help you to deal with stress.

NATURAL REMEDIES

The following remedies may help to provide welcome pain relief from headaches.

ACUPUNCTURE This treatment stimulates the flow of energy through your body to relieve pain and reduce the frequency of headaches.

CHIROPRACTIC Relieves muscular tension in the head, neck, and shoulders and corrects posture to stop the pain of headaches.

REFLEXOLOGY This works on the spinal reflex areas of the foot to reduce tension in the spine.

HERBAL REMEDIES

- For tension headaches, drink rosemary or lime blossom tea.
- For fatigue headaches, sip chamomile tea.

AROMATHERAPY

Try these essential oils for relief from headaches.

- Add a few drops of lavender, peppermint, or bergamot essential oils to a carrier oil and massage into the back of your neck.
- Add eucalyptus, spearmint, sweet marjoram, or basil essential oils to a vaporizer.
- Add several drops of peppermint, grapefruit, or rosewood essential oils to a nice warm bath.

HOMEOPATHIC REMEDIES

The homeopathic remedy you select will depend on the type of headache you have.

Belladonna 30C: Take two tablets three times daily for a throbbing, pulsating headache.

Nux vomica 30C: Take two tablets three times daily for a headache triggered by food or drink.

Arnica 30C: Take two tablets four times daily for a headache caused by trauma or injury.

CALL YOUR DOCTOR

Although most headaches don't require medical attention, you should see your doctor if:

- You have frequent headaches (on more than 15 days of the month)
- Your headache comes on suddenly and is extremely painful
- You have a stiff neck, high temperature, a rash, nausea, or vomiting
- You start having headaches after an accident or head injury
- You feel weak, numb, confused, or you have slurred speech
- You have disturbed vision.

IMMEDIATE RELIEF

To bring instant relief, apply a hot facecloth to your forehead or neck and hold it there for a few minutes.

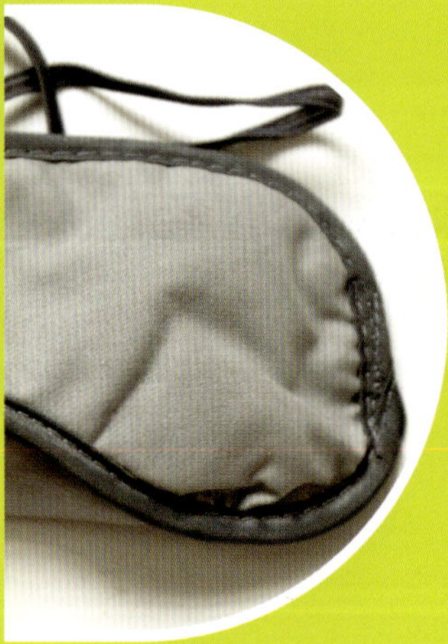

Migraine

Migraines are severe, throbbing headaches, which may last just a few hours or even several days. They can be triggered by a number of different factors, such as stress, dehydration, tiredness, smoking, chocolate, cheese, red wine, or orange juice. Anyone can experience migraines, but they are more common among women than men.

SYMPTOMS

- ▷ Intense pain on one side of the head, or at the front of the head
- ▷ Nausea or vomiting
- ▷ Visual disturbances, such as partial loss of vision or flashing lights
- ▷ Sensitivity to light, sound, or smells
- ▷ Stomachache
- ▷ Feeling hot or cold, or sweating

Did You Know?

It is not clear what causes migraines. It is thought that blood vessels in the brain become narrower, temporarily restricting blood supply. When they widen again, this causes a severe headache.

PREVENTION

In order to prevent migraine attacks, it helps if you can identify the factors that trigger them, so that you can try to avoid them.

- Keep a diary of when your migraines occur, the symptoms you have, how long they last, and anything you ate beforehand.
- Eat regular meals. Fluctuating blood sugar levels caused by eating irregularly can trigger migraines.
- Avoid dehydration by getting plenty of fluids.
- Establish a regular sleeping pattern; try to go to bed and get up at the same time each day.
- Try to manage your stress levels.
- Getting regular exercise may help to prevent migraines.

CONVENTIONAL TREATMENTS

Many people find they are able to manage their migraines by keeping away from the things that cause them. In the event of a migraine attack, it helps to lie down in a quiet, dark room. Over-the-counter remedies, such as acetaminophen or ibuprofen, help to relieve symptoms. Triptan medicines work by constricting blood vessels in the brain. Your doctor may also prescribe antivomiting medicines or nonsteroidal anti-inflammatory drugs (NSAIDs).

NATURAL REMEDIES

Try the following natural remedies and therapies to reduce the severity of migraines.

NUTRITIONAL MEDICINE Migraines could be related to low levels of magnesium. Good food sources of this mineral include spinach, nuts, seeds, and whole-grain cereals.

ACUPUNCTURE This may be effective in reducing the frequency of migraines by using needles to stimulate the flow of energy through the body.

AROMATHERAPY Add a few drops of rosemary essential oil to a bowl of steaming hot water. Cover your head with a towel, lean over the bowl, and inhale the steam for 10 minutes.

HERBAL REMEDIES

Taking the following herbs may help to relieve the symptoms of migraines.

- Take 380 milligrams of feverfew once or twice daily.
- Take 60 milligrams of butterbur two to four times a day.

HOMEOPATHIC REMEDIES

The remedy will depend on the type of pain:

Bryonia 30C: Take two tablets three times daily for sharp pain in the forehead or back of the head, which may be accompanied by either nausea or vomiting.

Natrum muriaticum 30C: Take two tablets four times daily for a beating pain in the head that is made better when lying down in a dark room.

Lachesis 6C: Take two tablets three times daily for migraine which is triggered by food or drink.

CALL YOUR DOCTOR

You should see your doctor if:

- You have a sudden, severe headache for the first time, especially if you are over 50 years old
- You can't seem to do anything to relieve your symptoms
- You are having frequent migraines (daily or weekly)
- You experience fever, vomiting, or a rash
- You keep having stiffness, numbness, or tingling on the same side of your body.

Quick Fix

For some migraine sufferers, drinking two or three glasses of cold tap water at the first signs of an oncoming migraine may be sufficient to prevent it.

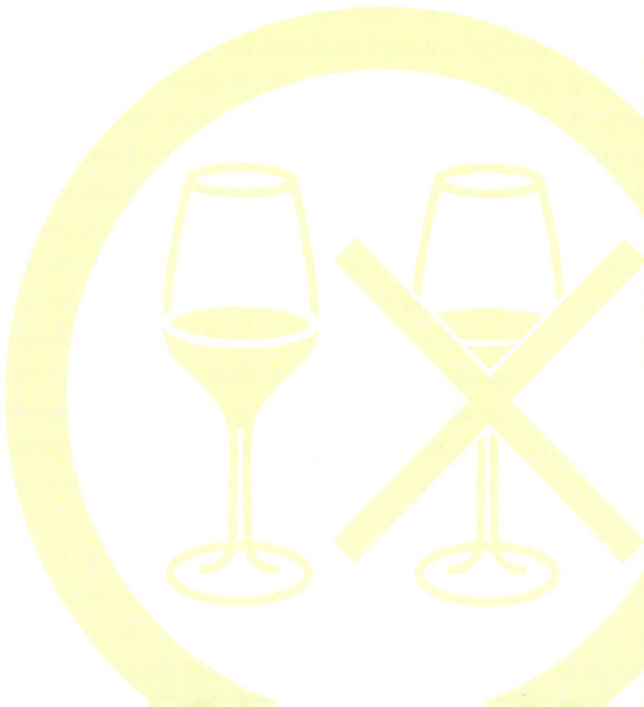

Fatigue

Fatigue is characterized by tiredness and exhaustion, which can have either a physical or an emotional cause. People may experience fatigue due to sleeping difficulties, stress, anxiety, being overweight or underweight, too little exercise, or pregnancy. Sometimes fatigue can be so severe that it interferes with normal day-to-day life.

SYMPTOMS

- Physical or mental tiredness
- Weakness and lack of energy
- Palpitations (irregular or rapid heartbeat)
- Feeling faint
- Breathlessness
- Difficulty concentrating and making decisions
- Lack of motivation
- Depression

Did You Know?

Lack of physical activity can cause fatigue. If you don't exercise regularly, your level of fitness falls, so when you do need to be active, you get tired more easily.

PREVENTION

Lifestyle changes, such as having a good diet, getting more exercise, and getting more sleep, should help to prevent fatigue.

- Eat plenty of fruits, vegetables, and protein to maintain your energy levels. Don't skip meals because this will lead to fluctuating blood sugar levels and cause fatigue.
- Try to avoid sugary foods, such as cakes and cookies. These will cause a surge in blood sugar levels, which will then drop quickly, leaving you tired and irritable.
- Get regular exercise. Aim for 30 minutes of moderate-intensity physical activity five days a week, but don't exercise just before going to bed.
- Try to find ways to cope with stress, and learn how to relax.
- Go to bed and get up at the same time each day, and don't take naps during the day.
- Don't eat a heavy meal before going to bed.
- Avoid caffeine, alcohol, and tobacco before you go to bed, and cut down on these substances in general.
- Try to do something relaxing before bedtime each night, such as taking a warm bath.

CONVENTIONAL TREATMENTS

People often find their fatigue improves by having a good rest, eating properly, and exercising. If fatigue is caused by an underlying medical condition, such as anemia or a thyroid disorder, appropriate treatment should relieve any associated tiredness.

NATURAL REMEDIES

You may find the following natural remedies are useful for combating fatigue and making you feel more energetic.

NUTRITIONAL MEDICINE Make sure your diet contains adequate amounts of the B vitamins, which are important for the release of energy from food. Good sources include meat, yeast extract, beans, and bananas.

AROMATHERAPY For an energizing, stimulating massage oil, try blending six drops of grapefruit and four drops of ginger essential oils with two tablespoons of jojoba oil.

ACUPUNCTURE Thin needles are placed at specific locations on your body in order to unblock the flow of energy and relieve fatigue.

HERBAL REMEDIES

You may like to try taking one of the following herbs to relieve fatigue and boost your energy.

- One to two milliliters of American ginseng extract three times daily.
- Four drops of gentian extract at least four times a day.
- 550 milligrams of ginger root twice daily.
- 500 milligrams of Siberian ginseng three times daily.

EXERCISE

Deep breathing exercises may relieve fatigue by releasing tension and improving oxygen circulation.

1 Lie on your back and relax with your knees bent.

2 Place one hand on your chest and the other on your stomach.

3 Breathe in deeply through your nose and exhale through your mouth.

NOTE Breathe in from your abdomen—you should feel your stomach rise higher than your chest. Continue this breathing exercise for a few minutes.

CALL YOUR DOCTOR

If you feel constantly tired and self-help measures don't seem to be working, consult your doctor. Fatigue can be caused by other conditions, such as anemia, asthma, thyroid problems, diabetes, malnutrition, infection, or chronic fatigue syndrome.

Caution

Don't drink high-energy carbonated beverages to relieve your fatigue. They are full of sugar and, after a brief blood sugar surge, you will feel even worse than you did before.

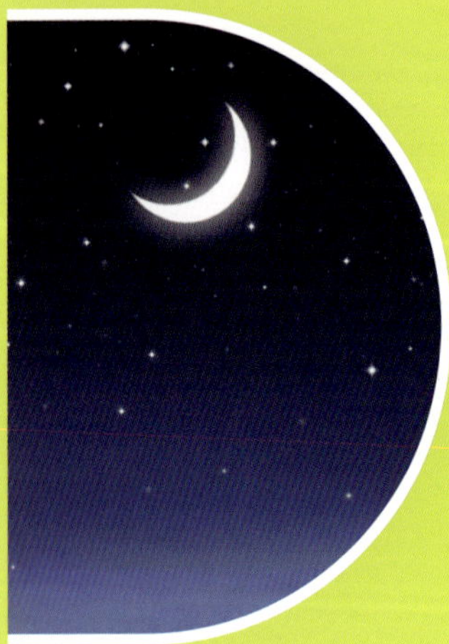

Insomnia

Most people will have trouble sleeping sometimes, but insomnia is a chronic sleep disorder, characterized by the frequent inability to fall asleep or stay asleep. This can go on for days, months, or even years. There are, however, things you can do to help yourself get a good night's sleep and wake up feeling refreshed the following day.

SYMPTOMS

- Difficulty getting to sleep
- Frequently waking in the night
- Waking early in the morning, and inability to get back to sleep
- Difficulty concentrating
- Irritability and tiredness

Did You Know?

There is no normal amount of sleep that is right for every individual. In general, most adults sleep for seven to nine hours each night, but older people tend to need less sleep, while children need a lot more.

PREVENTION

Simple changes to your evening routine can help you to sleep better. Prevention is better than cure, so try the following measures and see if they help.

- Don't take naps during the day.
- Make sure your bed is comfortable. Use thick curtains, blinds or shades, or an eye mask to block out light, and wear earplugs if noise disturbs you.
- Don't use the bedroom for activities unrelated to sleep, such as watching television, making phone calls, or eating.
- Make sure that you always go to bed and get up at the same time every day.
- Write down any worries you may have before going to bed.
- Do something relaxing every night before you go to bed, such as taking a warm bath.
- Don't eat a heavy meal late in the evening.
- Avoid coffee, tea, alcohol, or nicotine six hours before bed.
- Exercise regularly, but not within four hours of going to bed.
- Avoid checking the clock throughout the night. If you can't sleep, get up and do something else for a while.

CONVENTIONAL TREATMENTS

Treatment for insomnia involves addressing the cause of the disorder, such as reducing caffeine and alcohol intake. Sleeping pills, such as the benzodiazepines, ramelteon, zaleplon, and zolpidem, help aid sleep but are usually only for short-term use. Cognitive behavioral therapy may be recommended to help change your sleeping habits and negative thoughts about your insomnia.

NATURAL REMEDIES

There are many natural remedies you can try to help you sleep. Here are some options.

NUTRITIONAL MEDICINE Milk, eggs, turkey, chicken, and fish are good sources of the amino acid tryptophan, which is thought to have a calming effect and help to induce sleep.

ACUPUNCTURE This treatment calms your nervous system, relieves stress, and rebalances your energy, giving you a sense of deep relaxation.

REFLEXOLOGY Apply firm pressure to the top of the pad of your big toe to clear your mind and body in preparation for sleep.

HERBAL REMEDIES

To aid relaxation, try one of these popular remedies.

- Drink chamomile tea to soothe and calm you.
- Take one 450-milligram capsule of valerian root before bed to aid sleep.

AROMATHERAPY

Essential oils can calm and soothe and prepare you for a restful night's sleep.

- Place a drop of soothing lavender essential oil on a tissue, and put it under your pillow.
- Have a warm bath with a few added drops of marjoram, rose, or Roman chamomile essential oils to relax you before bed.
- Mix up to 15 drops of ylang ylang, sandalwood, or clary sage essential oils (you can create your own combination) with two tablespoons of jojoba oil and use it for a relaxing massage.

CALL YOUR DOCTOR

Insomnia can sometimes have an underlying cause, such as a physical or psychological medical condition. If it is persistent and is affecting your physical and mental health, you should see your doctor. After the appropriate treatment, your insomnia may go away.

Quick Fix

Lettuce has been used as a soporific since ancient times. Eat a lettuce sandwich before going to bed. Alternatively, a hot, soothing milky drink may help to relax you.

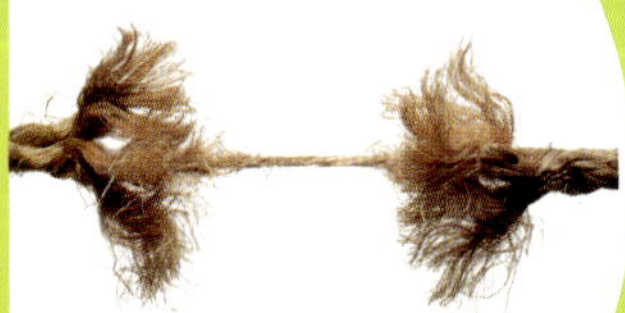

Stress

Stress is the mental or physical strain you experience when you are under pressure. This can be caused when you are faced with situations that you find difficult to handle. Common causes of stress include a wide range of factors, such as work pressures, money problems, relationship and family issues, and bereavement.

SYMPTOMS

- Anxiety, depression, frustration, or tearfulness
- Loss of control
- Difficulty concentrating
- Behavioral changes
- Headaches and other aches and pains
- Difficulty sleeping and restlessness
- Changes in appetite
- Sweating
- Nervous twitching, or pins and needles
- Palpitations (rapid or irregular heartbeat), breathlessness, or dizziness
- Constipation or diarrhea

Did You Know?

When under stress, your body releases chemicals, including cortisol, adrenaline, and noradrenaline. These chemicals build up and produce the emotional and physical symptoms that we associate with stress.

PREVENTION

Identifying the things that make you stressed and learning how to cope with them in a different way is the key to preventing the symptoms of stress. You also need to look after your physical and mental health.

- Learn some relaxation techniques to calm you down and relieve muscle tension.
- Make an effort to do things you enjoy. See your friends, read a book, listen to music, or do whatever makes you happy.
- Write down the things that are making you feel stressed; this can help you work out ways of organizing and prioritizing your responsibilities.
- Talk to someone about how you feel; this can give you a new perspective on the things that are troubling you.
- Eat a healthy, balanced diet with plenty of fruits and vegetables.
- Limit your alcohol and caffeine intake, and don't smoke.
- Exercise regularly.

CONVENTIONAL TREATMENTS

Learning how to handle difficult situations, having a good work-life balance, and looking after your health are all important for managing stress effectively. Stress and anger management techniques, and talking therapies, such as cognitive behavioral therapy or counseling, can teach you how to deal with stress. Medication may be given to treat anxiety or depression if these are symptoms of stress.

NATURAL REMEDIES

For natural relief from stress, you can try taking the following therapies.

NUTRITIONAL MEDICINE Vitamin C is an antioxidant that may help reduce the physical and psychological symptoms of stress. Good sources include red and green bell peppers, oranges and other citrus fruits, kiwis, broccoli, strawberries, and Brussels sprouts.

AROMATHERAPY Blend nine drops of bergamot, three drops of geranium, and three drops of frankincense essential oils with four tablespoons of jojoba oil. Add one-quarter of this blend to a nice warm bath.

REFLEXOLOGY Massage the ball of your foot to help you relax, and gently tug your toes to release tension in your head and shoulders.

HERBAL REMEDIES

- Take 500 milligrams of Korean ginseng three times daily to help your body cope with the effects of stress.
- Green tea may help to reduce levels of stress hormones and promote relaxation.
- Take 450 milligrams of Valerian root daily to reduce tension, anxiety, and irritability and aid restful sleep.

HOMEOPATHIC REMEDIES

The following remedies may help to relieve the symptoms of stress.

Aconite 6C: Take two tablets four times daily for anxiety, restlessness, and trouble sleeping.

Arsenicum 6C: Take two tablets four times daily for worry with an upset stomach.

Phosphorus 6C: Take two tablets three times daily for anxiety and nervousness.

CALL YOUR DOCTOR

If you are having difficulty dealing with stress, call your doctor. Stress is a common problem, and a physician will be able to help you cope. It may also be necessary to run some tests to check that your symptoms are not due to another underlying medical condition.

IMMEDIATE RELIEF

If you are in a traumatic situation, an emergency, or you are feeling very stressed, take some Bach Rescue Remedy to calm you down.

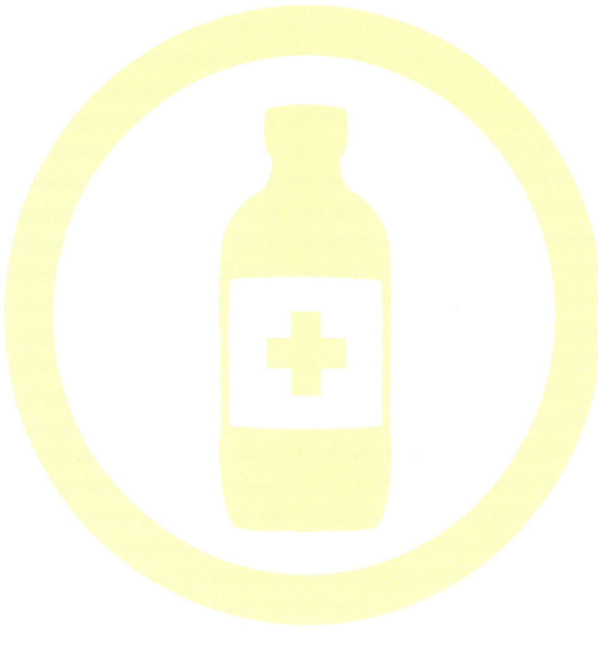

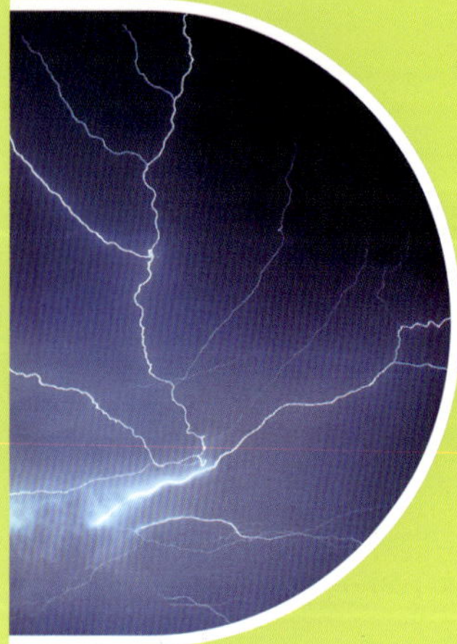

Neuralgia

Neuralgia is extreme nerve pain in the face or other parts of the body. Pain in the face may come on suddenly and last for a few seconds or minutes at a time, or pain in the body may last for days or even months. Neuralgia can be a difficult condition to live with—even smiling or the lightest touch of a breeze can cause pain.

SYMPTOMS

- Tingling, numbness
- Stabbing, shooting, shocklike pains in the face
- Pain in the mouth, teeth, and gums
- A burning, aching sensation
- Throbbing pains in the body
- Intense itching

Did You Know?

Trigeminal neuralgia is thought to be caused by blood vessels pressing on the trigeminal nerve, which runs through the face. Postherpetic neuralgia may be a result of nerve damage caused by shingles infection, and can occur in different parts of the body.

PREVENTION

To prevent pain from neuralgia, it helps to avoid the things that trigger an attack or make the pain worse.

- Wind and drafts can trigger pain, so avoid sitting near open windows or air-conditioning. When outside in breezy weather, protect your face with a scarf.
- Avoid very hot or cold drinks that can trigger pain. Drinking through a straw can help prevent liquid from causing pain in your mouth.
- Rough, synthetic, or tight clothing can aggravate your skin and cause pain. Try wearing loose clothing made from natural fibers, such as cotton.

CONVENTIONAL TREATMENTS

For trigeminal neuralgia, antiseizure medicines, such as Tegretol or Neurontin, are prescribed to numb pain and help settle nerve impulses. Some antidepressants have also been successful for relieving pain. If medication is ineffective, surgery may be recommended to release pressure on the trigeminal nerve. Postherpetic neuralgia is treated with painkillers, such as acetaminophen or codeine, or tricyclic antidepressants to reduce sensitivity to pain. Topical creams containing capsaicin (made from hot peppers), or lidocaine patches containing local anaesthetic may help to relieve pain.

NATURAL REMEDIES

The following natural remedies may be helpful.

NUTRITIONAL MEDICINE Eat more foods that are rich in the B vitamins, such as brewer's yeast, beans, and dairy products. These provide support for the nervous system.

AROMATHERAPY Place a few drops of calming lavender or chamomile essential oils in a carrier oil and massage into painful areas.

ELECTRO-ACUPUNCTURE This is similar to traditional acupuncture, but a low-frequency electric current (1 Hz) is passed down the needles.

HOMEOPATHIC REMEDIES

Treatment depends on the type of pain you have.

Kali phosphoricum 6C: Take four tablets three times daily for pain that is relieved by cold.

Belladonna 30C: Take two tablets three times daily for pain that suddenly comes and goes.

Magnesia phosphorica 6C: Take four tablets three times daily for pain that is relieved with warmth.

HERBAL REMEDIES

The following remedies may provide some relief.

- Take one or two milliliters passion flower tincture up to three times daily, to soothe and calm your central nervous system.
- Take one 150-gram capsule of St. Johns wort three times daily to reduce inflammation, or one milliliter of extract in water up to three times a day.
- Take 15 to 30 drops of wood betony two to three times daily; this has a calming, sedative effect.

CALL YOUR DOCTOR

If you suspect that you have neuralgia, see your doctor. Facial pain can also be caused by dental problems and sinus infection; these need to be ruled out before it can be ascertained whether or not neuralgia is responsible.

IMMEDIATE RELIEF

If your neuralgia is not aggravated by cold temperatures, you can place gel-filled cold packs in the freezer and hold them against painful areas to numb the pain.

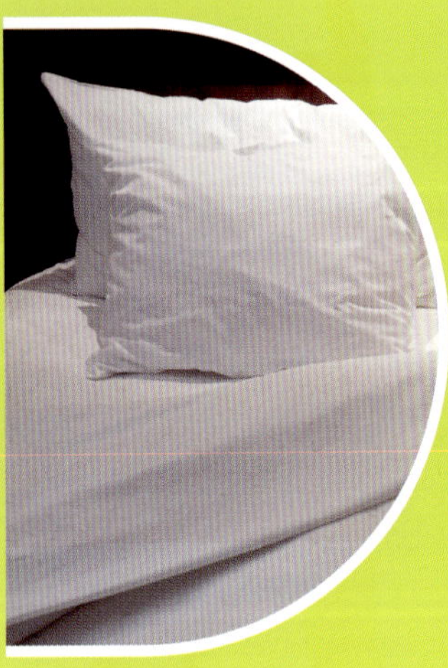

Chronic Fatigue Syndrome

Chronic fatigue syndrome (CFS) is long-term general weakness and muscle pain. Many people have symptoms that come and go, but for others, the condition is so debilitating and serious that they have to spend much of their time in bed, and they may end up wheelchair-bound.

SYMPTOMS

- ▷ Generally feeling unwell
- ▷ Physical and mental exhaustion
- ▷ Muscle aches and pains
- ▷ Poor memory and difficulty concentrating
- ▷ Difficulty moving
- ▷ Headaches
- ▷ Sleeping difficulties
- ▷ Sensitivity to light and sound
- ▷ Depression
- ▷ Painful lymph nodes
- ▷ Stomach problems
- ▷ Sore throat
- ▷ Dizziness and nausea
- ▷ Palpitations (rapid or irregular heartbeat)

Did You Know?

It is not clear what causes chronic fatigue syndrome. It may be triggered by viral infections, such as mononucleosis, a genetic predisposition, stress, depression, or trauma.

PREVENTION

There are positive things that you can do to help prevent the severity of the symptoms associated with chronic fatigue syndrome.

- Learn to manage your stress levels, and make time for relaxation.
- Eat a healthy balanced diet with plenty of fruits and vegetables. Be sure to include foods that release energy slowly, such as oats, whole-grain cereals, and beans.
- People with chronic fatigue syndrome are often sensitive to certain substances and foods, such as alcohol and caffeine, so try to avoid these.
- Keep a diary, so you can track how your energy levels change from day to day. This will help you to pace yourself better.
- Improve your quality of sleep by relaxing before bed each night. Go to bed and get up at the same time each day and try to avoid taking naps during the day.

CONVENTIONAL TREATMENTS

It is important for people to make sure they get the right balance of physical activity and rest that is suitable for them. Painkillers or antidepressants may be prescribed to relieve symptoms. Cognitive behavioral therapy is a talking treatment that helps people to cope with the effects of chronic fatigue syndrome. Supervised, graded exercise therapy aims to increase physical activity slowly, and tailors exercise duration and intensity to your own limits.

NATURAL REMEDIES

You may find the following natural remedies helpful, depending on your symptoms.

NUTRITIONAL MEDICINE Take 100 milligrams Coenzyme Q10 per day for healthy cell function and energy production.

AROMATHERAPY Add 12 drops of rosemary and 18 drops of bergamot essential oils to a spray bottle containing six tablespoons of distilled water. Use as a reviving, energizing air freshener.

ACUPUNCTURE This stimulates your body's energy to relieve fatigue, boost your immune system, and help you sleep better. See a qualified practitioner.

HERBAL REMEDIES

- Take 500 milligrams Korean ginseng three times daily to help increase stamina, relieve stress, boost immune function, and improve concentration.
- Mix one milliliter of echinacea extract in a little water two to five times daily to boost your immune system and reduce the risk of infection.
- Take 470 milligrams of astragalus three to six times daily to strengthen your immune system and reduce inflammation.

HOMEOPATHIC REMEDIES

The following remedies may help relieve symptoms. Take whichever is appropriate for you.

Arsenicum 6C: Take two tablets four times daily when feeling cold and weak.

Gelsemium 6C: Take two tablets four times daily when feeling physically tired with heavy, aching muscles.

Pulsatilla 6C: Take two tablets four times daily for aches and pains and when feeling emotional.

CALL YOUR DOCTOR

If you suspect that you have chronic fatigue syndrome, you should consult your doctor, who will be able to help you manage your condition. It may be necessary to conduct some tests to rule out other conditions that have similar symptoms to chronic fatigue syndrome, such as kidney disease, anemia, or thyroid problems.

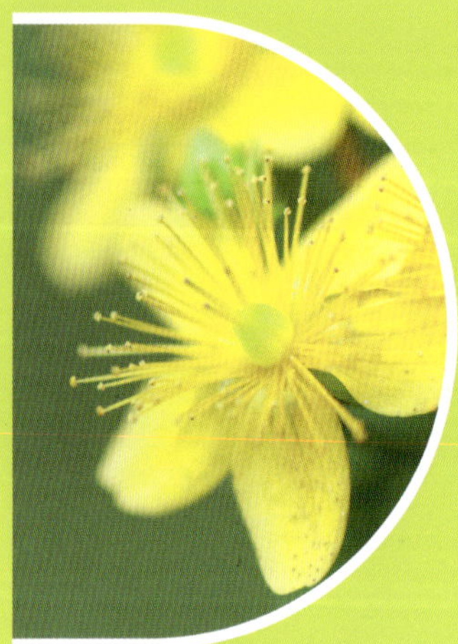

Depression

Depression is a mental illness that is characterized by feelings of sadness and hopelessness lasting for more than two weeks. Depression interferes with everyday life, preventing people from getting on with the things they would normally do. Symptoms can be psychological, social, or physical, and can affect anyone at any age.

SYMPTOMS

- ▷ Feeling low, with negative thoughts about the future
- ▷ Little interest in doing things you used to enjoy
- ▷ Anxiety and low self-esteem
- ▷ Inability to concentrate
- ▷ Trouble making decisions
- ▷ Irritability
- ▷ Unable to cope with normal things
- ▷ Feelings of guilt
- ▷ Trouble sleeping
- ▷ Tiredness and lack of energy
- ▷ Aches and pains
- ▷ Lack of appetite and weight loss (but sometimes weight gain)
- ▷ Loss of libido
- ▷ Social inactivity, work, and home life problems
- ▷ Thoughts of self-harm

Did You Know?

People with a family history of depression have an increased risk of experiencing depression themselves. Depression can also be triggered by life events, such as bereavement or loss of employment.

PREVENTION

A healthy lifestyle is important for preventing depression. The following can be helpful.

- Eat a balanced diet with plenty of fresh fruits and vegetables. Try to avoid sugar highs and lows, caused by foods such as cakes, cookies, and chocolate.
- Exercise regularly. Exercise will help you feel better about yourself and get you out of the house.
- Don't drink excessively. Men should drink no more than two drinks per day and women no more than one drink a day.
- Avoid recreational drugs, such as cannabis and cocaine; these will probably make you feel worse.
- If you smoke heavily, try to cut down or, better still, quit altogether.
- Make an effort with social relationships—with friends, family, and work colleagues.
- Keep up with your interests and hobbies.
- Learn how to deal with stress and relax.

CONVENTIONAL TREATMENTS

For mild depression, self-help measures, such as self-help books, an exercise program, or local support groups, may be all you need to recover. If depression is more severe, there are antidepressants, such as SSRIs (selective serotonin reuptake inhibitors), which alter levels of chemicals in the brain to improve mood. Psychological treatments, such as cognitive behavioral therapy, interpersonal therapy, or counseling, may also be recommended.

NATURAL REMEDIES

You may like to try the following treatments alongside conventional remedies.

NUTRITIONAL MEDICINE A lack of omega-3 fatty acids in the diet (found in cold-water fish, flaxseeds, and walnuts) may contribute to symptoms of depression. If your diet is lacking, consider taking an omega-3 supplement.

ACUPUNCTURE This treatment frees up the body's energy, increases the production of "feel good" chemicals in the brain, and promotes relaxation.

AROMATHERAPY Aromatherapy massage with essential oils, such as orange, sandalwood, or lavender, can help aid relaxation and relieve symptoms of depression.

HERBAL REMEDIES

Here are some herbal remedies that you might find useful in treating depression.

- St. John's wort may be as effective as antidepressants. Take 300 milligrams three times daily.
  NOTE St. John's wort can interfere with other medications, so check with your doctor if necessary.
- Try taking 60 milligrams of ginkgo biloba daily to relieve symptoms.

EXERCISE

Research shows that exercise is an effective way of treating depression and boosting self-esteem. It is thought to work by increasing levels of serotonin (a neurotransmitter in the brain) and endorphins (the body's natural painkillers). Try doing 30 minutes of physical activity, such as running, brisk walking, or aerobics three to five times a week. You may need to work up to this, depending on your fitness level. Also consider other types of exercise, such as weight training, yoga, or tai chi.

CALL YOUR DOCTOR

In severe cases of depression, early diagnosis is important. If you are feeling depressed and the symptoms persist and do not improve as time passes, you should call your doctor or seek professional advice and counseling.

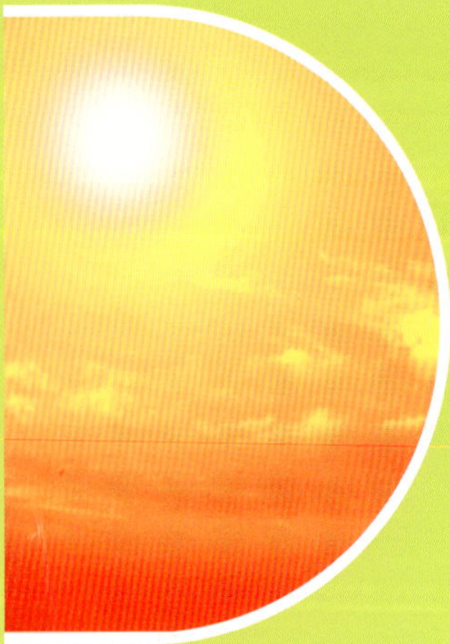

Seasonal Affective Disorder

Seasonal affective disorder (SAD) is a type of depression experienced by people during the winter. Symptoms occur repeatedly at the same time each year, and improve over spring and summer. As with other types of depression, SAD affects normal daily life and can be debilitating.

SYMPTOMS

- Feeling low and unhappy
- Irritability and tearfulness
- Stress, anxiety, and low self-esteem
- Lack of motivation
- Little interest in things you used to enjoy
- Difficulty concentrating and making decisions
- Lack of energy
- Spending more time sleeping
- Feelings of guilt
- Increased appetite (especially for carbohydrates) and weight gain

PREVENTION

You can help prevent symptoms of SAD by getting as much exposure to natural light as possible. You may also benefit from some lifestyle changes.

- Try and get outside for a short walk each day, whatever the weather.
- Make sure your indoor environment is as bright as possible, and try to sit near a window.
- Exercise regularly, outside if possible. Exercise increases the level of serotonin (the "feel good" hormone) in the brain. Aim for 30 minutes of moderate to vigorous physical activity five times a week.
- Eat a healthy, well-balanced diet with plenty of fresh fruits and vegetables. Eating properly can have a profound effect on your mood.
- Try to reduce your stress levels, and learn how to relax.

Did You Know?

It is not clear what causes SAD, but it is thought to be related to a lack of sunlight during the winter months. Reduced sunlight decreases the production of serotonin, a chemical in the brain, which is found to be low in people with depression.

CONVENTIONAL TREATMENTS

Antidepressants, such as selective serotonin reuptake inhibitors (SSRIs), increase the level of serotonin in the brain and improve mood. Talking therapies, such as cognitive behavioral therapy, counseling, or psychotherapy, may be recommended. Light therapy involves sitting beside a light box (a special lamp that emits bright light). This imitates natural sunlight and stimulates the production of serotonin, while reducing the production of melatonin (a hormone that induces sleep).

NATURAL REMEDIES

The following remedies may help you to feel better and relieve the symptoms of SAD.

AROMATHERAPY For an energizing and stimulating air freshener, add 18 drops of orange and 12 drops of grapefruit essential oils to a spray bottle containing six tablespoons of distilled water.

REFLEXOLOGY Try massaging the pads of the big toes. These areas correspond to the parts of the brain responsible for regulating mood.

ACUPUNCTURE This treatment regulates energy flow and rebalances your body to relieve the symptoms of depression.

HEALING FOODS

The following nutrients may help to reduce symptoms.

- The body needs tryptophan to make serotonin. It occurs in chicken, dairy products, eggs, fish, nuts, and seeds. It can also be taken as a supplement in the form of 5-hydroxytryptophan (5-HTP).
- Vitamin D is important. You get this from the action of sunlight on your skin, but it is also found in oily fish, eggs, and fortified foods.
- Omega-3 fatty acids are found in oily fish, flaxseeds, and walnuts.

HERBAL REMEDIES

You may find the following herbs and supplements useful for treating SAD.

- Take 300 milligrams of St. John's Wort three times daily to treat mild to moderate depression.
- Take 1,000 milligrams Korean ginseng three times daily to reduce stress and improve your mood.
- Take 500 milligrams of dl-phenylalanine (DPLA) daily to stimulate the production of "feel good" chemicals in your brain.
- Lemon balm is a natural antidepressant—drink it as a tea or use it in salads and soups.
- Many culinary herbs are uplifting and stimulating, so try to cook with them every day. Choose from basil, parsley, mint, thyme, rosemary, sage, ginger, and cinnamon.

CALL YOUR DOCTOR

If you think that you have seasonal affective disorder, you should call your doctor, who will be able to advise you about helpful treatments.

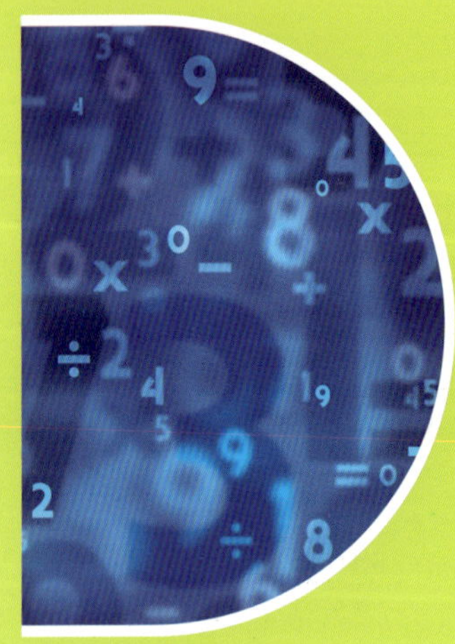

Dementia

Dementia is characterized by emotional, mental, and physical deterioration caused by damage to the brain. Symptoms of dementia can develop suddenly or more slowly over a long period of time, and the risk of dementia increases as you get older. There are different ways of treating the symptoms and improving quality of life.

SYMPTOMS

- Difficulty concentrating and planning things
- Memory loss and confusion
- Short attention span and lack of motivation
- Depression
- Personality, mood, and behavioral changes
- Delusions or hallucinations
- Incontinence
- Muscle weakness, stiffness, or paralysis
- Slow and unsteady movements
- Trembling in arms and legs
- Sleeping difficulties
- Aggression and frustration
- Difficulty communicating

Did You Know?

There are different types of dementia, including Alzheimer's disease, vascular dementia, dementia with Lewy bodies, and frontotemporal dementia. Each type of dementia affects the brain in different ways.

PREVENTION

To prevent dementia in later life, it helps to keep physically and mentally active. There are other factors to consider regarding your general health and well-being. Pay attention to the following.

- Eat a healthy balanced diet with plenty of fruits and vegetables.
- Limit foods that are high in saturated fat.
- Reduce your salt intake to no more than two-thirds of a teaspoon a day (remember that processed foods often already include salt, or sodium).
- Don't drink alcohol excessively. Men should have no more than two drinks a day, and women no more than one.
- Maintain a healthy body weight—obesity can cause high blood pressure.
- Get regular exercise to maintain good circulation.
- Avoid smoking.

CONVENTIONAL TREATMENTS

If you are diagnosed with dementia, a health care plan will be drawn up, and treatment options to manage your symptoms will be discussed. Psychological treatments include cognitive stimulation, behavioral therapy, reality orientation therapy, multisensory stimulation, and exercise therapy. Medications may be helpful, such as acetylcholinesterase inhibitors (AIs) or antipsychotics.

NATURAL REMEDIES

The following natural remedies may help to relieve the symptoms of dementia.

AROMATHERAPY Add a few drops of calming lavender essential oil to a vaporizer to relieve stress, agitation, and depression.

HERBAL REMEDIES Take 60 milligrams of ginkgo biloba twice daily to support the central nervous system, increase blood circulation to the brain, and improve memory.

MUSIC THERAPY Despite the deterioration of mental function associated with dementia, people with the condition are often able to enjoy music. Music therapy can reduce agitation and improve mood, thus enhancing quality of life.

Nutritional Supplements

The following supplements may help slow the advancement of dementia.

- Phosphatidylserine may improve memory and concentration, increase awareness, and relieve depression. Take 100 milligrams three times daily.
- Vitamin E is an antioxidant important for the protection of cell membranes. Take a daily supplement.
- Coenzyme Q10 is an antioxidant important for normal cell function. Take 100 milligrams each day.
- Omega-3 fatty acids support the heart and blood vessels, protect cell membranes and enhance mental function. Take a omega-3 fish oil supplement each day.
- The B vitamins are important for the healthy functioning of the brain and nervous system.
- Zinc is important for good mental function. Take a daily supplement that includes zinc.

HOMEOPATHIC REMEDIES

The following remedies may provide some support, depending on the symptoms.

Alumina 6C: Take two tablets four times daily for sluggishness and staggering.

Argentum nitricum 30C: Take two tablets three times daily for loss of control and trembling.

Cicuta 6C: Take two tablets four times daily for strange or violent behavior.

CALL YOUR DOCTOR

Call your doctor if you suspect that you or your partner may have some of the symptoms of dementia. Symptoms associated with dementia can be caused by other conditions, such as anemia, diabetes, kidney problems, thyroid disorders, or vitamin B_{12} deficiency, so you need to get an accurate diagnosis.

Relaxation and Meditation Techniques

Relaxation and meditation are two important ways of relaxing the body and releasing stress and tension. They have been used in Eastern health systems for thousands of years to help people maintain a healthy body and mind and cope more efficiently with stress. Both relaxation and meditation are easy to learn—here are some ways in which you can incorporate them into your daily life.

MUSCLE RELAXATION TECHNIQUE

Relaxing all the muscles in your body is a great way of releasing tension and stress. You can do it at any time of the day, but it's particularly good at night just before going to bed, as it can help you drift off into a deep sleep once your body is fully relaxed.

1. Lie down flat on your back, wearing loose clothing, and cover yourself with a light blanket. Close your eyes and become aware of your breathing. Take a deep breath and slowly breathe out. If you're breathing fast, try to slow down your breathing into a steady rhythm, pausing briefly as you exhale and before you take another breath.

2. Start by focusing on the muscles in your legs and feet. Tense and hold the muscles in your left foot for a few seconds, then release. Repeat by tensing and releasing the muscles in your left calf and left thigh, before repeating the sequence with your right leg and foot.

3. Next, clench each of your fists in turn and release them, wiggle your fingers, then let them relax. In turn, tense the muscles in your arms and each buttock, then release them.

4. Move on to your shoulders, lifting them up, then lower them back down. Gently move your neck from side to side to release tension, then focus on your face. Raise your eyebrows and move your mouth for a few seconds, then release to your relaxed state.

5. All the major muscles in your body should now be relaxed. Continue to lie still, breathing slowly, and enjoy the relaxed feeling. When you're ready, open your eyes and slowly get up.

SIMPLE OBJECT MEDITATION

Meditation is good for clearing the mind, relieving stress, and aiding relaxation. It can also help you think more clearly. Meditating regularly, for a few minutes each day, can have positive effects on your health.

1. Choose a quiet place and find a comfortable chair to sit on. Put your arms by your side or in your lap. Find an object to focus on—it could be a lit candle, a picture, a photograph, a vase of flowers, or a piece of art.

2. Breathe slowly and deeply, inhaling through your mouth and exhaling through your nose. Focus your attention on the object.

3. It's natural for your mind to wander, but when it does, bring it back to the object of your meditation and your breathing. Stay still, keep breathing, and relax. If you feel like closing your eyes, then do so.

4. Continue with your meditation until you feel ready to end. Open your eyes and slowly get up.

Men's Health Problems

We hear far more about women's health than men's in the media, and, traditionally, many men have been reluctant to take preventive measures, adopt self-help remedies, or consult their health-care professional when they do experience problems. However, many men today, especially young ones, not only value good health, physical fitness, and general well-being, but also equate it with their sexual health and virility, and they're not prepared to suffer in silence anymore.

With the exception of shaving problems, most exclusively male health disorders relate to their sexual health and reproductive organs. Serious reproductive health issues include impotence (erectile dysfunction), infertility, and prostate problems (enlarged prostate and prostate cancer).

A healthy lifestyle plays a big part in preventing these problems, and regular exercise, not smoking or taking recreational drugs, drinking alcohol in moderation, good stress management, maintaining a healthy weight, and eating a diet that is rich in fruits, vegetables, and omega-3 oils are all helpful. They will also increase your life expectancy and reduce the likelihood of heart disease, high blood pressure, diabetes, and high cholesterol. And, as you get older, it becomes even more important to monitor your weight, diet, cholesterol levels, alcohol consumption, and overall fitness to maximize your chances of staying healthy for as long as possible.

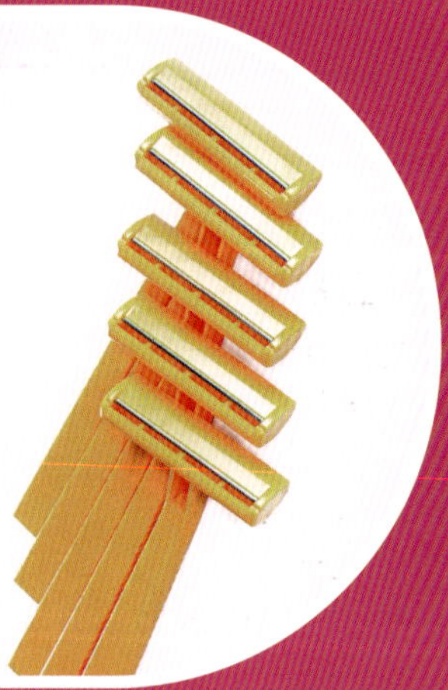

Shaving Problems

Some men are prone to shaving problems, while others can suddenly develop irritated skin after years of problem-free shaving. Fortunately, there are plenty of things you can do to prevent bad reactions and to treat them successfully with commercial products and natural remedies if they do occur.

SYMPTOMS

- ▷ Sore raised lumps and bumps
- ▷ Dry, irritated skin
- ▷ A red "razor" rash on the skin
- ▷ Ingrown hairs

Did You Know?

Shaving problems are most common among men of African descent with curly facial hair—about 80 percent are affected at some time or another. The hairs curl under and grow into the follicle, causing red bumps, which are tender and can lead to scarring.

PREVENTION

The most effective way to prevent shaving problems is to shave correctly.

- Rub your face and neck briskly with a facecloth before shaving to remove dead skin cells and lift the hairs. Alternatively, use an exfoliating facial cleanser or scrub to open the pores of the skin.
- Always use a sharp razor blade to avoid catching your skin.
- Go with the grain, shaving in the direction in which your hair grows naturally—this creates less pull on the hairs and minimizes skin irritation.
- If you are prone to shaving problems, use a specially formulated razor for sensitive skin.
- Do not shave too close; you'll be less likely to cut your skin and will avoid ingrown hairs, when the hair curls and grows back into the skin.
- Never stretch or tighten the skin excessively when shaving; try to keep it relaxed.
- For preference, use a razor with disposable blade cartridges and change them regularly.
- Use a shaving gel or cream to minimize friction and irritation.
- If you find that using an electric razor is irritating your skin, switch to wet shaving, or vice versa. Alternate between the two to minimize irritation.
- Avoid highly scented shaving products and harsh aftershaves containing alcohol, which can actually dry, sting, and irritate the skin. It is better to use a moisturizer after shaving.

CONVENTIONAL TREATMENTS

To treat shaving rashes and inflammation, you can use a hydrocortisone cream but be careful and only apply it sparingly and not for long periods. If the rash does not clear up, see your doctor.

NATURAL REMEDIES

There are many self-help treatments that you can try for razor burn, including drinking chamomile tea. Eating plenty of fresh fruits and vegetables containing vitamin C will help to clear it up quickly.

HERBAL REMEDIES Choose a shaving cream or gel with added aloe vera to soothe sensitive skin. If your skin is sore after shaving, apply pure aloe vera gel to the affected area or pat your face with a little soothing witch hazel. Calendula (marigold) cream can also be effective in treating shaving rashes.

AROMATHERAPY Aromatherapy shaving oils can be beneficial for men with sensitive skin—avocado and lemon oils are commonly used in these products.

HOMEMADE REMEDIES

Some of the kitchen ingredients in your refrigerator can be used to soothe irritated skin and bring welcome relief. Try the following:

- Cut a few thin slices off a cucumber and place on the irritated skin for a few minutes.
- Mash up some ripe avocado and apply to sore patches of skin for instant relief. Let sit for a few minutes and then wash off.

CALL YOUR DOCTOR

Most shaving rashes and problems clear up by themselves, but if they persist over a period of time you may have an allergy or an infection and should seek your doctor's advice.

Quick Fix

You can try rubbing in some baby rash cream after shaving—it's soothing, moisturizing, and is unlikely to irritate your skin.

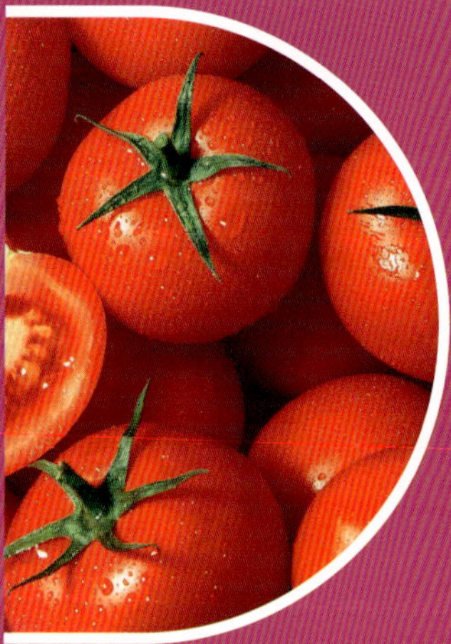

Prostate Problems

The prostate is a walnut-size sex gland, located under the bladder and encircling the urethra. Its function is to supply chemicals that are important in producing semen. However, it can become swollen, inflamed, enlarged, or even infected, especially in men over 50 years old. As they grow older, the prostate gland may enlarge due to an overgrowth of cells, thereby putting pressure on the urethra.

SYMPTOMS

- Slow, reduced urination
- Need to urinate more frequently
- Delay in starting to urinate
- Dribbling and weak flow of urine
- Sensation that bladder is not completely emptied
- Incontinence
- Possible urine infections

Did You Know?

The risk of prostate cancer increases if you are over 50 years old, have a family history of the disease (or of breast or ovarian cancer), are of African descent, or obese. The symptoms are similar to those for an enlarged prostate but may include pain or burning while urinating, passing urine more often, and pain or stiffness in the pelvis, hips, and lower back.

PREVENTION

There is a lot of conflicting advice on how to prevent prostate problems, especially prostate cancer. This disease develops slowly—and often invisibly without any symptoms—making it difficult to diagnose in many men. For a healthy prostate, follow the advice listed below.

- Eat a healthy diet that includes plenty of fresh fruits, green leafy vegetables, and omega-3 oils (found in salmon, mackerel, and other cold-water oily fish and flaxseed oil), which reduce the risk of cancer.
- Watch your weight and don't overeat, especially fatty foods.
- Cut down your alcohol intake, and choose wine and beer instead of hard liquor, which can irritate the prostate.
- Try to eat foods that contain zinc (the prostate contains more zinc than any other organ in the body). Meat, liver, seafood, wheat germ, brewer's yeast, pumpkin seeds, eggs, and mushrooms are all good sources.

- Eat tomatoes or tomato products every day. The lycopene in tomatoes is a natural oxidant and some researchers think that it can help reduce swelling of the prostate gland.
- Drink plenty of fluids, especially water, but not later in the evening before going to bed.
- Reduce your consumption of caffeine—it's a diuretic. Switch to green or herbal tea and decaf coffee, and avoid caffeinated cola drinks.
- Quit smoking—as well as all its other detrimental effects on health, nicotine irritates the bladder.

CONVENTIONAL TREATMENTS

If you have an enlarged prostate, your doctor may prescribe medication, such as alpha-blockers to increase the flow of urine, and/or 5-alpha-reductase inhibitors to reduce the size of your prostate. Surgery may be another option.

NATURAL REMEDIES

Relaxation, regular exercise, and a healthy diet are all important factors in treating an enlarged prostate.

- Try to relax in a warm bath for at 20 minutes at least once a day to reduce swelling.
- Make love frequently and always ejaculate completely to remove prostatic fluid.

HERBAL REMEDIES

- If urination is difficult, try taking a cleansing diuretic, such as chamomile tea.
- Stinging nettle may help to reduce prostate symptoms—you can make it into a tea or take it in capsule or extract form.
- Supplements of dried nettle root, hydrangea, saw palmetto, and pygeum may all be helpful in reducing swelling.

HOMEOPATHIC REMEDIES

Homeopathy may have a role to play but you should always consult a qualified homeopath and discuss your symptoms before taking homeopathic medicines. The most common remedies for prostate problems are Chimaphilia, Conium maculatum, Hepar sulphuris, Staphysagria, and Thuja. Seek professional advice on which remedy is best for your symptoms.

CALL YOUR DOCTOR

If you suspect that you may have an enlarged prostate or are experiencing any problems with urination, especially if you are over 50 years old, you must consult your doctor immediately.

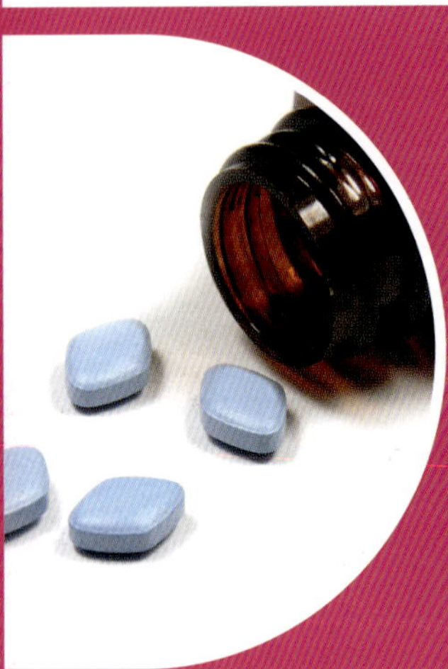

Impotence

Impotence (or erectile dysfunction) is the inability to achieve or sustain an erection that enables penetration and satisfactory sexual relations. This problem is relatively common, and 50 percent of all men over the age of 40 experience it at some time or another. There are a number of reasons for impotence, ranging from physical problems affecting blood supply to the penis to psychological ones, such as anxiety, depression, and stress.

SYMPTOMS

▷ Failure to achieve or sustain an erection

Did You Know?

Although many men experience impotence, most of them are embarrassed and suffer in silence; only about 10 percent of them seek medical or professional help. The good news is that 95 percent of men can be treated successfully.

PREVENTION

The ability to achieve an erection can be influenced by many psychological and physical factors, but lifestyle and the quality of your relationship play an important role. If there are no serious underlying health issues or a physical reason for your problem, you may want to consider the following possibilities.

- Eating a healthy diet that is low in saturated fats and contains all the essential nutrients for good health can be helpful. Make sure you get your daily portions of fruits and vegetables as well as omega-3 oils (found in oily fish and flaxseeds), which improve blood flow.
- Do you exercise enough? Regular exercise will improve blood flow, make you feel more energetic, and is a good way to relax and decrease stress. Working out in the gym, or going for a run, cycle, or even a brisk walk can all help to put your worries and problems in perspective and make you feel better about yourself.
- Take a candid look at your alcohol intake: too much alcohol can affect sexual performance, so limit your consumption to a maximum of two drinks per day.
- Some alternative practitioners think that too much caffeine can affect erectile function, so try cutting out regular cola, coffee, and tea and opting for decaf instead.

- There is evidence that smoking can affect a man's capacity to achieve a lasting erection. Nicotine constricts blood vessels, so quit smoking.
- Examine your life and your relationships to see if there are any areas that might be stressful and making you feel anxious, guilty, or depressed. Try to resolve any conflicts with your partner, family members, or work colleagues. Are there positive steps you can take to improve your lifestyle, reduce worries or stressful situations, and make you feel generally more content and relaxed?
- To help prevent impotence, do not be afraid to discuss your worries openly with your partner. With their support, you can avoid misunderstandings and overcome your problem.
- Some medications can have an effect on the capacity to achieve a sustained erection. These include some prescribed medicines for high blood pressure, heart problems, and depression.

CONVENTIONAL TREATMENTS

The best-known medicine for treating impotence is Viagra, but your doctor can prescribe other similar medicines. These all work by relaxing the blood vessels in the penis, so more blood flows into it, thereby creating an erection. Talking therapies, such as cognitive behavioral therapy, may be preferable to medication.

NATURAL REMEDIES

Some natural therapies may be helpful, including herbal medicine and acupressure.

ACUPRESSURE Governing vessel 20, a point on top of the head halfway between the ears, is recommended for treating impotence.

HERBAL REMEDIES

- Ginkgo biloba helps to boost blood flow and you could try taking 40 to 80 milligrams three times a day. However, don't take more than the recommended dose because there may be an increased risk of serious side effects.
- Ginseng is believed to enhance vitality and sexual function; take up to 150 milligrams three times daily.
- Evening primrose oil is recommended for healthy blood vessels, so you could try taking a daily supplement.

CALL YOUR DOCTOR

If you have problems achieving an erection and this has been the case for at least a couple of months, call your doctor. The condition is nearly always treatable. Impotence may also be linked to other health conditions, including poor cardiovascular fitness, coronary heart disease, diabetes, Parkinson's disease, and hormonal imbalance. Early and accurate diagnosis is important, so get it checked.

Caution

Viagra is not suitable for everyone and it can have unpleasant side effects, so never buy it from friends or over the Internet. Only take it if prescribed and monitored by your doctor.

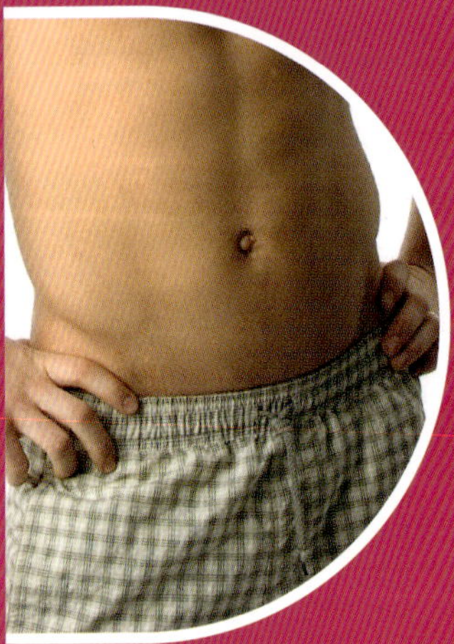

Fertility Problems

You may have a fertility problem if you have been having sexual intercourse with your partner for more than twelve months without using any contraception and she has not conceived. Male infertility is usually caused by abnormal semen, damaged testicles, or a blockage during ejaculation. There are several reasons for abnormal semen, including a very low sperm count, decreased sperm mobility, and abnormally shaped sperm.

SYMPTOMS

- Failure to conceive
- Possible pain or swelling inside the scrotum

Did You Know?

About 85 percent of couples having regular unprotected intercourse at least three times a week will conceive naturally within 12 months.

PREVENTION

You can increase your chances of conceiving by making sure that both you and your partner are in good health and are following the advice below.

- Eat a healthy diet and watch your weight—being seriously overweight or obese with a BMI of over 29 can affect your fertility, making it more difficult to conceive.
- Keep your alcohol intake to a minimum—no more than the recommended two drinks a day maximum. Too much alcohol can damage the quality of your sperm.
- If you smoke, quit. Smoking cigarettes can affect your fertility.
- Have intercourse at least three times a week so it is more probable that you won't miss your partner's fertile days in the monthly cycle, which are usually halfway between her periods.
- Wear loose-fitting underpants made of cotton or natural fiber; tight underpants can increase the temperature within your scrotum, reducing fertility.
- Some conventional and herbal medicines can affect sperm production, so check with your doctor if you are taking medication and avoid a Chinese herb called Tripterygium wilfordii.
- Try to relax and not to worry about the time it's taking to conceive. Stress can reduce your sex drive and limit sperm production.

- Recreational drugs, such as marijuana or cocaine, can also affect male fertility, so don't take them.
- Some recent studies have suggested that excessive laptop computer use and carrying a cell phone in your pants pocket while speaking on an earpiece may damage sperm, but this is not proven. However, you may want to check the safety standards in your workplace if you use a computer for long periods or work with potentially hazardous chemicals.

CONVENTIONAL TREATMENTS

The treatment for male infertility will depend on the cause of the problem. The available options include medications to improve fertility and assisted conception. Your doctor may arrange for you to have a male fertility test, such as a sperm count. If you have a blockage in your testicles that prevents you ejaculating sperm normally (epididymal blockage), you may need surgery to correct it.

NATURAL REMEDIES

Improving your quality of life and cutting out all the unhealthy elements in your diet and daily routine is a natural way to improve your chances of you and your partner conceiving.

NUTRITIONAL MEDICINE Zinc is especially beneficial in aiding healthy functioning of the male reproductive system. You can include foods that are rich in zinc in your daily diet—pumpkin seeds, mushrooms, seafood, meat, liver—or take a daily supplement.

HERBAL REMEDIES

- Saw palmetto, astragalus root, and tribulus are often used to treat male infertility.
- Ginseng is thought to increase sperm motility and you can try taking a supplement of 100 to 200 milligrams per day.

HOMEOPATHIC REMEDIES

The following remedies are used to treat male fertility problems. Use the appropriate one for your symptoms.

Sepia 6C, for low sex drive.

Medorrhinum, for impotence.

CALL YOUR DOCTOR

If you and your partner have been trying to conceive for a year without any success, make an appointment to see your doctor. You should go sooner if you have had an STI (sexually transmitted infection), such as chlamydia, or have received treatment for cancer and are concerned about your fertility.

Traditional Chinese Medicine

As the name suggests, traditional Chinese medicine (TCM) is one of the world's oldest medical systems and it has been used for thousands of years. It is based on a holistic approach and uses a combination of therapies, including acupuncture, Chinese herbal medicine, and tuina, a form of massage.

KEY IDEAS

At the heart of traditional Chinese medicine is the belief that the body should be treated holistically. Instead of starting with a symptom and looking for a particular disease or illness that is causing it, traditional Chinese medicine practitioners diagnose an individual pattern of symptoms.

Practitioners believe that a series of meridians run throughout the body, which help qi, or life energy, to flow through. Other key concepts include yin and yang, which represent certain organs of the body and the five elements—fire, wood, water, metal, and earth—that relate to symptoms and parts of the body.

When identifying the pattern of illness and the treatment or herbal remedy that could help, a practitioner makes their assessment by looking at yin, yang, and the five elements.

ACUPUNCTURE

A full medical history is taken by an acupuncturist and, as well as conventional details, they will test your pulse and look at your tongue, because it's believed that the tongue can hold important information about your health.

The meridian system is central to the work of an acupuncturist, who uses fine needles to stimulate the acupoints that exist on the channels throughout the body. It does not usually hurt, and the needles are left in place for a few minutes or in some cases up to an hour; they work by stimulating or suppressing the flow of qi.

A special herb called moxa is often used, too, particularly in instances where the acupuncturist needs to create heat over a certain point. The herb is burned over the acupuncture point for a short time.

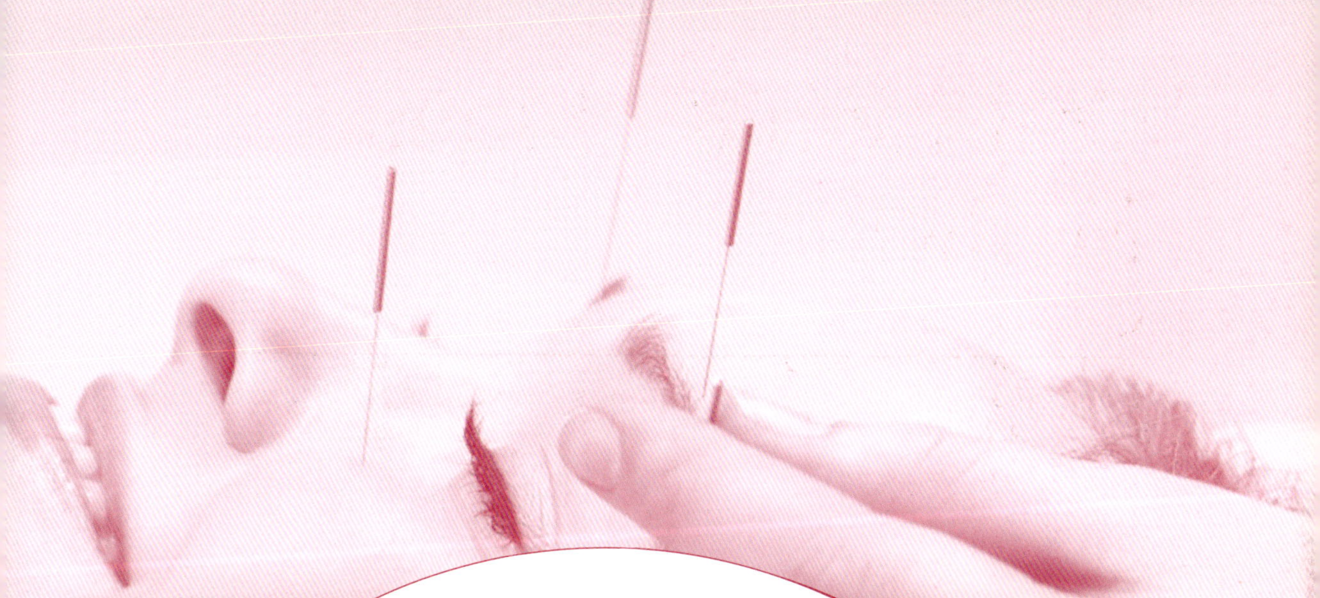

CHINESE HERBAL MEDICINE

Chinese herbal medicine is often practiced on its own or in conjunction with other aspects of Chinese medicine. For example, it is not unusual for an acupuncturist to also prescribe you herbs to take between sessions to continue your healing and treatment at home.

After taking notes on your medical symptoms, and analyzing your tongue and pulse, herbal remedies are prescribed. Herbs are classified according to whether they are sweet, sour, pungent, bitter, salty, hot, or cold. Mixtures of herbs are tailored to individual needs and may be taken as teas, powders, pills, creams, or lotions.

It is important to find a qualified Chinese herbal medicine practitioner and to never try taking herbs without proper advice, because some can cause serious side effects if used inappropriately.

TUINA

Tuina is a therapeutic form of Chinese massage. Like acupuncture, it focuses on using the meridians and points where qi typically gets stuck to release discomfort and aid healing.

As with other forms of traditional Chinese medicine, a full case history is taken and a practitioner will identify a pattern of symptoms before working out how best you can be treated.

Women's Health Problems

A woman's body changes as she progresses from puberty and adolescence through her child-bearing years to menopause and old age, and specific health problems are associated with these different stages in her life. During her reproductive years, there are also monthly variations in hormone levels in the body, which can also affect her physical and psychological health.

This chapter focuses on some of the things that go wrong, and how to treat them with conventional, self-help, and natural remedies. There is also practical advice on preventing common health problems and, as always, the emphasis is on the essential components of a healthy lifestyle: diet, weight control, exercise, relaxation and stress management, quitting smoking, and not drinking more alcohol than the recommended guidelines.

By being well informed, you can take preventive action to protect your health, recognize and respond quickly to symptoms when they occur, and treat your problem with natural or conventional remedies. Self-examination and listening to your body can help alert you to the early-warning signs of poor health.

Your sexual health is important for your well-being, self-esteem, and your relationship with your partner. The most common health problems associated with the reproductive system are difficulties with menstruation (premenstrual syndrome, pain, and irregular or heavy bleeding), pregnancy, and menopause. For many women, vaginal discharge, infection, and thrush can be debilitating and recurring. As well as conventional medical wisdom, there are many tried and tested natural home remedies that offer effective treatment or relief from the symptoms of these women's health conditions.

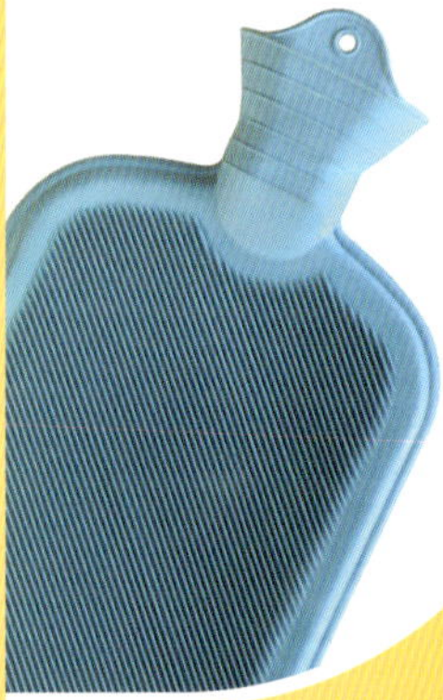

Premenstrual Symdrome (PMS)

Premenstrual syndrome, or PMS, is a term covering a wide range of symptoms that many women experience, to varying degrees, during the week or two before a period. For some women, these symptoms can become so severe that they seriously affect their quality of life.

SYMPTOMS

- Depression, tearfulness, and anxiety
- Irritability
- Insomnia
- Sugar cravings and increased appetite
- Fatigue
- Fluid retention and weight gain
- Confusion and forgetfulness
- Lack of concentration
- Clumsiness
- Swollen, bloated abdomen
- Breast tenderness
- Headaches

PREVENTION

- Avoid alcohol in the week or two weeks before a period is due, because it can exacerbate symptoms.
- Cut down on caffeine-containing drinks and sip herbal teas instead.
- Drink plenty of water.
- Avoid sugary foods that can cause blood sugar peaks followed by dips. Eat regular, small healthy meals and snacks to keep blood sugar levels as level as possible.

CONVENTIONAL TREATMENTS

Your doctor might prescribe hormone treatments, such as the combined birth-control pill, estrogen or progesterone-only pills, or intrauterine devices, to help balance your hormones. Antidepressants, such as one of the selective serotonin reuptake inhibitors (SSRI), may be offered to treat depression. Diuretics, such as spironolactone, can be prescribed for water retention. Gonadotrophin-releasing hormone (GnRH-a) analogs might be offered for severe PMS; they stop your normal cycle and plunge you into a temporary menopause.

NATURAL REMEDIES

There are several natural remedies you can try to tackle PMS symptoms.

FLOWER REMEDIES Australian Bush Flower's She Oak and Women's Essence help to balance hormones.

AROMATHERAPY Clary sage essential oil helps lift the mood and balance your hormones, while fennel can be used to treat water retention. Jasmine may ease depression and anxiety, and juniper is excellent for bloating.

HERBAL REMEDIES

- The best-known herbal treatment is evening primrose oil. It's especially good at improving mood, lessening breast pain, and easing sugar cravings. You may need to take it for three months before the effects are seen.
- Agnus castus is a hormone-balancing herb that can help to even out mood swings and irritability, as well as easing breast tenderness.
- St. John's wort is useful for women who get very depressed and anxious, but check with your doctor first if you take any other medication.

HOMEOPATHIC REMEDIES

A homeopath would treat you constitutionally, but you could try one of the following remedies.

Nux vomica 30C, if you crave sweet or fatty foods and are irritable.

Natrum mur 30C, if you are sad and irritable, have fluid retention, swollen breasts, and migraines.

Pulsatilla 30C, if you are feeling tearful, have painful breasts, and a tendency to irregular periods and nausea.

Sepia 30C, if you crave sweet or salty foods, are tearful, depressed, and/or generally irritable.

HEALING FOODS

- Magnesium deficiency can be a contributory factor in PMS. Take a daily supplement.
- Vitamin B6 is useful for counteracting the emotional effects of PMS. Take a daily supplement contain this vitamin.
- Soy-based foods, such as soy milk, soy yogurt, soybeans, and tofu, contain phytoestrogens, which mimic the action of estrogen in the body and can help to balance the body's estrogen levels when eaten regularly.

CALL YOUR DOCTOR

Most women find their own solutions to dealing with their PMS, however annoying the symptoms, but if it becomes severe and affects your well-being to such an extent that it interferes with your everyday routine, you should seek help and see your doctor.

Quick Fix

When you are about to explode with temper, drink 10 drops of avena sativa (oat straw) in a glass of water. It's a potent source of vitamin B6 and works almost instantly to calm you down and reduce irritability.

Heavy Bleeding

Heavy periods (menorrhagia) can be dangerous if they make you anemic, and they can seriously affect the quality of your life. If you turn down invitations during your period because of worrying about flooding, it's time to take action.

SYMPTOMS

- Heavy and/or prolonged periods
- Can be accompanied by pain, nausea, diarrhea, and dizziness

PREVENTION

- Low levels of essential fatty acids, iron, zinc, and vitamins A, C, and K are all linked to menorrhagia, so it's worth taking supplements.
- Avoid hot baths during your period, because these may make the bleeding worse. Don't take aspirin-containing medicines for the same reason.

CONVENTIONAL TREATMENTS

Your doctor might prescribe a hormone treatment, such as a progesterone-releasing IUD, or the birth-control pill. Tranexamic acid medication taken for the first four days of a period can help to reduce blood loss in many cases.

NATURAL REMEDIES

Heavy periods can be caused by your liver not eliminating old hormones efficiently, so any remedies that stimulate liver function can be helpful.

AROMATHERAPY Fennel, geranium, and rose oils are used to regulate periods and blood flow.

HERBAL REMEDIES

- Take milk thistle tablets or tincture, and drink dandelion tea or coffee to improve liver function.
- The hormone-balancing effects of agnus castus tincture can be helpful.
- Lady's mantle has an astringent effect on the uterus, drying up excretions. You can take it as a tea or a tincture.

HOMEOPATHIC REMEDIES

Chamomilla 30C, for heavy periods with cramping; blood may look dark or clotted.

Lycopodium 30C, for long, heavy periods accompanied by digestive upsets.

Veratrum album 30C, for heavy periods, cramping, and feeling exhausted.

CALL YOUR DOCTOR

You should seek medical advice if your complexion looks very pale, you are unusually tired, you find it hard to walk up hills you would normally manage without a problem, or if you experience heart palpitations. All these can be symptoms of anemia.

Period Pain

Period pain (dysmenorrhea) can range from a mild, dull ache in the lower abdomen to a sharp pain that is so severe it causes you to pass out. The pain is usually caused by cramping of the muscles of the uterus.

SYMPTOMS

- Pain in the lower abdomen
- Lower back pain
- Nausea and vomiting
- Diarrhea
- Dizziness and fainting

PREVENTION

- Eat a balanced diet, including three servings of oily fish a week. If you don't like fish, take a supplement of omega-3 essential fatty acids, because dysmenhorrhea is much worse for those who have low levels of essential fatty acids.
- Keep life as stress-free as you can during your periods.
- Get gentle exercise and plenty of sleep.

CONVENTIONAL TREATMENTS

There are plenty of over-the-counter painkillers, but avoid any containing aspirin, which could increase bleeding. Mefenamic acid is often prescribed to treat painful periods; it has a mild anti-inflammatory action as well as painkilling effects.

NATURAL REMEDIES

A traditional remedy is to soak cheesecloth in castor oil, then wrap it in plastic wrap before placing it on your lower abdomen. Put a hot water bottle on top and relax for half an hour. This decongests the uterus and relaxes the muscles.

HERBAL REMEDIES

Take wild yam capsules to reduce painful spasms. Cramp bark tincture is an effective antispasmodic and muscle relaxant.

NUTRITIONAL MEDICINE

- Vitamin E has been shown to relieve menstrual cramps in 70 percent of women within two menstrual cycles.
- Magnesium has a beneficial effect on painful periods and lower back pain.

CALL YOUR DOCTOR

If your symptoms are severe, call your doctor. You may be referred for tests to rule out other possible causes of the pain, such as endometriosis.

Caution

If you take painkillers to ease your symptoms, be careful not to exceed the maximum daily dosage, as stated on the package instructions.

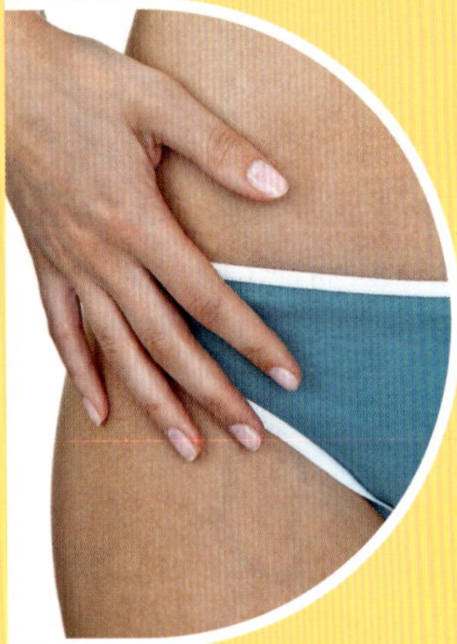

Thrush (Candida)

Thrush is an infection caused by a yeast (fungus) known as *Candida albicans*, which occurs naturally in the digestive tract, skin, and vagina. Under normal circumstances, it is kept under control by other "friendly" bacteria in the body, but it can overgrow after taking antibiotics, when you're rundown, or if you take hormones, such as the birth-control pill.

SYMPTOMS

- ▷ Itching of the vulva
- ▷ Soreness and irritation of the vulva
- ▷ Pain or discomfort during sex or urination
- ▷ Odorless vaginal discharge, usually thin and watery or thick and white
- ▷ Oral thrush affects the mouth, causing white patches that are red and sore underneath

PREVENTION

- A healthy diet that is low in sugar can help to prevent thrush; sugar feeds the candida fungus.
- Wear cotton undergarments, which can help the area to "breathe" and prevent overheating.
- Avoid wearing tight-fitting clothing, such as tights, swimsuits, exercise clothes, or pants for long periods of time, because this can cause irritation.
- Alcohol can contribute to an increased risk of thrush, as can bubble baths, so try to avoid them if you are prone.

CONVENTIONAL TREATMENTS

Thrush is normally treated with antifungal medication, such as fluconazole or itraconazole. Medication can be taken orally or as pessaries, and topical creams can be used for the sore parts of your vulva.

Did You Know?

Stress can also exacerbate the problem of thrush, as can natural hormonal changes (around the time of your period, for example).

NATURAL REMEDIES

Thrush can be treated with a wide range of natural remedies. A healthy diet is very important, and you should also eat plenty of yogurt with live cultures, which is full of healthy bacteria. Take a probiotic regularly, particularly if you have recurrent thrush. Look for one that contains at least four million bacteria per dose; acidophilus is a good choice.

NUTRITIONAL MEDICINE Vitamin C helps your body to form collagen, which maintains the structural integrity of your vagina, making infestations and infections less likely. It also works to boost your immune system. The B vitamins are often deficient in women with chronic yeast or bacterial infections. Take vitamin supplements with vitamins C and B daily.

HERBAL REMEDIES

- Calendula tincture has antimicrobial properties, and it is useful to combat vaginal infections and infestations, and promote healing. Echinacea will boost your immune system, making it easier for your body to fight off invaders.
- Increase your intake of fresh, raw garlic or take garlic capsules. One of the ingredients in garlic, known as allicin, can prevent the overgrowth of yeast.
- Goldenseal tincture contains a substance called berberine, which stimulates the immune system and combats yeast and bacteria.
- Pau d'arco has immune-boosting properties, and is also antifungal; take as a tincture or decoction.

AROMATHERAPY

- Tea tree oil is ideal for treating fungal infections. Buy tea tree pessaries to insert in your vagina, or add 5 to 10 drops to your bath water.
- Lavender oil can help to destroy fungi; use in your bath water, or place a few drops on a clean moist washcloth and wash the area regularly.
- Thyme oil boosts immunity and can also help to fight yeasts.

HOMEOPATHIC REMEDIES

For vaginal thrush, you can try one of the following:

Pulsatilla 30C, for cloudy or watery discharge that causes smarting and soreness.

Graphites 30C, if the vagina is sore, with small ulcers on the labia.

Calcarea 30C, if there is vaginal itching, yellow or milk discharge, and increased itchiness around periods.

Oral thrush may respond to one of the following:

Borax 30C, at the first sign of an outbreak.

Capsicum 30C, for sore, hot patches.

Arsenicum 30C, for burning pains, canker sores, and feeling worn out.

CALL YOUR DOCTOR

If your vaginal discharge has an unpleasant odor, you probably have a viral or bacterial infection instead of a fungal infestation. Call your doctor for an accurate diagnosis.

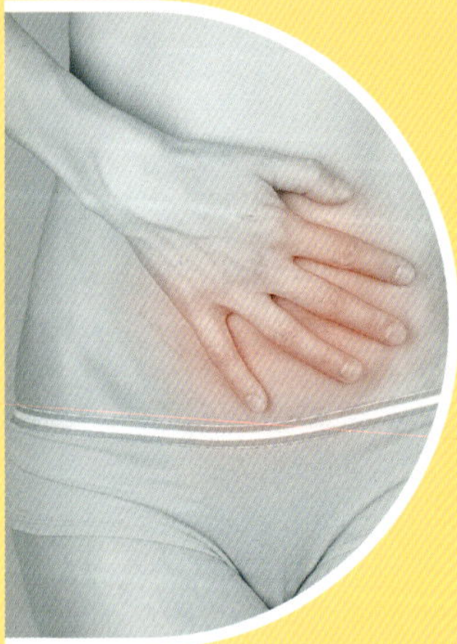

Fibroids

Fibroids are benign tumors that grow in and around the uterus. They are fed by estrogen, so they tend to occur in women of child-bearing age and decrease in size after menopause. Many women do not even realize that they have them, but, for others, fibroids can cause a host of troublesome and potentially dangerous health problems.

SYMPTOMS

- Heavy, prolonged periods, which can lead to anemia
- Acute pain during periods
- Abdominal pain and bloating
- Discomfort during sex
- More frequent urination; waking several times a night to urinate
- Constipation
- Pain in the lower back and legs
- Can cause infertility or complications during pregnancy

PREVENTION

One in four women has fibroids and most do not have any associated problems, but if the growths get very large, or are in an awkward position, they will become symptomatic. You can help to avoid them growing huge by doing the following things.

- Don't let yourself get overweight.
- Don't drink too much alcohol.
- Make sure you get enough exercise.
- Eat only organic dairy produce and meat to avoid ingesting the artificial hormones that are routinely fed to farm animals.

CONVENTIONAL TREATMENTS

Your doctor may prescribe hormone treatments, either as a progesterone coil or the birth-control pill. Tranexamic acid is commonly prescribed to deal with heavy periods, while mefanemic acid can be effective in treating period pains. In severe cases, you may be recommended to have injections of Gonadotropin-releasing hormone agonist (GnRH-a), which temporarily stops your menstrual cycle and can bring on some menopausal symptoms. Alternatively, there are a number of surgical procedures used, with hysterectomy at the extreme, and nonsurgical procedures, such as MRI-focused ultrasound treatment or uterine artery embolization.

NATURAL REMEDIES

A useful homemade remedy is to make a castor oil pack to help relieve congestion in the womb.

HERBAL REMEDIES

- Herbs that strengthen the liver, such as milk thistle tablets or tincture, will help it to eliminate old hormones from the blood.
- Agnus castus is useful for hormone balance. Take 25 drops of tincture in a glass of water every morning, or as prescribed by your herbalist.
- Lady's mantle can be effective at reducing excessive bleeding and lowering estrogen dominance, as is chaste tree. Take them as a tincture or in teas.

AROMATHERAPY

- Ginger oil is a powerful circulation stimulant, and it improves liver function. Put a few drops in the bath, or use in massage.
- Marjoram can help to relieve cramping and discomfort.
- Rose oil helps to ease tension. It also has mild hormone-balancing properties and is believed to work as a uterine tonic.

CALL YOUR DOCTOR

If you are worried that you may have fibroids, call your doctor. Most cases do not require medical intervention, but if the symptoms are severe and troublesome, you may need medication or surgery.

NUTRITIONAL MEDICINE

- Eat foods containing phytoestrogens, such as soybean products, lentils, and chickpeas, which can help to reduce excessive levels of estrogen in your blood.
- Reduce your intake of saturated fat but get plenty of essential fatty acids from eating oily fish, nuts, and seeds.
- Make sure you include plenty of fiber in your diet to ease constipation. Choose whole-grain products, brown rice, and oats, as well as plenty of fruits and vegetables.
- Dark chocolate with at least 80 percent cocoa is a good source of iron for those who are worried about anemia, or take a daily teaspoonful of molasses.
- Vitamins A, B, and C, plus zinc, calcium, magnesium, and iron are all essential for hormone balance. Choose a good-quality multivitamin supplement that contains them all.

HOMEOPATHIC REMEDIES

There are dozens of remedies that could be appropriate, according to your individual constitution and symptoms, of which the following may be useful:

Calc carb 30C, for fibroids causing heavy bleeding, fatigue, or chills

Sabina 30C, for fibroids causing lower-back pain and heavy bleeding with clots

Phosphorus 30C will help with heavy bleeding and clots.

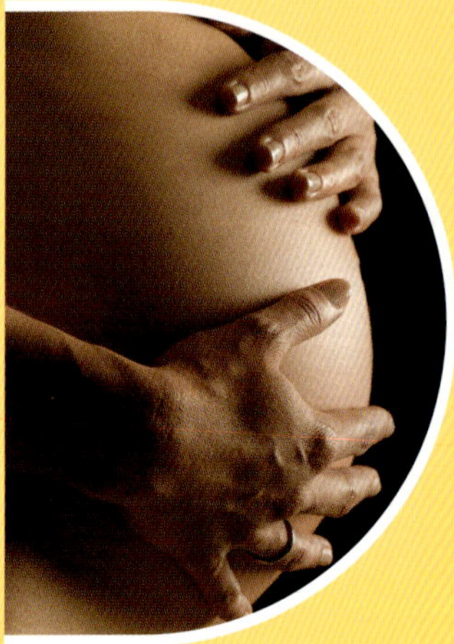

Pregnancy Health Problems

Many women sail through their pregnancy without any uncomfortable symptoms, while others seem to be plagued constantly. Symptoms are caused by many factors, such as changing hormones and the impact they have on your body, as well as the extra demands of your growing baby.

SYMPTOMS

- Nausea (morning sickness)
- Fatigue
- Heartburn
- Edema (swelling) of the feet, ankles, and face
- Backache
- Headaches
- Breast tenderness
- Sleep difficulties
- Constipation and hemorrhoids
- Mood swings

PREVENTION

A healthy diet, with plenty of fresh, whole foods, will help to make sure that your body has the fuel it needs to operate at optimum level and provide your baby with everything it needs to grow and develop.

- Gentle, regular exercise has been shown to reduce symptoms by improving circulation and by increasing endorphins, the "feel-good" hormones.
- Relaxation and restful sleep can also help, because many symptoms are exacerbated by fatigue.
- It's also important to drink plenty of water, because dehydration can make symptoms worse.

CONVENTIONAL TREATMENTS

Most doctors are reluctant to prescribe medication to pregnant women unless strictly necessary. However, in extreme circumstances you may need some medical intervention. Acetaminophen is considered to be safe during pregnancy for any related aches and pains. Fiber supplements may be recommended for constipation.

NATURAL REMEDIES

Many natural remedies are available to treat problem ailments and symptoms during pregnancy. If you are unsure as to their safety, consult your doctor.

FLOWER REMEDIES Olive is ideal for exhaustion. Use Walnut to relieve anxiety and mood swings. Impatiens helps when you are feeling irritable.

HERBAL REMEDIES

- Ginger is a traditional remedy for morning sickness and can be taken in pill form or added to foods or drinks. You can also chew crystallized or candied ginger.
- Slippery elm powder mixed with water or milk will protect the mucous membranes lining your digestive system and ease symptoms.
- Nettle tea can reduce leg cramps, hemorrhoids, and swelling.
- Dandelion root tea or coffee has a strong effect on your liver, which can help to ease digestive symptoms and hormone imbalances. The leaf is a mild diuretic, which can reduce water retention.

AROMATHERAPY

- Lavender oil can be added to a bath to encourage restful sleep, or dabbed neat on your temples to soothe headaches.
- Have a warm (not hot bath) about 30 minutes before bedtime, and add 8 to 10 drops of Roman chamomile oil to encourage sleep.
- Lemon oil can be inhaled to ease morning sickness.

NUTRITIONAL MEDICINE

- Vitamin B6 deficiency has been linked with morning sickness, so take a regular B-complex supplement.
- Fiber is important in preventing constipation and making sure that the vitamins and minerals from the food you eat are assimilated by your body. Psyllium or ispaghula husks (plantain seeds) are effective unblockers and safe during pregnancy.
- If you experience edema, include plenty of natural diuretics in your diet, such as asparagus, pumpkin, onions, grapes, beets, parsley, green beans, pineapple, and garlic.

HOMEOPATHIC REMEDIES

Treatment will be based on your individual symptoms, but the following remedies may be helpful.

Ipecacuanha 30C, for morning sickness characterized by continuous nausea and vomiting.

Symphoricarpus 30C, for morning sickness made worse by food and any type of motion.

Nux vomica 30C, for constipation, with a frequent urge to pass a bowel movement, but only managing a little a time; also itching, bleeding hemorrhoids.

Sulfur 30C, for constipation with hemorrhoids that itch and burn and are worse for heat.

CALL YOUR DOCTOR

If you are worried about any health problems or unfamiliar symptoms that you may experience during your pregnancy, make an appointment to see your doctor or mention it to your healthcare provider at your regular checkups.

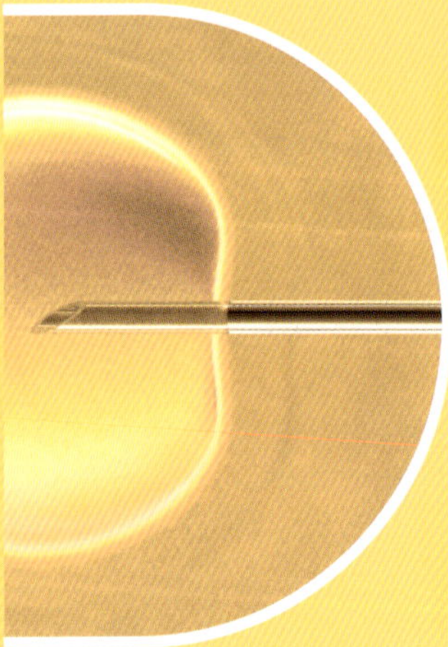

Infertility

Infertility is a general diagnosis given when you are unable to conceive after 18 months of unprotected sex. Many cases are treatable, particularly when the cause is established. Common causes include endometriosis, ovulation problems, poor egg or sperm quality, polycystic ovaries, tube blockages (male or female), or sperm allergy. However, most cases of infertility are unexplained.

SYMPTOMS

- Inability to conceive

PREVENTION

- Both you and your partner should eat a healthy diet, which is crucial to a successful pregnancy and a healthy baby, and can help to balance hormones that may be at the root of the problem.
- Avoid drinking alcohol and coffee, which can reduce your fertility by half.
- Smoking has also been linked with infertility in women, and can even bring on an early menopause. If you are a smoker and trying to conceive, quit smoking now.
- Eat organic food whenever possible to avoid consuming the environmental estrogens that are found in some pesticides used on many vegetables and fruits.

Did You Know?

About one in six couples has difficulty conceiving. Research indicates that women's fertility begins to decline in their late twenties, and men's in their late thirties.

CONVENTIONAL TREATMENTS

There are a number of options available, including assisted fertilization and medication. Your treatment will be undertaken according to the cause of your infertility. Some options include:

- Intrauterine insemination (IUI), a procedure that puts your partner's sperm directly into your uterus using a fine catheter
- IVF (in vitro fertilization), which involves placing a fertilized egg into your uterus, usually after taking medication
- Stimulatory medication (such as clomiphene) can encourage several eggs to mature at a time
- Follicle-stimulating hormone (FSH), which makes the ovaries begin the process of ovulation
- Human menopausal gonadotropin (hMG), which is used for women who don't ovulate due to problems with their pituitary gland
- Bromocriptine is often used for women who have trouble ovulating because of high levels of the hormone prolactin.

NATURAL REMEDIES

There are many natural remedies that you can try to help maximize your chances of conception.

NUTRITIONAL MEDICINE

- Vitamin B6 can help women who have trouble conceiving, whereas vitamin B12 is useful for men. Take in a daily supplement.
- Zinc is crucial for successful fertilization, and it also reduces the risk of miscarriage. Both you and your partner should take a daily supplement.
- Eat plenty of essential fatty acids (in nuts, seeds, oily fish). Consider taking a fish oil supplement.
- Vitamin E is a powerful antioxidant and can increase fertility in men and women.
- Vitamin C encourages the production of healthy sperm.

HERBAL REMEDIES

- Agnus castus helps to restore hormonal balance and increases fertility—take in tincture form.
- Lemon balm can help to reduce the impact of stress, which may be at the root of the problem. Take as an infusion.
- False unicorn root is traditionally used to regulate the ovaries—look for it in tincture form.

AROMATHERAPY

- Rose oil is frequently used to treat fertility problems. Use for massage or in the bath.
- Geranium has estrogenic properties and can help to balance your hormones.
- Melissa (lemon balm) helps to regulate your menstrual cycle and is also very relaxing.

HOMEOPATHIC REMEDIES

Your treatment will be constitutional, working to address anything that may be causing fertility problems. Some commonly used remedies include:

Sepia 30C, for irregular or absent ovulation
Aurum 30C, for low sex drive and depression
Phosphorus 30C, when stress is causing problems
Sabina 30C, when you have recurrent miscarriages
Silica 30C, which is an overall remedy to boost your chances of becoming pregnant.

CALL YOUR DOCTOR

Consult your doctor if you haven't had any success conceiving after trying for a year. You may be referred to a specialist in fertility treatment.

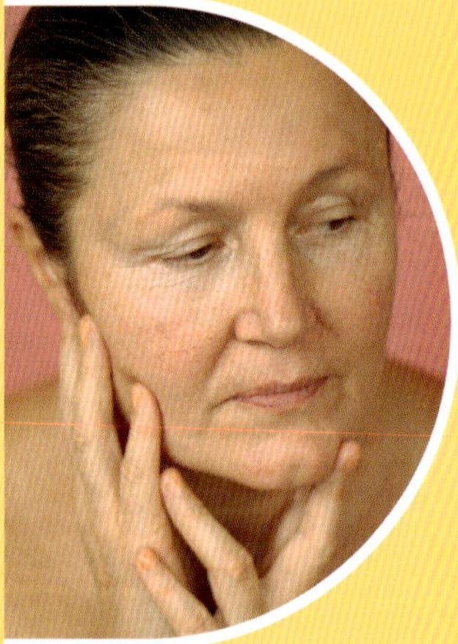

Menopause

The hormonal and biological changes that lead up to the cessation of menstrual periods can cause a number of physical and emotional symptoms that vary from woman to woman. Most get through it without recourse to medical treatments, but there's no need to suffer in silence, because there are a number of natural remedies to try.

SYMPTOMS

- Hot flashes and night sweats
- Mood swings
- Depression and anxiety
- Weight gain
- Insomnia
- Headaches
- Tiredness and lack of concentration
- Vaginal dryness
- Loss of skin elasticity
- Increased frequency of urination
- Reduced sex drive

Did You Know?

The adrenal gland can help to balance your hormones during the period leading up to and after menopause, as long as you are not too stressed. This is a good time to take up relaxation therapies, such as yoga or tai chi, which can help to maintain muscle strength, improve breathing, and alleviate stress.

PREVENTION

- Hot flashes can be triggered by eating spicy foods, drinking alcohol or caffeine-containing drinks, or hot climates, so avoid these.
- Wear light natural-fiber clothing and try to keep rooms cool, especially the bedroom.
- Exercise regularly and eat sensibly to keep your weight under control.
- Avoid sugar-laden foods that cause blood sugar peaks and troughs that affect your emotions.
- Use plenty of moisturizer on your skin, reapplying throughout the day.

CONVENTIONAL TREATMENTS

Hormone replacement therapy (HRT) can be taken as a pill, cream, gel, or skin patch. It provides estrogen to replace the falling natural levels. Clonidine may be prescribed to treat hot flashes and night sweats. Your doctor might even suggest taking antidepressants or sleeping pills if you have severe problems with depression or insomnia.

NATURAL REMEDIES

Many women prefer to treat the annoying symptoms of menopause with a range of natural treatments instead of resorting to conventional medicine. There are many over-the-counter remedies available in pharmacies and health food stores.

FLOWER REMEDIES Impatiens is ideal for mood swings and irritability, while Walnut is perfect for this time of life. Cherry Plum helps when you are feeling irrational or ready to explode.

NUTRITIONAL MEDICINE Regularly eating foods containing phytoestrogens, such as soybean products, can significantly reduce menopausal symptoms. Eating a well-balanced diet with plenty of essential fatty acids from oily fish, nuts, and seeds, and a full range of vitamins and minerals is vitally important.

HERBAL REMEDIES

- Black cohosh is the best-known treatment, and in several tests it has emerged as being at least as effective as HRT in treating menopausal symptoms (see cautionary note).
- Drink sage tea to combat hot flashes and night sweats. Keep a cup of cold tea by your bedside to sip during the night as required.
- St. John's wort is extremely effective at combating depression and anxiety, and it can also boost your sex drive. Consult a qualified professional before taking it if you are on any other medications.
- Dong quai, licorice, sage, and yarrow can help to counteract hot flashes and night sweats. Blend tinctures together, if you prefer.

CALL YOUR DOCTOR

If gentle natural remedies do not appear to be working and your symptoms are severe, consult your doctor.

AROMATHERAPY

- Lavender, marjoram, and Roman chamomile can be added to the bath to soothe anxiety and irritation and to encourage restful sleep.
- Clary sage helps to balance hormones, which can ease symptoms.
- Anise, fennel, and angelica oils all contain estrogen-like substances that can provide relief from many menopausal symptoms. Use two or three drops in the bath.

HOMEOPATHIC REMEDIES

Treatment should be constitutional but the following remedies are commonly used.

Sepia 30C helps with hot flashes, a low libido, irritability, and feelings of weakness.

Lachesis 30C helps with hot flashes that feel like a rush of blood to the head, headaches, and left-sided pain.

Pulsatilla 30C is great for tearfulness, irritability, and symptoms that seem to change constantly.

Caution

Don't take black cohosh if you have any liver problems. Talk to your doctor about this.

TOP 20 Aromatherapy Oils

Aromatherapy uses aromatic essential oils, extracted from plants, to promote good health and treat many common ailments. The essential oils can be used in massage, baths, warm compresses, steam inhalations, sprays, and vaporizers. For massage, a few drops are added to a carrier oil, such as sweet almond, grapeseed, jojoba, or sunflower oil.

1 BERGAMOT

Scent Citrus, fresh

Used for Calming, healing; depression, stress; acne, boils, psoriasis; colds, coughs

2 CEDARWOOD

Scent Woody

Used for Stimulating, toning; eczema; dandruff

3 CHAMOMILE (ROMAN)

Scent Pungent

Used for Calming, soothing; insomnia, stress; skin irritations and inflammations, acne; digestive problems; children's ailments; headaches; sprains and strains

4 CYPRESS

Scent Spicy, balsamic, sweet

Used for Astringent; chest infections; dandruff; varicose veins; eczema; cramp; hemorrhoids

5 EUCALYPTUS

Scent Camphor, woody

Used for Antiseptic; colds, flu, catarrh, sinusitis, upper respiratory tract infections; muscular pain; headaches; chicken pox, shingles

6 FRANKINCENSE

Scent Balsamic, sweet

Used for Calming, soothing; promotes skin healing; asthma; coughs, bronchitis

7 GERANIUM

Scent Floral, sweet

Used for Relaxing, calming; hormonal imbalance, premenstrual syndrome, menopause; acne, eczema; depression, stress; headaches; cramp; hemorrhoids; varicose veins

8 GINGER

Scent Spicy

Used for Stimulating, warming; muscle aches and pains; digestive problems, nausea, motion sickness, constipation, indigestion, heartburn; arthritis, rheumatism

9 LAVENDER

Scent Sweet, floral

Used for Calming, sedative, antiseptic; insomnia, stress, depression; burns; acne, eczema; backache, muscular pain, sprains and strains; nausea; catarrh, sinusitis, colds, coughs, chest infections; dandruff

10 LEMON

Scent Refreshing, citrus

Used for Astringent, antiseptic; warts, verrucae, athlete's foot; bad breath; flu

11 LEMONGRASS

Scent fresh, citrus

Used for Sedative, antiseptic; fatigue, chronic fatigue syndrome, stress; insect repellent, restless legs; digestive problems, constipation; acne

12 MANDARIN

Scent Fresh, fruity, citrus

Used for Relaxing, calming, refreshing, gentle, safe; suitable for babies

13 MARJORAM

Scent Herby, sweet, camphor

Used for Calming, antiseptic; chest infections, coughs and colds; constipation, flatulence; headaches; insomnia; muscular pain, backache; arthritis, rheumatism

14 NEROLI

Scent Sweet, floral

Used for Calming, sedative; stress; insomnia; diarrhea, irritable bowel syndrome; premenstrual syndrome

15 ORANGE

Scent fresh, citrus

Used for astringent, uplifting; constipation; stress

16 PEPPERMINT

Scent Minty, fresh

Used for Stimulating, decongestant; catarrh, sinusitis, coughs, colds, chest infections; headaches; nausea

17 ROSEMARY

Scent Herby, fresh

Used for Invigorating, refreshing, antibacterial, decongestant; backache, muscular pain, sprains and strains; catarrh, sinusitis, coughs, colds; headaches, dandruff

18 SANDALWOOD

Scent Sweet, woody

Used for Calming, soothing, anti-inflammatory, antiseptic; skin problems, eczema; sore throats, coughs, colds, chest infections, sore throat

19 TEA TREE

Scent Fresh, spicy

Used for Antifungal, antiviral, antibacterial, antiseptic; boosting immune system; warts, verruca; acne, boils, dermatitis; bad breath, gum disease; insect bites; cuts; colds, coughs, sinusitis, sore throat, tonsillitis; fainting, fever

20 YLANG YLANG

Scent Exotic, floral

Used for Sedative, soothing, antidepressant; depression; premenstrual syndrome

Children's Health Problems

Babies and children experience rapid physical growth and emotional development. Their fast-growing bodies require healthy nutrients and exercise, and they also need to develop a wide range of everyday skills, mobility, and social behaviors. As they grow and develop individually, they will not only pass many milestones but will also come into contact with common health problems and infectious childhood illnesses. This is perfectly natural and your child needs to be vaccinated against some diseases, such as mumps, measles, rubella, and whooping cough, and exposed to a range of minor infections and viruses in order to build up immunity.

Even the common cold or a cough is distressing for babies, and it is always sensible to err on the side of caution and consult your doctor if you are worried or in any doubt. The younger your baby or toddler is, the more vigilant you must be in spotting the symptoms of poor health or illness and taking action or seeking medical advice as soon as possible—your child cannot tell you what is wrong or describe the location and nature of the pain. Especially in their first year, when their immune system is not well-developed, children are particularly susceptible to infections, and fevers, dehydration, and breathing difficulties are potentially more serious, so don't adopt a "wait-and-see-how-it-is-in-the-morning" policy—act fast and play safe.

Not all health problems are a cause for concern. All babies will experience teething problems, diaper rash, and sleepless nights to a lesser or greater degree, and many of these problems can be treated with some traditional self-help measures or natural remedies and a large pinch of common sense.

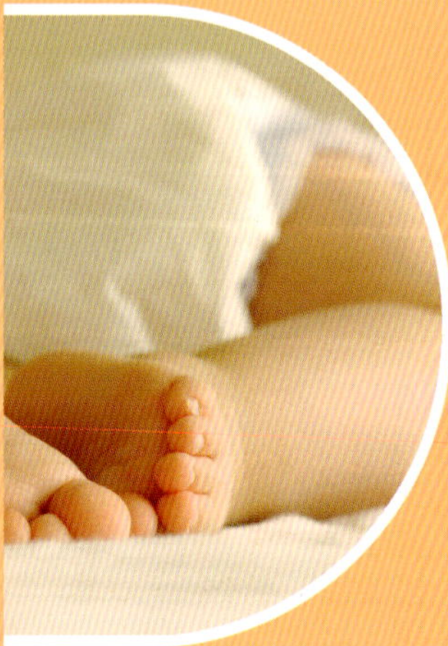

Diaper Rash

Diaper rash is caused by contact with either urine or feces, which makes the skin produce less protective oil and, therefore, provide a less effective barrier to additional irritation. Friction may also exacerbate this distressing condition, which can be painful and may make your baby irritable and prone to waking up during the night.

SYMPTOMS

- Redness in the diaper area, sometimes spreading up to the abdomen or down your baby's legs
- Redness may be blotchy, spotty, or appear as a uniform, raised red rash covering a large area
- White patches on the diaper rash may indicate thrush (candida), a type of fungal infection
- In a candida rash, the skin may be inflamed with extra spots around the edges

PREVENTION

Although most babies will get diaper rash at some time or another, there are many things you can do to try to prevent it from occurring.

- Change your baby as soon as the diaper becomes wet or soiled. Use a barrier cream, such as zinc oxide, which will protect his/her skin from coming into contact with feces and urine.
- If your baby is prone to diaper rash, you might consider using disposables some of the time because they tend to be better than reusable diapers at keeping urine away from the skin.
- If you prefer using reusable diapers, put them through an extra rinse cycle to be sure that there are no traces of detergent.
- Avoid using soap or other detergents on the diaper area. Rinse carefully with clean water at each diaper change.
- Let your baby spend as long as possible without wearing diapers to let the area dry and heal.

CONVENTIONAL TREATMENTS

Your doctor will recommend changing your baby more frequently and allowing periods of time without a diaper. In severe cases, an ointment containing a mild corticosteroid may be prescribed to suppress the inflammation. This might be prescribed in combination with an antifungal medicine to kill any candida present.

HERBAL REMEDIES

- Rub a little calendula (marigold) ointment onto the cleaned diaper area to soothe and to reduce inflammation.
- Powdered goldenseal can be applied to a cleaned diaper area before you put on the diaper.
- Give your baby plenty of soothing drinks, such as very diluted, cooled chamomile tea, to reduce the acidity of the urine. There are many herbal formulas available for newborn babies, but make sure there isn't any sugar in the preparation. If you are breast-feeding, continue to do so, making sure that your baby remains well hydrated and that his/her urine is not too concentrated.

HOMEOPATHIC REMEDIES

Homeopathic remedies may be helpful, but see a homeopath if your baby experiences regular rashes in the diaper area, or if you suspect thrush.

Rhus tox 6C: Use for an itchy, blistered rash.

Sulfur 6C: This may be appropriate if the skin is dry and scaled.

Merc sol 6C: This can help to reduce the acidity of the urine.

Cantharis 6C: Use when the urine is scalding and the skin is raw.

CALL YOUR DOCTOR

Any diaper rash that does not heal within a week or so should be seen by a doctor. Rashes that are accompanied by white patches, sores, or yellow spots should also always be investigated.

Flower Remedies

Rescue Remedy cream may be gently massaged into the affected area to reduce inflammation and ease any pain or itching. A few drops of Rescue Remedy on the pulse points will help to calm down a baby who is distressed.

Aromatherapy

- A drop of lavender or rose oil in a peach kernel carrier oil can be gently rubbed into the diaper area. Use this to protect against diaper rash as well as heal it.
- A drop of oregano or thyme oil in a light carrier oil, such as olive oil, can be used to discourage thrush.

Traditional Remedies

- Egg white can be painted on the baby's sore skin; let it dry before putting on a diaper. This will encourage the skin to heal and prevent additional irritation.
- You can spread yogurt with live cultures on the diaper area to soothe it and prevent thrush from occurring in the skin folds.
- Some people swear that using powdered cornstarch or arrowroot instead of talcum powder is soothing to a baby's skin.
- Blend a little baking soda with some warm water and use to wash your baby's skin in the diaper area.

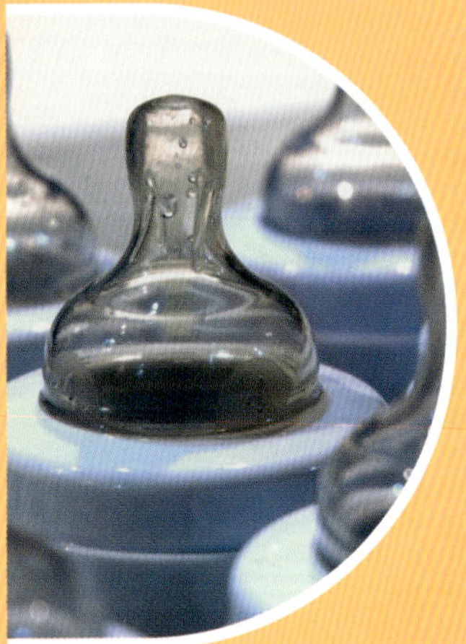

Infant Colic

Colic is characterized by apparently unending frantic crying, usually at around the same time of the day or night. Your baby's legs will be drawn up to the abdomen, and he may appear to be in severe pain. Excessive crying causes him to swallow air, which can lead to abdominal bloating and exacerbate the problem. Most cases of colic resolve themselves at around three or four months of age.

SYMPTOMS

- Seemingly endless crying, usually at the same time of day or night
- Legs drawn up to abdomen
- Belching and other symptoms of gas
- Abdominal bloating
- Arched back

Did You Know?

The causes are unknown, but colic may be linked with contractions of the colon, an intolerance to formula (if bottle-fed) or the mother's diet (if breast-fed), or simply excessive air that is gulped in during repeated bouts of crying. There is some evidence that a difficult birth can lead to colic.

PREVENTION

- If you are bottle-feeding, consider changing the brand of formula—you can ask your doctor about hypoallergenic or lactose-free formulas. You can also purchase anticolic feeding bottles, which reduce the amount of air that your baby takes in while feeding. Burping your baby several times during feeding may also help, as well as giving a massage before a feed.
- If you are breast-feeding, avoid eating dairy produce for a few days to see if this helps. Your baby could have an allergy or intolerance that is making him or her react to something in your milk. Other foods to be avoided are very spicy dishes, citrus fruits, gas-producing foods (beans, cabbage, etc.) and sugar, all of which may make your baby uncomfortable.
- Some mothers who breastfeed their babies find that abstaining from eating onions and garlic helps to prevent colic.

CONVENTIONAL TREATMENTS

There are a variety of over-the-counter antispasmodic medicines that may be suggested for your baby. Simethicone drops, which is used to relieve trapped air, may help. Babies over three months can be given acetaminophen to ease discomfort.

NATURAL REMEDIES

You may need to experiment to find out which natural remedies work best for your baby.

HERBAL REMEDIES Because colic in babies is exacerbated by tension, relaxing herbs are often suggested—used in the bath, or infused, cooled slightly, and drunk from a bottle. Chamomile, lemon balm, and limeflower are most effective. A warm bath with an infusion of dill, fennel, marshmallow, or lemon balm will usually soothe a colicky baby.

FLOWER REMEDIES Rock Rose flower essence is excellent for distress and fright, and Rescue Remedy can be used to calm and help to reduce any spasm. Place a drop or two on your baby's pulse points.

Aromatherapy

- A gentle massage of the abdominal area with one or a blend of essential oils of chamomile, dill, lavender, or rose, will help to ease symptoms and calm a distressed baby. Try massaging before feeding. A drop of each in a warm carrier oil, such as grapeseed, should be adequate.
- Try a drop of lavender or chamomile oil in a warm bath just before evening feeds.

HOMEOPATHIC REMEDIES

Make sure you use the appropriate homeopathic remedy for the symptoms presented.

Chamomilla 30C is useful for babies who seem better when they are held.

Pulsatilla 30C is suggested for babies who are better in the fresh air, and when they are rocked.

Cuprum metallicum 30C is appropriate when your baby's stomach rumbles, and fingers and toes are curled in discomfort.

CALL YOUR DOCTOR

Colic is distressing for you as well as your baby, and you may well find it difficult or even impossible to comfort your screaming child. However, colic is rarely a serious problem and if your baby is healthy, putting on weight, and sleeping well, you need not worry. If your baby begins to resist feeding or is experiencing vomiting, diarrhea, or a fever, you must contact your doctor and get professional medical advice.

Teething

Babies get their first teeth between four and six months of age, but there can be problems with teeth coming through until they reach two or three. The majority experience some discomfort, which can range from being clingy and fractious to dribbling, loosened stools, and problems sleeping.

SYMPTOMS

- Irritability and fussiness as the gums become sore
- Drooling
- Coughing or gagging, as a result of extra saliva
- A rash on the chin
- Gnawing and biting everything put into the mouth
- Rubbing cheeks and pulling ears, because the pain travels to the ear area and around the jaw
- Mild diarrhea
- A slightly raised temperature
- Poor sleep
- A runny nose

PREVENTION

You can't do much to prevent the discomfort, but you can make your baby more comfortable by offering a cool teething gel to gnaw on, or a washcloth soaked in freezing cold water. Rub the gums with a clean finger.

CONVENTIONAL TREATMENTS

Use a gentle teething gel to rub into the gums, but many contain acetaminophen, so don't use them at the same time as any oral doses for pain relief.

NATURAL REMEDIES

AROMATHERAPY A few drops of chamomile and lavender essential oils can be added to the bathwater to calm a distressed baby.

FLOWER REMEDIES Rub a little Rescue Remedy directly into the gums, or apply to pulse points if your baby is crying inconsolably. A few drops at nighttime will encourage sleep, as will a few drops of lavender oil on a handkerchief tied to the head of the crib.

HOMEOPATHIC REMEDIES

- Chamomilla is standard for teething, and 6C can be taken as required up to six times a day to ease symptoms and relieve the distress.
- Homeopathic teething granules are also available, and they will help to ease the symptoms.
- If your baby has bright red cheeks and a high fever, offer Belladonna, 6C.

HERBAL REMEDIES

Syrup made from the marshmallow root will soothe inflamed gums, and a few teaspoons can be added to your baby's meals. You can also offer infusions of chamomile or fennel to calm and soothe.

CALL YOUR DOCTOR

High fever and vomiting are not symptoms of teething. Always see your doctor without delay if your baby seems unwell.

Catarrh

This is overproduction of thick phlegm by the mucous membranes of the air passages. Inflammation of the membranes, as a result of a cold or flu, is the usual cause, but other triggers include passive smoking, inhalation of dust, chronic sinusitis, upper respiratory tract infection, or allergy.

SYMPTOMS

- ▷ A blocked and stuffy nose.
- ▷ An excessive discharge of mucus from the nose, or down the back of the throat
- ▷ An irritating, persistent cough
- ▷ Headaches or facial pain

PREVENTION

- Be sure that your house is free of dust and smoke.
- Chronic catarrh is a common symptom of food allergy, so assess your child's diet carefully (see pages 148–149).

CONVENTIONAL TREATMENTS

Antihistamine or steroid nasal sprays, cough suppressants, decongestants, and acetaminophen are the usual conventional remedies for treating pain. Antibiotics are used to treat any bacterial infection.

NATURAL REMEDIES

If the problem is recurrent, it's worth getting an individual opinion from a qualified practitioner.

HERBAL REMEDIES Herbs such as golden rod and elderflower are anticatarrhal and astringent. Take them as an infusion, several times each day.

AROMATHERAPY Eucalyptus, chamomile, and mint oils are decongestant and expectorant. Rub into the child's chest and temples in a light carrier oil, such as grapeseed, or place several drops in a vaporizer and encourage your child to inhale.

NUTRITIONAL MEDICINE

- Beta-carotene helps to strengthen mucous membranes of the respiratory system; choose red, orange, and yellow fruits and vegetables.
- Cut down on mucus-forming foods, such as dairy produce.

HOMEOPATHIC REMEDIES

Choose the most appropriate remedy for the symptoms presented.

Arsenicum 30C, for thick, yellow discharge that makes the nose and the surrounding area sore.

Pulsatilla 30C, for yellow or green catarrh that is not painful; accompanied by weepiness.

Natrum muriaticum 30C, for catarrh like raw egg white, with a dry nose and loss of taste and smell.

CALL YOUR DOCTOR

If the catarrh becomes thick and yellow or green, call your doctor to rule out an infection.

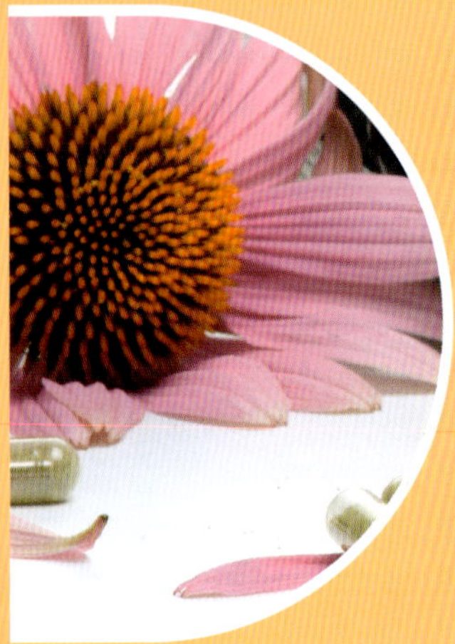

Colds

The common cold is an infection of the upper respiratory tract, which may be caused by any one of up to 200 strains of virus. These are spread either by inhaling droplets coughed or sneezed by others, or more probably by direct contact when your child touches something that has been touched by someone with the virus. The incubation period is from one to three days, after which symptoms start to occur, and most colds run their course in 3 to 10 days.

SYMPTOMS

- Running or stuffy nose
- Headache
- Sometimes a cough
- Sometimes throat discomfort
- Fevers of up to 102°F in infants and children
- General malaise

PREVENTION

Small children are more susceptible than adults to the viruses that cause colds and flu because their immune systems are immature. Don't be surprised if your children seem to contract every cold they come into contact with. Keeping their immune system strong by feeding a healthy diet and making sure that they get plenty of sleep can help. Teach them to wash their hands regularly with hot soapy water.

CONVENTIONAL TREATMENTS

In conventional medicine, colds are usually treated with rest and fluids, in addition to antihistamines, decongestants, and cough medicines as required. Acetaminophen or ibuprofen may be suggested to lower your child's temperature and relieve any pain.

Did You Know?

Babies and children can have a temperature of up to 102°F. Such a high fever in an adult would indicate flu, but it is less to worry about in children who become hotter faster.

NATURAL REMEDIES

Natural remedies work to heal a cold gently, while boosting your child's overall vitality.

FLOWER REMEDIES Rescue Remedy is the traditional way to soothe any distress—rub the cream into your child's chest area to calm them. Olive flower essence will help with fatigue.

HERBAL REMEDIES

- Goldenseal and elecampane are useful for clearing mucus from the lungs and nasal passages in chronic colds.
- Elderflower, drunk as an infusion, will reduce catarrh and help to decongest.
- Chamomile infusion will soothe an irritable child and help him to sleep. Chamomile also has antiseptic action, which will help to rid the body of infection, and it works to reduce fever and feverish symptoms.
- Herbs to strengthen the immune system, such as echinacea, can be taken throughout a cold, and in the period afterward to stimulate healing and prevent subsequent infection.

Aromatherapy

- Place your child's head over a steaming bowl of water with a few drops of added essential oil of cinnamon. Drape a towel over his head to make a tent, and let him sit there for four or five minutes to ease congestion. Be careful to make sure that the water is not boiling and that it cannot be knocked over.
- Try adding a few drops of lavender or tea tree oil to a warm bath to encourage healing and help to open up the airways.

HOMEOPATHIC REMEDIES

If your child gets recurrent colds, it would be a good idea to try a constitutional homeopathic treatment and perhaps consult a qualified practitioner. In the short term, however, the following remedies should help, according to the symptoms presented.

Aconite 30C in the first stages of a cold, particularly if it seems to have come on suddenly, after your child has been outside, for example.

Belladonna 30C, for colds with a high temperature, and great thirst.

Natrum muriaticum 30C, for watery colds, particularly if they are accompanied by cold sores.

Arsenicum 30C, for watery colds, especially if your child is prone to frequent colds.

Pulsatilla 30C is useful if your child is clingy and irritable, and when there is thick yellow discharge from the nose.

Bryonia 30C helps an irritable child who is thirsty and wants to be left alone.

CALL YOUR DOCTOR

Most colds can be treated at home with plenty of rest, regular fluids, and conventional over-the-counter medications formulated for children. However, if your child also has a sore throat or fever and it lasts for more than 48 hours, or if your baby has a fever for more than 24 hours or is struggling to feed, call your doctor without delay.

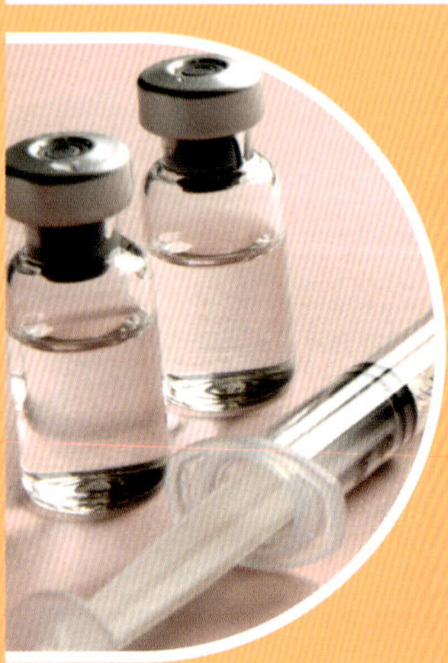

Infectious Childhood Illnesses

The majority of childhood illnesses are on the wane as a result of large-scale immunization, but children who have not been immunized, and even a proportion of those who have been vaccinated, can still contract these conditions, which include mumps, measles, and whooping cough.

PREVENTION

The MMR vaccine is offered to prevent the likelihood of acquiring mumps and measles; immunization against whooping cough (pertussis) is routinely offered to infants, and is given in three doses from two months of age. If you have any concerns about immunization, talk them over with your doctor.

CONVENTIONAL TREATMENTS

Drinking plenty of fluids and getting plenty of rest are the main recommendation for all these infectious childhood illnesses, as well as acetaminophen for pain relief and treating fever. Antibiotics are not prescribed unless there is a secondary infection. If whooping cough is diagnosed early enough, erythromycin can be given to reduce your child's infectivity to others and also to reduce the duration of the illness.

NATURAL REMEDIES

Many of the natural treatments for childhood illnesses are similar. Suggested remedies are given for each of the infectious diseases on the following pages.

FLOWER REMEDIES Rescue Remedy is excellent for calming a child who is frightened by any of the three illnesses (mumps, measles, and whooping cough). A few drops applied to the pulse points, or sipped in a glass of cool water, will help to soothe an upset child. Cherry Plum will help if there is serious spasmodic coughing, and Mimulus and Olive are good in the later stages of whooping cough.

CALL YOUR DOCTOR

If you suspect that your child may have any of these infectious diseases, you must call out a doctor to confirm the diagnosis.

Did You Know?

Mumps and measles are viral illnesses, whereas whooping cough is bacterial. Regardless of the cause, all of these diseases are highly infectious.

INFECTIOUS CHILDHOOD ILLNESSES

Mumps

This viral infection is highly contagious, and children are more commonly affected than adults. There is no cure for mumps and the aim of treatment is always to relieve the symptoms, which usually pass within two weeks.

SYMPTOMS

- Swollen salivary glands, producing a characteristic chipmunk appearance
- Fever and general malaise
- Headache
- Pains in the neck area

NATURAL REMEDIES

Try the following natural remedies to alleviate the symptoms of mumps.

HERBAL REMEDIES Red clover and marigold can help to reduce congestion and swelling. Add tinctures of these to any drink, or offer them to your child as a tea.

AROMATHERAPY Very gently massage the child's neck and jaw with one drop each of chamomile, eucalyptus, and lavender oils in six tablespoons of olive oil.

HOMEOPATHIC REMEDIES

If your child has not had mumps, the homeopathic remedy Phytolacca 30C can be taken during an epidemic to reduce severity of symptoms. If he does succumb, try the following.

Rhus tox 30C when the left glands are more severely affected than the right.

Belladonna 30C when there is high fever, shooting pains, and a bright red face and throat.

Merc sol 30C is useful when there is heavy sweating and a coated tongue.

Pulsatilla 30C may help to prevent orchitis, and is useful if fever continues.

CALL YOUR DOCTOR

If mumps is followed by a severe headache, stiffness, or fever, call your doctor immediately.

Caution

Teenagers and adults have a higher risk of developing complications, such as swelling of the testicles (in boys and men), hearing loss, meningitis, and encephalitis. Always consult your doctor.

INFECTIOUS CHILDHOOD ILLNESSES

Measles

Another highly infectious viral disease, measles can occasionally have serious complications and you should consult your doctor.

SYMPTOMS

- A rash characterized by flat, brown-red spots, which usually begins behind the ears and on the face
- High fever
- Swollen lymph nodes
- Little or no appetite
- Occasionally vomiting and diarrhea

NATURAL REMEDIES

Try the following natural remedies to alleviate the symptoms of measles.

HERBAL REMEDIES A compress of crushed ginger may be placed on the rash to encourage the release of toxins from the body. Heat it a little and wrap it in several layers of gauze to protect the skin.

AROMATHERAPY Lavender oil can be dropped on the bedclothes or on a handkerchief by the bed to calm. It can also be applied neat to spots to encourage healing. When there is a buildup of phlegm, a gentle chest massage with a few drops of tea tree oil in a light carrier oil base will help.

HOMEOPATHIC REMEDIES

In the short term, offer one of the following.

Aconite 30C and **Belladonna 30C,** for high fever.

Pulsatilla 30C when there is diarrhea, yellow discharge, and a cough.

Bryonia 30C when there is a hard, painful cough and a high temperature accompanied by thirst.

Stramonium 30C when there is a high fever, a red face, and convulsions.

CALL YOUR DOCTOR

With measles, you should call your doctor if the fever recurs several days after the spots have begun to heal.

Caution

Keep your child in a darkened room during an episode of measles. Many children are sensitive to bright light during measles, and their eyes can be damaged.

INFECTIOUS CHILDHOOD ILLNESSES

Whooping Cough

This is an infection of the lining of the respiratory tract. The name is derived from the cough, followed by an intake of breath that sounds like a "whoop."

SYMPTOMS

- A runny or snuffly nose for about a week
- Paroxysms of coughing, which can cause a blue or red face and bulging eyes
- There may be a whooping sound as the child draws breath between coughs
- Coughing fits may cause vomiting

NATURAL REMEDIES

Try the following remedies to alleviate the symptoms of whooping cough.

AROMATHERAPY Mix a few drops of lavender and chamomile oils in a light carrier oil and massage into the chest and back area to calm your child, and to relax tensed muscles. Tea tree, lavender, chamomile, and eucalyptus can be used in a vaporizer to help open the lungs.

HERBAL REMEDIES

- A few drops of thyme tincture can be taken to loosen and expel mucus.
- Elecampane is commonly used for children's coughs, and can be purchased in easy-to-use syrup form.
- After a bath, you can massage a little comfrey ointment into the chest and back to relax and expand the lungs.

HOMEOPATHIC REMEDIES

Treatment should be constitutional, but the following homeopathic remedies could be useful. Use the appropriate one for the symptoms.

Aconite 30C can be taken during an attack, or at the beginning of the illness.

Antimonium tartaricum 30C is particularly good when there is a rattling cough with gasping.

Drosera 30C is useful when the cough is made worse by lying down, and there are pains below the ribs.

Bryonia 30C is suggested when there is a dry, painful cough and vomiting.

Pertussin 30C may be given in one dose toward the end off the disease to prevent an "echo" effect.

CALL YOUR DOCTOR

Most cases of whooping cough in older children and adults can be treated at home, but you must call your doctor immediately if your child becomes blue around the lips. Babies are most at risk of developing complications and sometimes they are admitted to hospital for treatment.

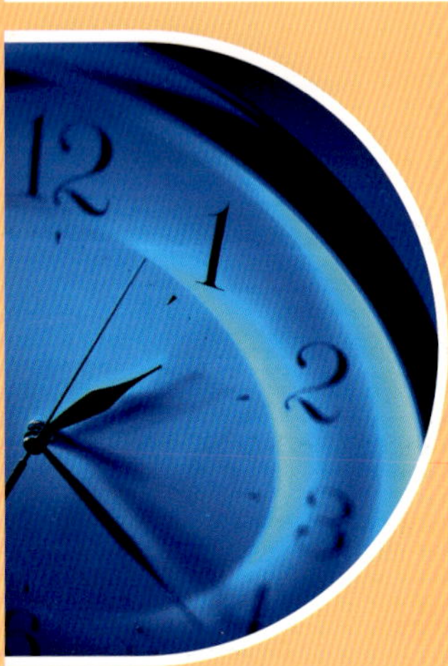

Sleep Problems

Many children have difficulty sleeping, experiencing nightmares or night terrors, sleepwalking or talking in their sleep, struggling to get to sleep, or waking in the early hours and being unable to settle again. Sleep is essential for a child's emotional and physical health and well-being, so it is important that you investigate the underlying causes of sleep disturbances before attempting treatment.

SYMPTOMS

- Waking up during the night
- Inability to fall asleep—or stay asleep
- Nightmares or night terrors
- Sleepwalking
- Talking in their sleep
- Sleep apnoea

Did You Know?

Doctors and psychologists estimate that about 30 percent of children will experience a sleep disorder at some point in their childhood. In many cases, the problems are only temporary, caused by illness, a change in routine, or even growth spurts.

PREVENTION

How you prevent sleep problems depends to some extent on your child's age. It takes babies a while to get into a regular pattern of sleeping and waking, and many parents expect them to sleep more than they actually need to, thereby creating a problem for themselves. Most toddlers and preschool children sleep between 10 and 12 hours per night.

- Do make sure that your child has plenty of regular exercise and fresh air, so that he is physically tired enough to fall asleep.
- A healthy diet that is low in processed food and sugar, focusing instead on good-quality proteins and whole grains, can help to prevent your child's blood sugar from soaring and dipping, which can exacerbate sleep problems.
- Establish a simple, reassuring bedtime routine and modify it as your child gets older. This should include: a bath, brushing teeth, a bedtime story, and a goodnight hug and a kiss. A favorite soft toy and soothing music or a warm milky drink may also be helpful in encouraging sleep.

CONVENTIONAL TREATMENTS

Your child will be treated according to the cause of any sleep problems, but most doctors are reluctant to offer medication except in severe cases. Behavioral modification is offered first.

NATURAL REMEDIES

There are several types of remedy to try, depending on the specific problem. A common-sense approach is to get your child into a relaxing bedtime routine (see Prevention opposite), so that going to bed becomes a pleasurable experience.

AROMATHERAPY A few drops of chamomile, geranium, rose, or lavender can be added to the bathwater to calm and soothe, or placed on a handkerchief by the bed. A gentle massage before bedtime, with a little lavender or chamomile blended into a light carrier oil, may ease any tension or distress.

HERBAL REMEDIES

- Vervain infusion is a gentle sedative and can help children fall asleep—particularly, if they are fighting it.
- An infusion of limeflowers is useful for children who are nervous and sensitive.
- A crying baby may be soothed with an infusion of chamomile, offered an hour or so before bedtime, or on waking in the night.
- A strong infusion of chamomile, hops, lavender, or limeflowers can be added to a warm bath to soothe and calm a baby or child.

HOMEOPATHIC REMEDIES

Remedies should be taken an hour before going to bed for up to 14 days. Repeat the dose if your child wakes in the night and cannot get back to sleep.

Calcarea 30C and **Antimonium tartaricum 30C,** for night terrors.

Colocynth 30C or **Bryonia 30C,** for constant crying.

Arsenicum 30C when your child wakes between midnight and 2 a.m., restless, worried, and apprehensive.

Rhus tox 30C when your child cannot sleep, is irritable, restless, and wants to walk around.

Aconite 30C, for restlessness and nightmares.

Pulsatilla 30C, for a weepy, clingy child.

Chamomilla 30C if sleep is disturbed by teething, or if your child cannot settle without being hugged, rocked, or patted to sleep.

Nux vomica 30C, for irritability, and after a busy day or too much food or fun.

CALL YOUR DOCTOR

If the sleep difficulties last longer than a couple of months, your child is very sleepy during the day, or seems distressed by chronic nightmares or night terrors, you should call your doctor.

Flower Remedies

- White Chestnut will be helpful for children with overactive minds.
- Offer Rock Rose for night terrors.
- Aspen is useful for fear of the dark, and Mimulus is good for other "known" fears.

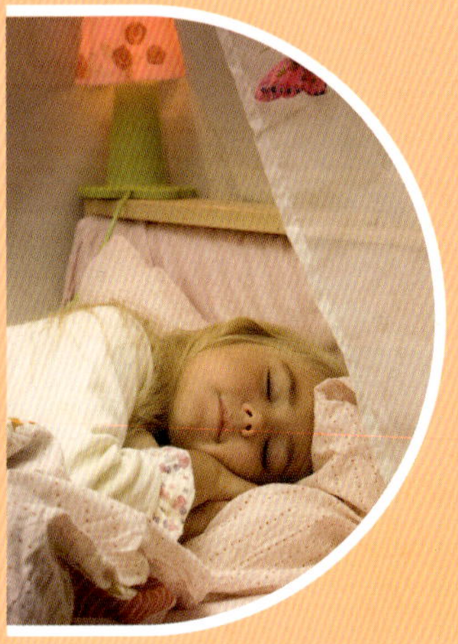

Bed-Wetting

Bed-wetting (enuresis) is not considered a problem until your child is at least five years old. Many children, boys in particular, are slow in getting the message that they should get up to use the bathroom at night, but that is no reflection on the state of their health—emotional or otherwise. Some children are naturally deep sleepers and may take several years to stay dry at night; many children manage it by the age of two or three.

SYMPTOMS

- Nighttime urination

Did You Know?

Bed-wetting almost always stops as children get older because their bladder capacity increases as they grow and they learn to wake up if their bladder is full.

PREVENTION

- Limit drinks in the hour or so before bedtime.
- Some parents find it helps to carry their children to the bathroom partway through the night.
- Reassure your child, because embarrassment can exacerbate the problem.
- Don't be tempted to carry on using diapers—it can be belittling for older children, and younger children will continue to wet them.
- A resumption of bed-wetting in children who have already established a pattern of dry nights is often caused by stress or trauma of some kind, such as moving house, changing schools, family problems, or even a new sibling. In most cases, the problem is resolved by the age of eight.

CONVENTIONAL TREATMENTS

Your doctor may prescribe antidepressants (not for depression, but because they have an impact on urination) and antidiuretic hormone medication (known as desmopressin), which concentrates the urine at night. A bedtime alarm (known as an enuresis alarm) can waken your child when he begins to urinate, giving him time to get to the bathroom. This has the impact of conditioning him to waken at the first signs of urination.

NATURAL REMEDIES

Treatment should be undertaken according to the likely cause of the enuresis.

HERBAL REMEDIES Offer St. John's wort in a cup of water and sweetened with honey, sipped throughout the day, to encourage control of the bladder. If the bed-wetting stems from an emotional upset or disturbance, infusions of vervain and lemon balm will relax and soothe.

HOMEOPATHIC REMEDIES

The following remedies may have some success.

Equisetum 30C when the wetting occurs during dreams.

Belladonna 30C when it occurs early in the night.

Kreosotum 30C when wetting occurs during dreams in early night, and deep sleep.

Causticum 30C, for wetting in first sleep, worse in clear weather, or when your child has a cough.

Plantago 30C when all else fails.

FLOWER REMEDIES

- Wild Rose if your child seems to drift through life.
- Walnut will help if the bed-wetting is brought on by change, such as a new house, school, or baby.
- Vervain may help if your child is stressed.
- Star of Bethlehem if bed-wetting is related to a trauma or shock.
- Mimulus, when the problem is linked to fear.

CALL YOUR DOCTOR

If your child is still bed-wetting at the age of five, consult your doctor. In some cases, physical illness can be at the root, including food allergies, diabetes, a urinary tract infection, constipation, and sleep apnoea. If your previously dry child wets the bed consistently for six months or more, there may be an underlying physical or emotional cause and it's worth seeking professional advice.

Self-Help Remedies

Try not to become angry with your child because this will only exacerbate the problem and affect their self-esteem. Instead, use a star chart and plenty of praise for dry nights, and don't comment if you find a wet bed. If your child is slightly older, you could suggest a sleepover at a friend's. Many children will not wet the bed under these circumstances, and it can help to break a long-term habit.

Caution

Never punish your child for wetting the bed, however troublesome it may be for you. This could lower their self-esteem and harm them psychologically. Try to be patient.

TOP 20 Healing Herbs

Safe and gentle herbal remedies can offer a holistic approach to healing and help maintain our well-being. Here are the top 20 healing herbs with information on their properties and which common ailments they can be used to treat.

1 ALOE VERA

Properties Antiseptic, blood purifier, laxative, purgative

Used for Acne and skin problems, burns, minor cuts, insect bites, digestive problems

2 BASIL

Properties Energy stimulant, respiratory decongestant, reduces mucus, aids digestion

Used for Fatigue, hay fever, headaches, insomnia, PMS, sinusitis

3 CHAMOMILE

Properties Carminative, anti-inflammatory, aids digestion, reduces mucus, calming

Used for Insomnia, stress, nervous tension, digestive problems, sore throat, colds, catarrh, asthma, eczema, teething problems in babies

4 COMFREY

Properties Tonic, demulcent, arrests bleeding, heals tissue, respiratory system, anemia

Used for Soothing coughs, bronchial inflammation, healing cuts and burns

5 DANDELION

Properties Diuretic, purifies blood, liver tonic, aids digestion, nutritive

Used for Anemia, constipation, fluid retention, diabetes, hepatitis, heart disease, excess weight

6 ECHINACEA

Properties Antibiotic, antiviral, antifungal, immune tonic, blood purifier, fever reducing

Used for Colds, flu, sore throats, acne, athlete's foot, kidney infections, candida and vaginal yeast infections

7 GARLIC

Properties Antiseptic, antibacterial, antifungal, blood purifier, circulatory stimulant, digestive stimulant

Used for Good digestion, lowering blood cholesterol, hypertension, heart disease, respiratory infections, strengthening immune system

8 GINGER

Properties Circulatory stimulant, antiseptic, analgesic, antispasmodic, expectorant

Used for Colds, flu, fever, nausea, and vomiting

9 GOLDENSEAL

Properties Antibiotic, astringent, blood purifier, laxative

Used for Treating inflammation and infection, colds, flu, catarrh, ulcers, nausea, colitis, IBS, gastroenteritis, urinary tract infections, boils

10 LAVENDER

Properties Sedative, cooling, antibacterial, aromatic

Used for Anxiety, stress, headaches, migraines, insomnia, stress, indigestion, coughs, colds, burns, stings, minor cuts, sunburn

11 LEMON BALM

Properties Calming, antibacterial, antidepressant, antiseptic, blood purifier and regulator, insect repellant

Used for Depression, easing menstrual cramping, digestive upsets, infections, fever, insect bites, wounds

12 MARSHMALLOW

Properties Astringent, anti-inflammatory, demulcent, blood purifier, nutritive

Used for Irritable bowel, colitis, kidney stones, urinary inflammations, coughs, catarrh, boils, abscesses, drawing splinters and pus

13 MEADOWSWEET

Properties Calming, antacid, antiseptic, anti-inflammatory, analgesic, diuretic, astringent, source of natural aspirin

Used for Gastritis and digestive upsets, arthritis, rheumatism, headaches, urinary infections

14 PLANTAIN

Properties Antibacterial, diuretic, blood purifier, astringent, demulcent

Used for Insects stings, cuts, abrasions, burns, eczema, IBS, cystitis, heavy menstrual bleeding, thrush, vaginal discharge, gum disease, fever

15 ROSEMARY

Properties Restorative, antiseptic, circulatory stimulant, blood regulator, aromatic

Used for PMS, depression, headaches, migraine, indigestion, constipation, arthritis, rheumatism, colds, flu, fever

16 SAGE

Properties Astringent, antiseptic, diuretic, stimulant, clears mucus

Used for Respiratory problems, ulcers, sore throat, hot flashes in menopause

17 ST. JOHN'S WORT

Properties Antidepressant, sedative, restorative, anti-inflammatory, tonic and pain relieving, soothing, antiseptic

Used for Wounds, inflammations, ulcers, sciatica, neuralgia, rheumatism, anxiety, depression, postoperative pain, period pain, burns, cuts, and scrapes

18 TEA TREE

Properties Antiseptic, antifungal, treating infections

Used for Acne, cold sores, insect stings and bites, warts, abscesses, gum and tooth infections, ringworm, athlete's foot, thrush

19 THYME

Properties Antiseptic, stimulant, respiratory cleanser, expectorant

Used for Colds, flu, coughs, bronchitis, sore throat, diarrhea, wounds

20 YARROW

Properties Anti-inflammatory, astringent, digestive tonic, blood regulator

Used for Fever, wounds, urinary problems, colds, flu, infections, excessive menstrual bleeding, cramping

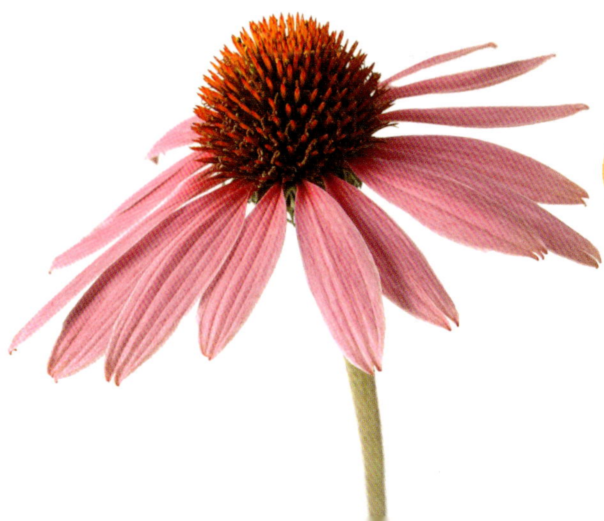

First Aid and Emergencies

You can treat most minor accidental injuries yourself at home with conventional treatments and first-aid measures or natural remedies. Featured in the following pages is practical advice on treating a wide range of problems, ranging from insect bites and stings to nosebleeds, splinters, and fainting. If you know how to treat them fast and effectively, you are less likely to develop complications and you can prevent the condition from getting worse and speed up the healing process.

However, if you have to deal with a serious accident or life-threatening injury, you must contact the emergency services immediately and, if necessary, carry out emergency life-saving first aid, such as resuscitation, which does not come within the scope of this book. It is a good idea to familiarize yourself with these techniques and go on a first-aid course to enable you to deal with emergencies if they arise.

Common sense and good judgment are essential, even when dealing with common injuries, and it is extremely important to stay calm, to reassure your patient, and protect them from additional danger. You should also have a first-aid box at home and keep it stocked up with conventional medications, bandages, dressings, and antiseptic creams as well as natural remedies, such as arnica cream, Bach Rescue Remedy liquid or cream, witch hazel, aloe vera gel, and marigold cream. Eucalyptus, lavender, and tea tree essential oils are also useful. Tweezers, scissors, and safety pins are essential items.

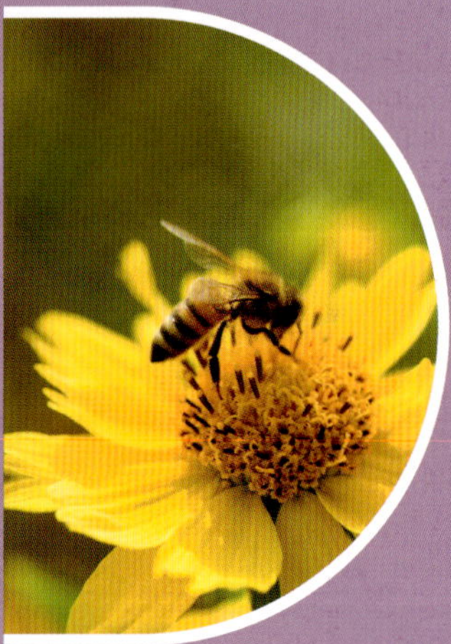

Bites and Stings

If your skin is punctured by an animal bite, you must act quickly because bite and puncture wounds can become infected if they are not treated promptly. Insect bites and stings are seldom serious, but they can trigger allergic reactions in some people. Conventional first aid and natural remedies can treat the problem and alleviate the symptoms. Snake bites from poisonous snakes need prompt emergy treatment; call 911 immediately.

SYMPTOMS

- Puncture marks in the skin
- Bleeding from wound
- Pain and swelling from snake bites
- Itching, pain, redness, and swelling from insect bites and stings
- In rare cases, an allergic reaction with difficulty breathing, pale and clammy skin, sweating, nausea, fainting, mental confusion—call 911 to get immediate emergency help

Did You Know?

Rattlesnakes, copperheads, water moccasins, and coral snakes are poisonous snakes found in the United States, except in Maine, Alaska, and Hawaii. Gila monsters and Mexican beaded lizards are also poisonous. Not all bites release poisonous venom, and a snake or lizard can still have dangerous venom to inject in another bite.

PREVENTION

You can't prevent bites and stings from happening, but you can minimize their likelihood.

- If you live in an area where there are snakes, wear pants and do not go barefoot in the summer. If you hear a rattlesnake, do not approach it. If you hike in areas with rocks and boulders, be careful of snakes sunbathing on them in hot weather.
- If mosquitoes are commonplace, use an insect repellent. You can buy nontoxic natural products as well as chemical repellents. Cover up any exposed skin.
- If you are traveling to a tropical country where malaria is a problem, seek medical advice before you go. You can take antimalaria medication. Be sure to sleep under a mosquito net and check that all doors and windows have insect-proof screens.
- Don't use strongly perfumed cosmetics and deodorants; they can attract insects.
- Check there are no wasp nests in your yard.
- Keep your tetanus injections up to date.

FIRST AID

The conventional remedies for dealing with bites and stings are as follows.

ANIMAL BITES Wash the wound carefully with soap and warm water. Pat dry with a clean tissue, then cover with a sterile dressing or bandage. For wounds with severe bleeding, using a clean pad or dressing, apply direct pressure to the wound to control the bleeding. Cover it with a sterile dressing and bandage and seek medical attention immediately. You may need an antitetanus vaccination or antirabies injections.

SNAKE BITES If you are bitten by a snake, stay calm. Symptoms may appear from within minutes to hours. If you know or think the snake could be poisonous, keep the bitten area as still as possible and seek immediate medical attention by calling 911. Try to remember what the snake or lizard looked like to help identify the type. You can treat a nonpoisonous bite at home by gently washing the bite and applying a bandage.

INSECT BITES Most gnat and mosquito bites can be treated locally with soothing calamine lotion or antihistamine cream. Or apply a cold compress and take painkillers, such as acetaminophen. For severe swelling, your doctor may prescribe oral steroids. If you have a severe allergic reaction, seek immediate medical assistance.

JELLYFISH STINGS If you are stung by a jellyfish, remove any visible stings and treat with calamine lotion or antihistamine cream. Apply cut tomato slices or sit in a warm bath.

INSECT STINGS If the sting is visible, try to remove it with a clean finger or tweezers. Wash with soap and warm water and apply a cold compress to reduce the swelling. If the sting is painful, take acetaminophen or another painkiller. If the pain and swelling persist for 48 hours, seek expert medical help. If you experience a severe allergic reaction, seek emergency help immediately—you may be experiencing life-threatening anaphylactic shock.

NATURAL REMEDIES

There are many traditional remedies for insect bites.

- Cut a clove of garlic and rub onto the skin surrounding mosquito bites, or blend a crushed clove with honey and apply to bites and stings.
- Rub a slice of raw onion onto flea bites and bee and wasp stings.
- Make a paste with baking soda and vinegar and dab onto bee stings.
- Make a paste with salt and vinegar and dab onto wasp stings.

AROMATHERAPY Apply a drop of undiluted lavender oil to the insect bite or sting.

HERBAL REMEDIES

- Apply the soothing sap of the aloe vera plant or a little gel to the insect bite.
- Rub the affected area with some plantain leaves or lemon balm.
- For bee and wasp stings, bathe with an infusion of sage or marigold.

HOMEOPATHIC REMEDIES

The remedy used will depend on the symptoms.

Apis mel 30C, for burning and rapid swelling from bee and wasp stings and insect bites, take one tablet every hour for three doses.

Ledum palustre 30C, for immediate swelling from animal and insect bites and stings, take one tablet hourly for three doses.

CALL YOUR DOCTOR

If you are bitten by a snake or develop a severe reaction to an insect sting, call 911 and seek emergency care immediately. If you are bitten by an animal or have a severe reaction to an insect bite, call your doctor.

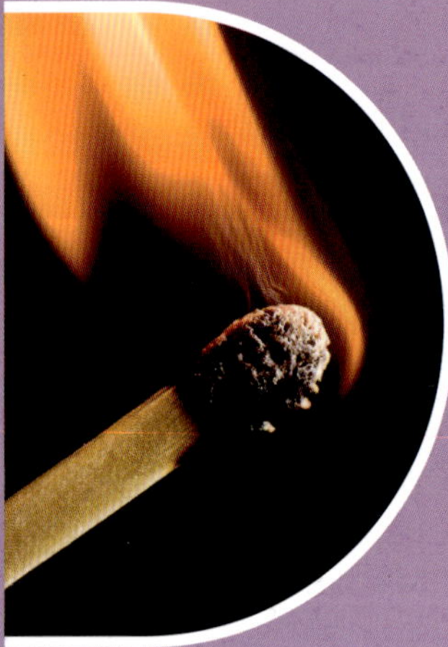

Burns and Scalds

Burns are damage to the skin's tissues, caused by dry heat (fire), corrosive chemicals, electricity, radiated heat (from the sun), or friction. Scalds are caused by moist heat (hot liquids or steam). Both burns and scalds are treated in the same way with first-aid measures, although natural remedies may be used to relieve pain and speed up healing.

SYMPTOMS

- Sore, red skin
- May be blisters (pockets of clear fluid)
- Pain and swelling
- In severe cases, skin may be broken, severely blistered, or charred (black) with intense pain

Caution

- Do not try to remove any clothing that may be stuck to burned skin.
- Do not burst any blisters that form.
- Do not apply cream, ointment, or butter to the burn.
- Do not attempt to cool it with ice.

PREVENTION

To minimize the risk of burns and scalds, be aware of potentially dangerous situations and substances and follow common-sense safety guidelines.

- Always be careful when filling hot water bottles, pouring boiling water out of kettles, and handling hot liquids.
- Use coiled safety cables on electric kettles and never leave any wires and cables hanging down within reach of young children.
- Never put your hand over steam.
- Be especially careful when using deep fryers.
- Be careful when handling chemicals or electrical wires. Always unplug appliances and turn off the electric current before tackling do-it-yourself jobs.
- Protect open fireplaces with a sturdy fireguard.
- Wear a strong sunscreen in hot, sunny weather to protect your skin from burning.

FIRST AID

The conventional advice for dealing with minor burns and scalds is to treat them immediately without delay.

1 Stop the burning process by dousing the flames with water or smothering them in a blanket.

2 Remove any jewelry or clothing near the burned skin but not if it is sticking to the burn. If it has been soaked in boiling water, hot fat, or chemical agents and is not sticking to the burned area, you should remove it.

3 Cool the burn with cold or tepid water for at least 10 minutes, or until the pain stops. You can do this by immersing the burned area in cold water or holding it under a running water.

4 Cover the burn with plastic wrap, a clean plastic bag, or clean, nonfluffy material to protect it from infection.

5 Keep warm if the burn is extensive to prevent your body temperature from dropping and hypothermia.

NOTE For burns to the mouth and throat, sip some cold water.

NATURAL REMEDIES

Severe burns should always be treated by a medical professional, but there are some natural remedies that may be helpful for healing minor burns after the first aid measures outlined above.

HERBAL REMEDIES When healing is underway, you can soothe minor burns with aloe vera sap or gel. Alternatively, smooth in a little calendula ointment. Diluted witch hazel promotes healing and helps prevent infection.

AROMATHERAPY Apply a drop of undiluted lavender oil to minor burns where there is no blistering or broken skin after immersing the area in cold water and patting it dry.

HOMEOPATHIC REMEDIES

The remedy used will depend on the symptoms.

Aconitum 30C, for initial trauma and shock.

Cantharis 30C, for raw burns with severe pain and possibly blisters.

Urtica urens 30C, for red skin with minor stinging.

CALL YOUR DOCTOR

You can treat most minor burns yourself at home but severe burns will require immediate medical attention. These include the following:

- Burns affecting an extensive area with seriously blistered skin
- Burns to the mouth and throat, which cause swelling and inflammation
- Deep burns with broken, charred skin
- Chemical and electrical burns.

NOTE Pregnant women, babies, and young children should also see a doctor.

Self-Help Remedies

- Always keep the burned area clean and dry.
- If the burn is extensive, drink additional fluids to prevent feeling dehydrated.
- Eating foods that are good sources of vitamin C (citrus fruits, strawberries, tomatoes, bell peppers, and leafy green vegetables) and zinc (pumpkin seeds, mushrooms, seafood, meat, eggs) will promote repair of damaged skin tissue. Or you can take supplements.

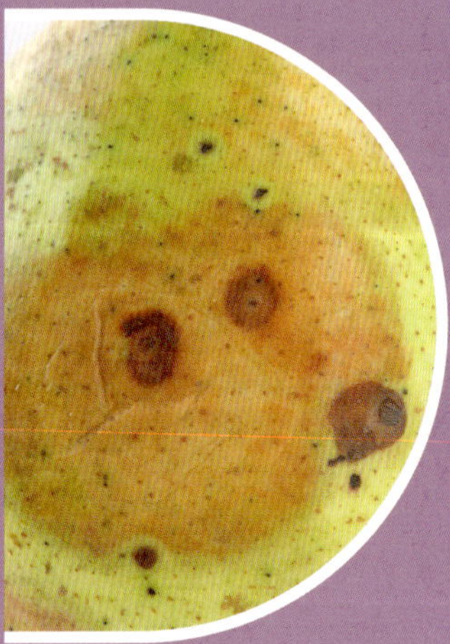

Bruises

A bruise is a discolored area of skin caused by damaged tiny broken blood vessels leaking blood underneath into the dermis. It is usually caused by a blow or pressure and gradually fades as it heals. Severe bruising and swelling of the eye socket and eye lids is known as a black eye.

SYMPTOMS

- Blue, purple, or black patch of skin
- Fades to yellow or green before disappearing
- Pain, tenderness, and swelling
- Movement may be restricted

PREVENTION

You can't prevent bruising, but if you have a tendency to bruise easily and frequently you should take extra care to avoid bangs, falls, and other injuries.

FIRST AID

Treat a bruise as soon as possible after injury to minimize the swelling and bruising.

1 Apply an ice pack to the bruised area. A bag of frozen peas is ideal for this—first wrap it in a cloth or towel. Keep it in place with a bandage or cloth. Cooling the area with ice packs will help limit the bleeding under the skin.

2 Alternatively, apply a cold compress—soak a towel or washcloth in cold water, wring it out, and apply to the bruise, changing it every 10 minutes for 30 minutes.

3 Elevating the bruised limb, especially if it is a leg or foot, may promote healing.

4 If necessary, take a painkiller, such as ibuprofen.

Did You Know?

You may have a tendency to bruise more easily if you are slim and don't have much padding and fat covering your arms and legs.

NATURAL REMEDIES

Bruises usually respond well to old-fashioned, natural remedies. Some people believe that the best remedy for a black eye is to hold a raw steak against it.

HERBAL REMEDIES Apply a cold compress soaked in an infusion of comfrey or rue; or gently smooth some comfrey, chickweed, or arnica lotion or cream into the bruised area. Or you can rub some aloe vera gel or sap into the bruise.

AROMATHERAPY Add two drops each of chamomile and lavender essential oils to some ice-cold water and use as a compress.

SELF-HELP REMEDIES For a black eye or any other form of bruising, drink several glasses of pineapple juice daily. It contains enzymes that help to speed up healing. Apply a vitamin E cream to the bruised skin.

HOMEOPATHIC REMEDIES

The remedy used will depend on the symptoms.

Arnica 30C, for all bruising.

Ledum palustre 30C, for dark bruises that feel cold and black eyes with swollen skin.

Bellis perennis 30C, for deep bruising and sore muscles.

Aconite 30C, for shock after the blow of a black eye.

CALL YOUR DOCTOR

Most bruising is minor and does not need medical attention, but you should consult your doctor for any of the following:

- You have two black eyes, which may indicate a fractured skull
- Bruises appear for no apparent reason without injury
- You have a tendency to bruise easily and often
- Bruising is accompanied by severe pain and difficulty moving.

NOTE There may be an underlying medical condition that is causing unexplained bruising, possibly linked to blood clotting or liver problems, so have it checked without delay. In addition, not all bruises are visible. Deep, internal bruising after an injury or accident may cause pain and swelling; if in doubt, always check with your doctor.

Quick Fix

If you hit your skin, injure yourself, or at the first sign of a bruise appearing, quickly rub in some arnica cream.

Caution

- Never rub or vigorously massage the bruise—this will only make it worse.
- Never apply arnica cream to broken skin.

Cuts and Grazes

You can treat most minor cuts and grazes yourself. They may bleed and feel painful at the time, but they will soon heal. However, deeper cuts with greater blood loss may damage blood vessels, nerves, and tendons below the skin.

SYMPTOMS

- ▷ Bleeding and pain
- ▷ Surface layer of skin is scraped off (graze).

PREVENTION

Obviously, you cannot prevent cuts and grazes from happening occasionally, but you can be extra careful when you are using sharp kitchen knives, saws, axes, and gardening implements. A lot of accidents involving cuts occur in the home and yard.

FIRST AID

1 Stop any bleeding by applying pressure to the cut with a clean, dry towel or cloth.

2 Wash the cut area under running tap water or bathe with warm water to clean the wound and remove dirt.

3 Gently pat dry with a clean towel.

4 Cover with a sterile dressing or bandage.

NATURAL REMEDIES

Cuts and grazes have been treated with natural therapies and remedies for centuries.

HERBAL REMEDIES Chamomile, echinacea, calendula (marigold), or St. John's wort cream may aid the healing process for cuts and grazes.

AROMATHERAPY When cleaning a cut or graze, add antiseptic lavender or tea tree oil to the warm water. To speed up healing, apply diluted essential oil of lavender or cloves.

HOMEOPATHIC REMEDIES

The remedy used will depend on the symptoms.

Hypericum 30C, for all deep and painful wounds, especially with dirt.

Ledum palustre 30C, for clean puncture wounds and cuts.

Calendula 30C, for profuse bleeding and probable infection.

CALL YOUR DOCTOR

Seek medical help in the following instances:

- You have a deep wound and cannot stop the bleeding after applying direct pressure for 10 minutes. It may need stitches.
- The cut is contaminated with substances you can't remove, such as glass.
- It becomes infected and painful with swelling, redness, and pus.
- It will not close and opens up when you move.

NOTE Keep your tetanus injections up to date.

Self-Help Remedies

- To bathe cuts and grazes, add ordinary table salt to the warm water—it is a good disinfectant.
- Blend a spoonful of honey with a crushed garlic clove and smear over cuts and grazes before covering with a clean dressing.

Nosebleeds

Nosebleeds (epistaxis) are rarely serious and may be caused by minor injuries, infections, illness, or cold weather. When the tiny blood vessels inside the nose rupture—perhaps due to cracked, dry mucous membranes—your nose bleeds.

SYMPTOMS

- Bleeding from the nose
- Usually from one nostril but may be both
- Flow of blood may be heavy or light

PREVENTION

You cannot prevent nosebleeds from happening, but you can make them less probable by not picking your nose or blowing it too hard.

FIRST AID

1 Sit down, leaning forward.

2 Breathing through your mouth, pinch the fleshy end of your nose (just above your nostrils) between your thumb and index finger. Hold for 10 to 20 minutes, until the bleeding stops.

3 Wipe away any blood from around the nose and mouth with cotton balls moistened with water.

NOTE Don't lie down—the blood will drain down the back of your throat.

Did You Know?

Nosebleeds are more common when you are pregnant because the increased blood supply in your body makes the tiny blood vessels in the nose more susceptible to rupture. You may also get them if you are taking aspirin or anticoagulants (such as warfarin) or have a blood disorder.

NATURAL REMEDIES

The traditional natural approaches to dealing with nosebleeds are listed below. Applying an ice pack or cold sponge may help stop the bleeding.

HERBAL REMEDIES When the bleeding stops, plug the nostril with a cotton ball soaked in witch hazel.

HOMEOPATHIC REMEDIES

The remedy used will depend on the symptoms.

Ferrum phos 30C, for bright red blood that oozes from the nose.

Phosphorus 30C, for nosebleeds in children and when blowing the nose.

Sabina 30C, for a general tendency to nosebleeds.

Arnica 30C, for nosebleeds resulting from a blow to the nose.

CALL YOUR DOCTOR

If the bleeding continues for more than 30 minutes and will not stop, you should seek medical attention. Likewise, if it is accompanied by shortness of breath or palpitations, or you vomit from swallowing blood. Consult your doctor if you have frequent nosebleeds—more than once a week—for no apparent reason; they may be a symptom of an underlying medical condition, such as high blood pressure.

Fainting

Fainting is a brief loss of consciousness, caused by a sudden drop in blood pressure or abnormally low blood sugar levels. Emotional shock, stress, anxiety, exhaustion, standing for too long, dehydration, and heat can interrupt temporarily the supply of blood to your brain, causing you to faint.

SYMPTOMS

- ▷ Brief loss of consciousness
- ▷ May be preceded by feeling giddy, unsteady, and light-headed
- ▷ Feeling weak, cold, sweaty, or clammy
- ▷ Feeling nauseous
- ▷ Confusion
- ▷ Blurred vision
- ▷ A slow pulse
- ▷ May result in a fall

PREVENTION

You can minimize the risk of fainting by making sure you eat regular meals, drinking sufficient liquid (especially in hot climates), avoiding stuffy and overheated rooms, and not standing for long periods.

FIRST AID

1 If you feel faint, sit or lie down immediately to prevent a fall and subsequent injuries.

2 Ideally, lie on your back with your legs raised above the level of your heart. Support them with some cushions or whatever is handy.

3 Alternatively, if there is no room to lie down, sit with your head between your knees.

4 Loosen any tight clothing and, if indoors, ask someone to open the windows to let in fresh air.

5 When you regain normal consciousness, stay lying down for a few minutes before trying to get up. You may feel weak and confused for up to 30 minutes.

NATURAL REMEDIES

The old-fashioned remedy for fainting was smelling salts, and you can still buy these in pharmacies. After regaining normal consciousness, sip some weak green or Indian tea sweetened with honey.

HERBAL REMEDIES To aid recovery, drink some chamomile tea.

AROMATHERAPY Sniffing rosemary or tea tree oil may help to bring a person round.

FLOWER REMEDIES Take three to four drops of Rescue Remedy in water.

HOMEOPATHIC REMEDIES

Crush a tablet and put a few grains on the tongue.

Ignatia 6C, for sudden emotional shock.

Lilium tigrinum 30C, for becoming overheated.

Sepia 30C, for a general tendency to faint.

CALL YOUR DOCTOR

Isolated episodes are not a cause for concern, but if you have a tendency to faint, consult your doctor. There may be an underlying medical reason for the problem, such as diabetes or heart disease.

NOTE If the person does not regain consciousness, call an ambulance immediately.

Sprains and Strains

A sprain occurs when the ligaments around a joint, such as the wrist, thumb, ankle, or knee, are overstretched, twisted, or even torn. A strain is when the tissues or fibers that make up a muscle become overstretched or torn, usually due to a sudden movement. This is often referred to as "pulling a muscle."

SYMPTOMS

SPRAINS

- ▷ Pain and tenderness around the joint
- ▷ Swelling, inflammation, and bruising
- ▷ Inability to use a joint normally or put weight on it

STRAINS

- ▷ Sudden sharp pain and swelling in a muscle
- ▷ Bruising

PREVENTION

Many sprains and strains are sports injuries: minimize the risk by stretching. Regular exercise in the gym, cycling, swimming, walking, or whatever you enjoy will keep you fit and supple. If you are prone to sprained ankles, strap them up when you exercise and wear supportive sneakers. Don't wear really high heels.

FIRST AID

The acronym for the recommended treatment for sprains and strains is PRICE.

1 Protect the injured joint or muscle from getting worse with a support, if necessary.

2 Rest the injured area for at least 48 hours.

3 Ice packs should be applied to the injury to reduce the swelling for 15 to 20 minutes at a time. Repeat every three hours or so during the first couple of days.

4 Compression will limit movement and decrease swelling. Use a tubular, elastic, or crepe bandage.

5 Elevation of the injured area, especially a knee or ankle joint, will also reduce the swelling.

NATURAL REMEDIES

A warm bath will reduce the swelling and ease the pain—add a cup of Epsom salts or a spoonful of dry mustard.

HERBAL REMEDIES Make a poultice of comfrey or cabbage leaves and wrap around the injury in a towel or cloth. Let sit for 20 to 30 minutes. Rub in a little arnica, comfrey, or marigold cream.

AROMATHERAPY Add chamomile, cypress, eucalyptus, or rosemary oil to a carrier oil and massage gently into the affected area, or add a few drops to a warm bath.

HOMEOPATHIC REMEDIES

Choose a remedy according to the symptoms.

Arnica 30C, for bruising, pain, and shock on the first day.

Ledum palustre 6C, for sprains, especially ankles.

CALL YOUR DOCTOR

Because some sprains can be difficult to differentiate from a fracture, you must seek medical help if:

- The injured joint looks crooked or has unusual lumps and bumps
- The pain is severe and persistent
- You cannot put any weight on the injury or move it
- You experience numbness in the area.

NOTE Do not resume exercise until the injured joint is healed. Returning to a sports activity too soon may cause additional damage. If in doubt, check with your doctor or a sports fitness expert.

Heat Exhaustion

This is when body temperature rises to 98.6–104°F. It should not be confused with heatstroke, when your temperature rises above 104°F. Both conditions are more probable in hot, humid weather.

SYMPTOMS

HEAT EXHAUSTION

- ▷ Feeling hot, flushed, and sweating profusely
- ▷ Headache
- ▷ Feeling faint and dizzy
- ▷ Nausea and vomiting

HEATSTROKE

- ▷ Muscle cramps
- ▷ Rapid, shallow breathing
- ▷ Mental confusion
- ▷ Seizures or fits
- ▷ Loss of consciousness

PREVENTION

- Stay in the shade, out of the sun, especially in the middle of the day, and wear a sun hat.
- Wear loose-fitting, light cotton or linen clothes.
- Don't drink alcohol or caffeinated drinks but have plenty of cold drinks to stay hydrated.
- Keep your house cool.
- Don't leave babies, children, elderly people, or pets in parked cars in hot weather.

FIRST AID

Heat exhaustion leads to heatstroke if left untreated, so act fast.

1 Lie down in a cool place—preferably inside with a fan or air-conditioning. Loosen any tight clothing.

2 Drink plenty of water or a rehydration drink.

3 Sponge your face and body with cold water or take a cold shower or bath to cool down.

NOTE If heatstroke is suspected, call 911.

NATURAL REMEDIES

In cases of heat exhaustion, common sense is the best remedy but the following may aid recovery.

HERBAL REMEDIES You can relieve a fever and headache by adding half a teaspoon cayenne to half a cup of boiling water. Dilute with cold water and sip slowly. Eating a raw or cooked onion may also help bring relief and protection.

FLOWER REMEDIES Add a few drops of Rescue Remedy to a glass of water and drink three to four times a day or apply directly to the tongue.

HOMEOPATHIC REMEDIES

Choose a remedy according to the symptoms.

Belladonna 30C, for burning, hot, dry skin and dilated pupils.

Bryonia alba 30C, for a severe headache.

CALL YOUR DOCTOR

Most cases of heat exhaustion do not require medical attention, but heatstroke is a medical emergency and will require hospitalization. Elderly people, babies, children, and people with chronic health problems are most at risk of developing both conditions.

Sunburn

This is caused by the ultraviolet (UV) rays in sunlight. If you are fair skinned or have naturally blonde or red hair, you will have low levels of melanin—the pigment that protects your skin against burning and helps you to tan.

SYMPTOMS

- Red, sore, or painful skin
- Skin feels warm even in the shade
- May blister
- May peel or flake

PREVENTION

- Apply sunscreen with an SPF of at least 15 at regular intervals, even if you are dark or olive skinned—you can still experience sun damage.
- Use water-resistant sunscreen before and after swimming.
- Use a sunblock on your lips, nose, and areas that burn easily or where the skin is very thin.
- Cover up with light, loose clothing and a sun hat.
- Wear sunglasses with UV filters to protect your eyes and the delicate skin around them.
- Stay indoors or in the shade between 11 a.m. and 3 p.m., when the sun is at its strongest.

FIRST AID

1 Cool sunburned skin in a cool shower or bath, or sponge with some cold water and gently pat dry.

2 Apply an aftersun moisturizing cream.

3 If your skin is itchy and sore, smooth on some calamine lotion.

4 Drink plenty of water or nonalcoholic fluids to rehydrate your body.

5 If it's painful, take acetaminophen or ibuprofen.

6 If you go back into the sun, cover up and wear a hat.

NATURAL REMEDIES

To relieve mild sunburn, blend two parts cider vinegar and one part olive oil and apply to the affected areas.

HERBAL REMEDIES To soothe sore skin, apply aloe vera gel or some fresh sap. Calendula (marigold) cream is also soothing.

AROMATHERAPY Add a few drops of lavender, chamomile, or peppermint oil to a tepid bath

HOMEOPATHIC REMEDIES

Choose a remedy according to the symptoms.

Belladonna 6C, for red, sore, inflamed skin with throbbing headache.

Cantharsis 6C, for sunburn with blisters.

CALL YOUR DOCTOR

Unless the sunburn is severe or the blisters get infected, there is no need to seek medical advice.

Caution

You don't need to be in the sun to get sunburned. Beware of hazy days with high cloud and a breeze at the seaside or even light reflecting off snow.

Shock

This life-threatening condition, usually associated with accidents, may be caused by large blood loss, severe burns, or serious injuries. It is characterized by a dramatic drop in blood pressure and requires hospitalization. Less severe emotional shock may follow bad news or a scare, triggering anxiety or fainting.

SYMPTOMS

- Skin is pale, cold, and clammy
- Rapid, weak pulse
- Shallow, fast breathing
- Thirst
- Yawning and sighing
- Drowsiness and confusion
- Loss of consciousness

FIRST AID

For severe clinical shock, do the following:

1 Call an ambulance.

2 Lay the person down on their back with their legs slightly raised. Support them with cushions, pillows, or whatever is available.

3 Loosen any tight clothing.

4 Talk reassuringly but do not offer anything to drink or eat.

5 Check the person's pulse and breathing often. If he or she becomes unconscious, they may need resuscitation.

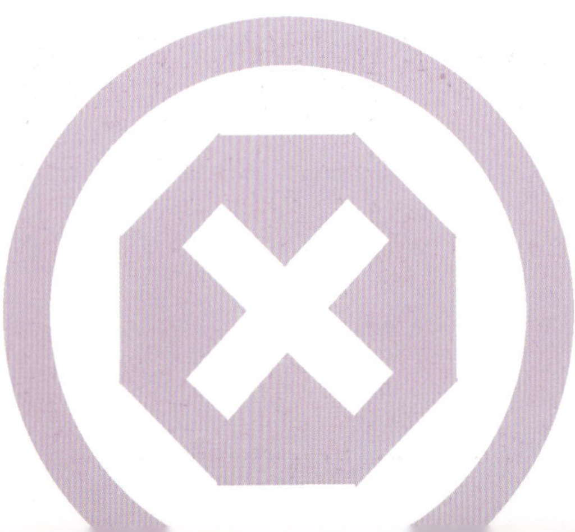

NATURAL REMEDIES

The traditional natural approach to dealing with lesser emotional shock is plenty of rest and relaxation.

HERBAL REMEDIES Sip a tea made with elderflower, rosemary, chamomile, or lemon balm.

AROMATHERAPY Add lavender, geranium, or chamomile oil to a carrier oil and use as a relaxing body massage or just work on the legs and arms.

FLOWER REMEDIES Take a few drops of Rescue Remedy in water at regular intervals.

NUTRITIONAL MEDICINE The B vitamins and zinc may be beneficial. Take a daily supplement or eat foods that are rich in these nutrients.

HOMEOPATHIC REMEDIES

The remedy used will depend on the symptoms.

Aconitum 30C, for a sudden scare, sweat, and rapid pulse.

Arsenicum album 30C, for great anxiety, restlessness, and weak pulse.

CALL YOUR DOCTOR

For severe clinical shock, you must get medical assistance immediately. For lesser emotional shock, it may help to talk to your doctor or a therapist.

Splinters

Splinters are usually thorns or very small fragments of wood, glass, or metal that become embedded in the skin, often when you are performing household chores or working in the yard. If the splinters are not removed, they can become infected and painful.

SYMPTOMS

- ▷ The end of the splinter may be visible
- ▷ Swollen and inflamed skin
- ▷ Discomfort and pain

FIRST AID

1 Wash the area around the splinter with warm water and soap. If the splinter is embedded deeply, soak it in warm water for 10 to 15 minutes.

2 Squeeze the splinter out by applying pressure on the skin to both sides.

3 If it does not budge, pull it out with tweezers, grasping the end firmly and extracting it at the same angle it went in.

4 If the splinter is stubborn or embedded deeply, tease it out with a sterilized needle.

5 If the wound bleeds, cover it with a bandage.

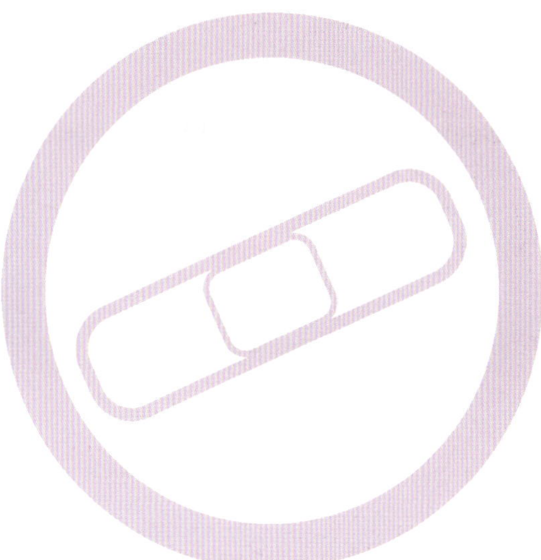

NATURAL REMEDIES

The traditional method of removing a splinter was to cover it with a hot bread poultice

HERBAL REMEDIES For deep splinters, rub some marshmallow, chickweed, or slippery elm ointment into the skin, then cover with a dressing or bandage for an hour to two to draw out the splinter. You can then remove it in the usual way with tweezers or a sterile needle, and dab with tea tree oil or vervain tincture.

AROMATHERAPY After removing a splinter, add a drop of antiseptic lavender oil to the skin.

HOMEOPATHIC REMEDIES Try using Silicea 6C to expel glass shards and splinters, but take it sparingly—no more than one tablet twice a day for a maximum of 14 days.

CALL YOUR DOCTOR

Splinters rarely merit medical attention, but if they are really deep under the skin or a finger nail and become infected, you may need to see a doctor. You may also want to consider being inoculated against tetanus.

Did You Know?

To sterilize a needle or tweezers, you can pass it through a gas or candle flame, being careful not to burn your fingers.

Motion Sickness

This term is used to cover a range of symptoms that may be triggered by traveling by sea, air, road, or rail. If you do have to go on a long journey or a sea crossing, there are conventional and natural remedies you can take.

SYMPTOMS

- ▷ Feeling unwell
- ▷ Dizziness
- ▷ Cold sweat
- ▷ Nausea and sickness

PREVENTION

To prevent motion sickness, you can buy over-the-counter pills or patches in most pharmacies. You must follow the instructions and take them before you set on your journey. You can also try the following.

- In a boat or car, get some fresh air. Go up on deck or open a window.
- Sit in the middle of a boat where it is more stable and moves less.
- Closing your eyes may help; otherwise, try fixing them on a distant object and focus on that.
- Don't eat or drink before traveling.

CONVENTIONAL TREATMENTS

There are over-the-counter and prescription medicines available for coping with motion sickness, including scopolamine, promethazine, and dimenhydrinate. The latter is an antihistamine. Don't give it to a child unless your doctor instructs you to.

NATURAL REMEDIES

One of the simplest remedies is just to suck some boiled licorice candies or eat a stick of licorice candy.

HERBAL REMEDIES Make a chamomile, black horehound, lemon balm, or licorice tea. Alternatively, put a couple of drops of tincture on your tongue.

AROMATHERAPY To settle an upset stomach, put a few drops of peppermint oil on a handkerchief and sniff frequently.

NUTRITIONAL MEDICINE Ginger supplements may help to prevent or alleviate the symptoms of motion sickness. Alternatively, steep some grated ginger in boiling water, then strain and sweeten with honey before sipping. Give children small pieces of crystallized ginger to nibble.

ACUPRESSURE You can try wearing an acupressure wristband; these are available from most health stores and pharmacies.

HOMEOPATHIC REMEDIES

The remedy used will depend on the symptoms.

Cocculus indicus 30C, for nausea and giddiness, worsened by watching moving objects.

Tabacum 30C, for nausea and headache, which improves in cold fresh air or with eyes closed.

CALL YOUR DOCTOR

If over-the-counter medication does not work or you are over 70, have a history of heart disease or liver or kidney problems, have an overactive thyroid, or are pregnant, consult your doctor.

Hangover

This term is used to cover all the symptoms associated with drinking too much alcohol. Excessive alcohol dehydrates the body, dilates the blood vessels in your head, and reduces blood sugar levels, causing a hangover.

SYMPTOMS

- ▷ Feeling tired
- ▷ Throbbing headache and dizziness
- ▷ Dehydration and thirst
- ▷ Sensitivity to noise and light
- ▷ Sweating and interrupted sleep
- ▷ Nausea and sickness
- ▷ Diarrhea
- ▷ Red, bloodshot eyes
- ▷ Shaking and tremors

PREVENTION

- Drink plenty of water as well as alcohol, alternating them if possible.
- Always try to eat a meal before drinking alcohol.
- Avoid dark-colored drinks, such as red wine, port, and brandy; drink white wine or clear liquors.

CONVENTIONAL REMEDIES

Drink plenty of water and isotonic drinks to counter dehydration. Take acetaminophen to ease headaches.

Did You Know?

Alcoholic drinks that are a darker color, such as red wine and port, may produce more severe hangovers, possibly due to the larger numbers of toxic "congeners" that they contain.

NATURAL REMEDIES

There are many traditional remedies for hangovers, including the "hair of the dog," but drinking more alcohol will only make your symptoms worse.

HERBAL REMEDIES Make a soothing cup of dandelion or kudzu tea.

AROMATHERAPY Relax in a warm bath to which you have added a couple of drops of juniper and fennel essential oils.

NUTRITIONAL MEDICINE Have a large glass of fruit juice to rehydrate you. Orange, grapefruit, and tomato juice all contain fructose, a natural sugar that helps your body to metabolize the alcohol faster. Sip some vegetable broth or clear chicken soup, or make a milk shake with a fresh banana, milk, and honey.

HOMEOPATHIC REMEDIES The remedy used to treat headaches associated with too much alcohol is Nux vomica 6C.

CALL YOUR DOCTOR

Most hangovers will get better within 24 hours. However, if you drink heavily and often wake up with a hangover, you have a serious problem, you should seek expert medical help.

NOTE Even the following day, you may still be over the legal limit for driving. In general, it is sensible not to operate any heavy machinery.

Glossary

Acupressure
In traditional Chinese medicine, pressure massage on the pressure points along the acupuncture meridians (the channels through which the body's motivating energy flows). Used to relieve tension-related ailments.

Acupuncture
Needles are inserted in the acupuncture points along the meridians running through the body to balance the flow of qi (pronounced "chee"), which is the vital motivating energy.

Alexander technique
A technique, developed by F. M. Alexander, for improving posture, balance, and respiratory function, and using muscles more efficiently.

Analgesics
Pain-relieving medicines, including simple analgesics for mild pain (aspirin, acetaminophen); anti-inflammatories for arthritis and muscular pain; and narcotic analgesics for severe pain (morphine).

Antibiotics
Medicines that destroy or inhibit the growth of bacteria in the body. They do not work against viruses.

Antihistamines
Medicines that counteract allergic symptoms produced when histamine is released in the body.

Anti-inflammatories
Drugs that reduce inflammation, as in arthritis, gout, and muscular problems. Include analgesics (see above), corticosteroids, and nonsteroidal anti-inflammatory drugs (NSAIDs).

Antiseptic
A substance that controls infection and helps prevent tissue degeneration.

Antispasmodics
Medicines or natural substances for relieving cramp and bowel spasms.

Aromatherapy
The use of aromatic essential oils, which are extracted from plants, to treat many common health problems and illnesses. Used in massage, diffusers, and inhalation.

Bach flower essences (remedies)
The 38 Bach flower essences (infusions of different plants) were developed by Dr. Edward Bach and are used to correct emotional imbalances that can threaten our health and to promote self-healing.

Chinese herbal medicine
A holistic branch of traditional Chinese medicine in which herbs are used to treat disease and health problems, by eliminating symptoms, rebalancing the body, and strengthening the individual. It emphasizes the interaction between the body, mind, and spirit.

Chiropractic
A form of manipulation whereby joints in the spine are manipulated to relieve not only back problems but also ones elsewhere in the body, because the spine carries the nerves to the rest of the body.

Cognitive behavioral therapy (CBT)
A term covering a number of talking therapies that are used to treat anxiety, depression, and other psychological problems. It was developed from cognitive therapy and behavioral therapy.

Demulcent
A soothing agent that protects mucous membranes and relieves irritation.

Detoxicant
A substance that eliminates or counteracts poisons.

Distillation
Process of extracting essences of plants by heating to vapor, condensing by cooling, and collecting the liquid.

Essential oils
Concentrated essences extracted from plants.

Expectorant
A substance that removes excess mucous from the respiratory passages.

Herbal medicine
An ancient holistic system of medicine, which uses the healing properties of medicinal plants to treat a wide range of health disorders and common diseases.

Homeopathy
A natural system of medicine whereby minute amounts of diluted substances are used to treat various medical conditions on the principle that "like cures like." A qualified homeopath will address the patient's personality as well as their symptoms before prescribing an appropriate remedy.

Hydrotherapy
The therapeutic use of water in treating a range of health problems. Utilizes hot, cold, and mineral baths; steam baths, vapor baths, and Turkish baths; inhalation therapy; and hot and cold compresses.

Massage
An ancient hands-on therapy that is used to: induce mental and physical relaxation; eliminate toxins from the body; improve muscle tone and circulation; and help the digestive system to function effectively.

Meditation
Used to promote relaxation and spiritual growth and enlightenment. It is believed to be beneficial to health, relieving stress and treating high blood pressure.

Naturopathy
A holistic, preventive therapy emphasizing the body's natural vitality and potential for self-healing. Encourages a healthy lifestyle, encompassing a natural, organic diet, relaxation, exercise, and hydrotherapy.

Osteopathy
A therapy that involves massage and manipulation of the joints, especially in the spine, to promote self-healing and correct skeletal misalignment.

Pathogen
An agent that causes disease, such as bacteria, viruses, fungi, and parasites.

Pilates
A system of body conditioning that improves posture, balance, alignment, flexibility, and breathing.

Reflexology
An ancient therapy using foot massage, in which the soles of the feet mirror the rest of the body and pressure is applied to specific points that correspond to other body parts and organs.

Traditional Chinese medicine (TCM)
A complete, integrated, holistic system of medicine, including acupuncture, acupressure, herbal medicine, and food cores. Aims to promote health by restoring harmony to the body and balancing yin and yang.

Yin and yang
The equal and opposite qualities of qi (see Acupuncture), the body's vital energy.

Yoga
An ancient Hindu system of exercises, postures, meditation, breathing, and relaxation, designed to promote physical, mental, and spiritual well-being by creating union between the body, mind, and spirit.

Useful Information

Accreditation Commission for Acupuncture and Oriental Medicine

Recognized by the U.S. Department of Education, a national acrrediting agency that fosters excellence in acupuncture and Oriental medicine education.
Tel: (301) 313-0855
www.ACAOM.org

Acupuncture Today

Online source that provides information on traditional Chinese medicine and acupuncture; it also provides an extensive list of national and state acupuncture organizations.
Tel (toll-free): (800) 359-2289
www.acupuncturetoday.com/abc

American Association of Naturopathic Physicians

Organization with a vision of a comprehensive healthcare system that incorporates the principles of naturopathic medicine, with every American having the right to choose a naturopathic practitioner.
Tel (toll-free): (866) 538-2267
Tel: (202) 237-8150
www.naturopathic.org

American Botanical Council

An independent, nonprofit research and education organization, the council works to provide the lay user with reliable information that can help with personal or professional interests, including making informed decisions for a healthier life through the responsible use of medicinal plants.
Tel: (512) 926-4900
abc.herbalgram.org/site/PageServer

American Cancer Society

A nonprofit organization that has worked relentlessly to save lives, helping people stay well, helping people get well, finding cures, and fighting back against cancer. Its website provides a wealth of information on cancer, including comprehensive details on complementary and alternative thearapies.
Tel (toll-free): (800) 227-2345
www.cancer.org

American Chiropractic Association

The largest professional association in the United States representing chiropractors, it promotes the highest standards of ethics and patient care, contributing to the health and well-being of chiropractic patients. Their website has a section for patients.
Tel: (703) 276-8800
www.acatoday.org/patients/index.cfm

American Heart Association

A nonprofit, voluntary health agency whose mission is to build healthier lives, free of cardiovascular diseases and stroke. They provide education and information through the use of a variety of publications and resources, including consumer and patient educational materials, cookbook, heart-healthy books, and scientific publications.
Tel (toll-free): (800) AHA-USA1
www.heart.org/HEARTORG

American Herbalists Guild

A nonprofit, educational organization serving professional herbalists specializing in the medicinal use of plants. Among their goals, the guild aims to promote diversity in herbal medicine; foster high standards of ethics and integrity in the education and

the practice of therapeutic herbalism; and to promote cooperation between herbal practitioners and other health care providers. The guild offers an online forum and a variety of publications.
Tel: (617) 520–4372
www.americanherbalistsguild.com

American Institute of Homeopathy

A trade association of medical and osteopathic physicians, dentists, and other healthcare providers dedicated to homeopathic medicine. Their website is intended as a resource for both the professional and the public.
Tel (toll-free): (888) 445–9988
www.homeopathyusa.org

American Podiatric Medical Association

A professional organization representing the nation's doctors of podiatric medicine (podiatrists). Podiatrists are physicians and surgeons who practice on the lower extremities, primarily on feet and ankles. The APMA's Web site provides information about how to find a podiatrist as well as health information related to feet and ankles.
Tel: (301) 589–9200
www.apma.org

American Urology Care Foundation

The official foundation of the American Uroloigcal Association (AUA), it is committed to promoting urology research and education to improve patients' lives; provides up-to-date educational materials.
Tel (toll-free): (800) 828–7866
Tel: (410) 639–3700
www.urologyhealth.org

Asthma and Allergy Foundation of America

A nonprofit patient organization dedicated to improving the quality of life for people with asthma and allergic diseases through education, advocacy, and research. Some of the educational materials they supply are available in Spanish.
Tel (toll-free): (800) 7–ASTHMA
www.aafa.org

Bach Flower Remedies

Provides information about the history of Dr. Edward Bach and his Flower Remedies, as well as information on the use of Bach Flower Remedies.
Tel (toll-free): (800) 214–2850
www.bachflower.com

Childbirth Connection

A national, nonprofit organization, their mission is to improve the quality of maternity care through research, education, advocacy, and policy. Programs place special emphasis on helping women to gain access to accurate information and supportive resources for making informed decisions about their care; to navigate the complex health care system; and to understand and exercise their legal maternity rights. Childbirth Connection produces a variety of materials, which are available on their website.
Tel: (212) 777–5000
www.childbirthconnection.org

Crohn's and Colitis Foundation of America

A nonprofit, volunteer-driven organization dedicated to finding a cure for Crohn's disease and ulcerative colitis and to improve the quality of life of children and

adults affected by these diseases. The foundation funds research at major medical institutions, conducts educational workshops and symposia, and provides information on their website.
Tel (toll-free): (800) 932–2423
www.ccfa.org

Food Allergy and Anaphylaxis Network

This organization's goal is to raise public awareness, provide education, and advance research on behalf of all those affected by food allergies and anaphylaxis. It provides emotional support, education, practical tips, and accurate medical information. A wide variety of information resources are available at the website.
Tel (toll-free): (800) 929–4040
www.foodallergy.org

Healthy Women

A nonprofit organization, it is the nation's leading independent health information source for women. Its core mission is to educate, inform, and empower women to make smart health choices for themselves and their families. It has a long history of providing unbiased, accurate health information and has earned the trust of consumers and healthcare providers.
Tel (toll-free): (877) 986–9472
www.healthywomen.org

Herb Research Foundation

This nonprofit organization has been educating the public, health practitioners, legislators, and the media about the health benefits and safety of herbs, drawing on a specialty botanical library containing hundreds of thousands of scientific papers on thousands of herbs and multiple online sources of clinical, pharmacological, chemical, and horticultural information. The foundation aims to encourage and support research into the benefits of herbs; to establish a solid scientific foundation for their use as foods and medicines; and to serve as a reliable source of information on the safe and appropriate use of medicinal plants and herbal products.
Tel: (303) 449–2265
www.herbs.org

Mental Health America

Country's leading nonprofit organization dedicated to helping all people live mentally healthier lives. A primary goal is to educate the general public about the realities of mental health and illness, from anxiety disorders to schizophrenia. Their Web site provides information on different mental health illnesses, where to find treatment and support groups, and on insurance.
Tel (toll-free): (800) 969–6642
In crisis tel (toll-free): (800) 273–TALK
www.nmha.org

National Center for Homeopathy

A national, membership organization for the promotion of homeopathy through education, publication, research, and membership services. By providing general education to the public about homeopathy and specific education to homeopaths, the organization helps to make homeopathy available throughout the United States.
Tel: (703) 548–7790
www.homeopathic.org

National Eczema Association

A nonprofit organization working to improve the health and quality of life of all persons living with atopic dermatitis/eczema through research, support, and education.
Tel (toll-free): (800) 818–7546
www.nationaleczema.org

National Psoriasis Foundation

A nonprofit, voluntary health agency dedicated to finding a cure for psoriasis and psoriatic arthritis and eliminating their devastating effects through research, advocacy, and education.
Tel (toll-free): (800) 723–9166
www.psoriasis.org

National Women's Health Network

A membership-based organization committed to advancing women's health, their website provides fact sheets about specific women's health topics and links to numerous other organizations decided to improving the health of women and girls.
Tel: (202) 682–2640
www.womenshealthnetwork.org

National Healthy Mothers, Healthy Babies Coalition

The American College of Obstetricians and Gynecologists (ACOG), the March of Dimes, the American Academy of Pediatrics (AAP), the American Nurses Association (ANA), the National Congress of Parents and Teachers, and the U.S. Public Health Service established this informal coalition to improve the quality of education related to prenatal and infant care. The website provides downloadable "fast facts" information on a number of health-care issues related to children.
Tel: (703) 837–4792
www.hmhb.org

NIH/National Center for Complementary and Alternative Medicine

This clearinghouse serves as the communications arm of the U.S. National Institutes of Health (NIH). It responds to inquiries on complementary and alternative medicine in English and Spanish, serving the public, patients, and health professionals by providing information; locating other information sources; and creating health information materials.
Tel (toll-free): (888) 644–6226
Tel (toll-free) TTY: (866) 464–3615
nccam.nih.gov

NIH/National Institute of Child Health & Human Development

Since it's establishement in 1962, the institute has supported the investigation of human development throughout the entire life process, focusing on understanding developmental disabilities, including intellectual and developmental disabilities (IDDs), and illuminating important events that occur during pregnancy. Its website provides information on childhood illnesses and diseases.
Tel (toll-free): (800) 370–2943
www.nichd.nih.gov/Pages/index.aspx

Reflexology Association of America

National organization that provides information on reflexology research and links to practitioners across the country.
Tel: (980) 234–0159
www.reflexology-usa.org

U.S. Pharmacopeial Convention

A scientific, nonprofit organization that sets standards for medicines, food ingredients, and dietary supplements manufactured, distributed, and consumed worldwide. USP's drug standards are enforceable in the United States by the Food and Drug Administration. It has a section on its website to provide basic information for consumers.
Tel (toll-free): (800) 227–8772
www.usp.org

Index